Keio University International Symposia for Life Sciences and Medicine Vol. 12
K. Kobayashi, E. Tsuchida, H. Horinouchi (Eds.)
Artificial Oxygen Carrier
Its Front Line

K. Kobayashi, E. Tsuchida,
H. Horinouchi (Eds.)

Artificial Oxygen Carrier

Its Front Line

With 75 Figures, Including 7 in Color

Springer

Koichi Kobayashi, M.D., Ph.D.
Chief Professor of Surgery
Division of General Thoracic Surgery, Department of Surgery
School of Medicine, Keio University
35 Shinanomachi, Shinjuku-ku, Tokyo 160-8582, Japan

Eishun Tsuchida, Ph.D.
Professor Emeritus
Department of Polymer Chemistry, Waseda University
3-4-1 Ohkubo, Shinjuku-ku, Tokyo 169-8555, Japan

Hirohisa Horinouchi, M.D., Ph.D.
Division of General Thoracic Surgery, Department of Surgery
School of Medicine, Keio University
35 Shinanomachi, Shinjuku-ku, Tokyo 160-8582, Japan

Library of Congress Control Number: 2004111703

ISBN 4-431-22074-7 Springer-Verlag Tokyo Berlin Heidelberg New York

Springer is a part of Springer Science+Business Media
springeronline.com

Printed in Japan

Typesetting: SNP Best-set Typesetter Ltd., Hong Kong
Printing and binding: Shinano, Inc., Japan

Printed on acid-free paper

Foreword

This volume of the *Keio University International Symposia for Life Sciences and Medicine* contains the proceedings of the 13th symposium held under the sponsorship of the Keio University Medical Science Fund. The fund was established by the generous donation of the late Dr. Mitsunada Sakaguchi. The Keio University International Symposia for Life Sciences and Medicine constitute one of the core activities sponsored by the fund, of which the objective is to contribute to the international community by developing human resources, promoting scientific knowledge, and encouraging mutual exchange. Each year, the Committee of the International Symposia for Life Sciences and Medicine selects the most significant symposium topics from applications received from the Keio medical community. The publication of the proceedings is intended to publicize and distribute the information arising from the lively discussions of the most exciting and current issues presented during the symposium. On behalf of the Committee, I am most grateful to the late Dr. Sakaguchi, who made the series of symposia possible. We are also grateful to the prominent speakers for their contribution to this volume. In addition, we would like to acknowledge the efficient organizational work performed by the members of the program committee and the staff of the fund.

Naoki Aikawa, M.D., D.M.Sc., F.A.C.S.
Chairman
Committee of the International Symposia
for Life Sciences and Medicine

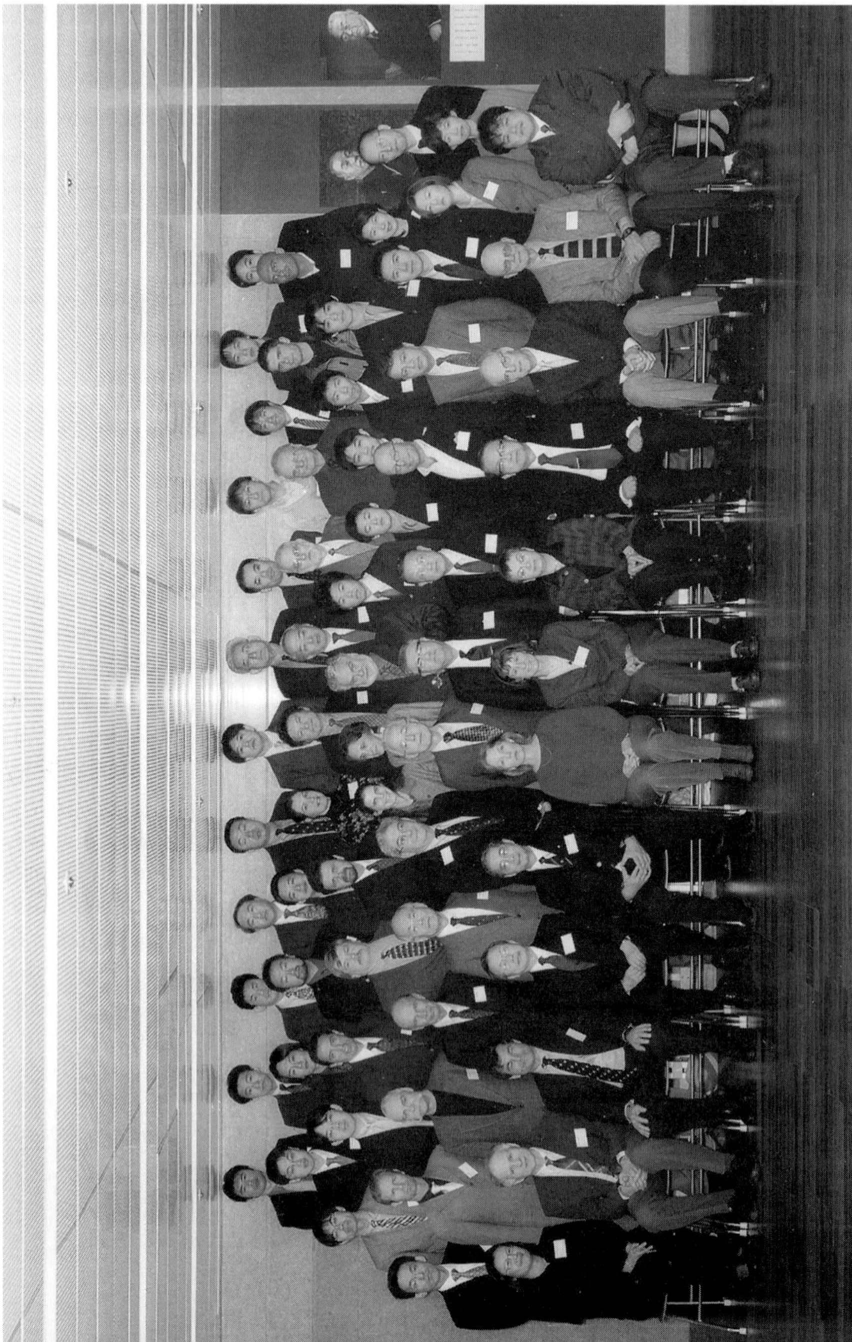

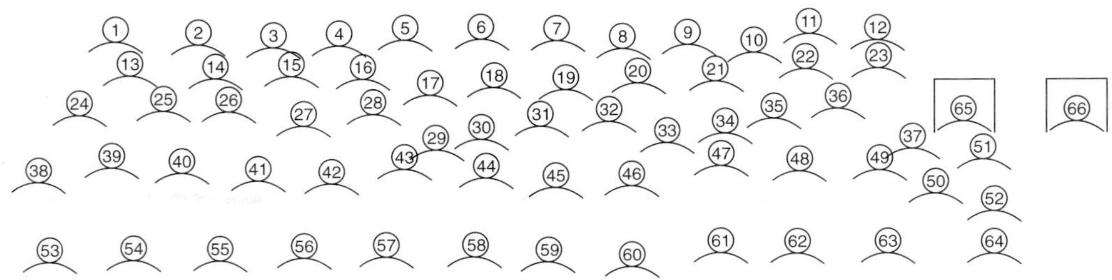

The 13th Keio University International Symposium for Life Sciences and Medicine

Speakers, chairpersons, and discussants at the symposium are identified in the photograph by numbers on the diagram.

1. Sou 2. Teramura 3. Izumi 4. Hirotsu 5. Watanabe 6. Fujimoto 7. Prof. Yonetani 8. Sakai 9. Ikeda 10. Abe
11. Yamamoto 12. Goto 13. Nakagawa 14. Atoji 15. Tajima 16. Takeoka 17. Dr. Krafft 18. Prof. Popel 19. Prof. Miyao
20. Tyssebotn 21. Prof. Kjellström 22. Wettstein 23. Contaldo 24. Kaneda 25. Komatsu 26. Dr. Briceño 27. Dr. Burhop
28. Prof. Simoni 29. Toussaint-Hacquard 30. Fronticelli 31. Prof. Bucci 32. Obata 33. Kubota 34. Okamura 35. Ando
36. Maekawa 37. Kamouchi 38. * 39. Prof. Erni 40. Dr. Baumler 41. Prof. Intaglietta 42. Dr. Yuasa 43. Prof. Greenburg
44. Prof. Shimizu 45. Prof. Takaori 46. Prof. Fukushima 47. Dr. Drobin 48. Dr. Alayash 49. Wang 50. Ms. Oguro
51. Horinouchi 52. Ms. Ohba 53. Dr. Tsai 54. Dr. Hahn 55. Prof. Zapol 56. President Prof. Kobayashi 57. Prof. Chang
58. Dr. Vandegriff 59. Dr. Baldwin 60. Dr. Silverman 61. Prof. Tsuchida 62. Prof. Winslow 63. Prof. Lundgren
64. Prof. Suematsu 65. Founder of Keio, Yukichi Fukuzawa 66. The first dean, Prof. Kitasato

*The editors regret that the name was unavailable.

Preface

Our understanding of blood has changed considerably since the Middle Ages, when it was regarded with a mixture of fear and superstition. The first successful human transfusion was done by James Blundell in 1818, and in the last century, since Karl Landsteiner discovered blood types, transfusion medicine has evolved to become one of the most important therapeutic modalities today, changing medical practice along the way. However, unexpected side effects such as bacterial and viral infections, immunological disorders, and mismatch transfusion compromise the beneficial results gained through transfusion.

Although every effort has been made to avoid these side effects, we know that blood transfusion still comes with the risk of infectious diseases and adverse reactions. Also, long-term storage and transportation of blood components is still a challenge.

To solve these problems, physicians and researchers have been searching for suitable artificial blood substitutes. The concept of an artificial oxygen carrier was advocated by Michael Heidelberger at the Rockefeller Institute in 1922. Thomas Ming Swi Chang invented the artificial cell in 1957 and demonstrated its medical potential. Since then, hemoglobin-based oxygen carriers have been the mainstream of research, with some even entering clinical application.

Biologically inert oxygen carriers such as perfluorochemicals were studied by Leland Clark in 1957, while Eishun Tsuchida synthesized an oxygen-carrying material using polymer chemistry in 1973. It is hoped that all these endeavors will bear fruit in the near future.

Research into artificial oxygen carriers has generated a spin-off in oxygen therapeutics. Because oxygen is a fundamental molecule in the body, this concept has changed therapeutic modalities. When we can understand gas biology in cells, tissues, and organs, we will be able to open a new era in medicine.

Research into artificial oxygen carriers at Keio University began in 1985 in collaboration with Eishun Tsuchida of Waseda University's Department of Polymer Chemistry when he developed a totally synthetic oxygen-carrying lipidheme vesicle. Since then, we have developed and evaluated several types of artificial oxygen carriers, assessing their safety, efficiency, and the reactions they generate. Of the techniques explored, we have chosen hemoglobin vesicles and lipidheme vesicles, which are nanocapsule-type artificial oxygen carriers, and the proteomics-type artificial oxygen carrier albumin-hemes as potential candidates for human use. We have been enthusiastically studying these materials and feel they have considerable potential.

Nevertheless, there are still many issues to be solved concerning medical, chemical, physical, industrial, and ethical problems. To enhance research activity, collaboration with international core facilities and conscientious discussion are necessary. In this book, cutting-edge research and development of artificial oxygen carriers are presented.

The Keio University International Symposium for Life Sciences and Medicine is supported by the Keio University Medical Science Fund, founded on donations from the late Dr. Sakaguchi and Mrs. Sakaguchi. I express my deepest appreciation to the founder, and thanks to all fund staff for their unstinting efforts.

Koichi Kobayashi, M.D., Ph.D.
Chairman
The 13th Keio University International Symposium for
Life Sciences and Medicine
Chief Professor of Surgery
Division of General Thoracic Surgery
Department of Surgery
School of Medicine
Keio University

Contents

List of Contributors

Opening Remarks

Professor Yuichiro Anzai
President, Keio University
Chairman, Keio University Medical Science Fund

Distinguished guests, ladies and gentlemen: On behalf of Keio University, it is a great pleasure to welcome all of you to the 13th Keio University International Symposium for Life Sciences and Medicine. I am particularly grateful to the distinguished medical scientists who have traveled such long distances to participate in this meeting.

The major subject of this year's symposium is "Research and Development of Artificial Oxygen Carrier: Its Front Line." As various advances have been made in the field of artificial oxygen carrier, I believe that it is an opportune time to hold a symposium at Keio University related to the subject. All speakers kindly accepted our invitation to contribute to this symposium, and I feel certain that this unique meeting will prove both exciting and successful.

Keio was founded in 1858 by Yukichi Fukuzawa and is the oldest university in the country. Fukuzawa was a pioneer in the modernization of Japan. He was a member of the very first mission of the Tokugawa Shogunate government to the United States in 1860 and to European countries in 1862. Before that time, Japan's doors to the outside world had been closed in a period of self-isolationism lasting almost 300 years. Fukuzawa realized during his visit to the United States and Europe that education and learning were crucially important and inevitable in the future of Japan. Keio has its origins in international exchanges; indeed, international exchanges such as this symposium have been one of the most important academic and social missions of Keio University since its foundation.

In the fall of 1994, Dr. Mitsunada Sakaguchi, an alumnus of the class of 1940 of our medical school, donated five billion yen, approximately 45 million dollars, to the university. He expressed the wish that his fund be used to encourage research in life sciences and medicine and to promote worldwide advancements in life sciences. We agreed with his proposal and thus launched the Keio University Medical Science Fund in April 1995. The International

Symposia for Life Sciences and Medicine have been organized as one of several projects supported by the fund. In 1999, Dr. Sakaguchi made an additional donation of two billion yen. With these funds, Keio University has established a new laboratory in the field of cell differentiation.

It is thus more than a pleasure, indeed it is an honor, for me to be able to meet the distinguished medical researchers and clinicians from world-renowned institutions who kindly gathered here, and to share in frank and valuable exchanges of views. I am also grateful for the efforts made by the organizing committee, chaired by Dr. Koichi Kobayashi, who has devoted himself to ensuring that this symposium is an auspicious and enjoyable event. I do hope that the meeting will prove a truly fruitful and productive one for you all.

Let me close by wishing everyone gathered here further success in your research and clinical work. Thank you very much.

Safety and Efficacy of Hemoglobin-Vesicles and Albumin-Hemes

K. Kobayashi[1], H. Horinouchi[1], M. Watanabe[1], Y. Izumi[1], Y. Teramura[2], A. Nakagawa[2], Y. Huang[2], K. Sou[2], H. Sakai[2], T. Komatsu[2], S. Takeoka[2], and E. Tsuchida[2]

Summary. Keio University and Waseda University have worked together on artificial O_2 carrier research for 20 years in close cooperation. Two candidate materials have been selected from the viewpoints of safety, efficacy, and cost performance. One is Hemoglobin-vesicles (HbV) and the other is albumin-heme (rHSA-heme). This chapter summarizes our video presentation that introduced the recent results of our research into HbV and rHSA-heme.

Key words. Blood substitutes, Oxygen carriers, Hemoglobin-vesicles, Albumin-heme, Oxygen therapeutics

Introduction: Keio-Waseda Joint Research Project

For human beings to survive, it is necessary to continuously deliver oxygen that is needed for the respiration of all tissue cells. Red blood cell, a so-called moving internal-organ, reversibly binds and releases O_2 under physiological conditions. From this point of view, red blood cell substitutes, or O_2-Infusions, are very important. In order to promote this research, we have emphasized that the establishment of basic science for macromolecular complexes and molecular assemblies is essential. We have systematically studied the Metal Complexes (synthetic heme derivatives) embedded into a hydrophobic cluster, and clarified that the electronic processes of the active sites are controlled by the surrounding molecular environment. Therefore, the reaction activity and its rate constant are observed as cooperative phenomena with the

[1] Department of Surgery, School of Medicine, Keio University, 35 Shinanomachi, Shinjuku-ku, Tokyo 160-8582, Japan
[2] Advanced Research Institute for Science & Engineering, Waseda University, 3-4-1 Ohkubo, Shinjuku-ku, Tokyo 169-8555, Japan

properties of the molecular atmosphere. In other words, the development of our O_2-Infusion has been based on "the Regulation of the Electronic Process on Macromolecular Complexes and Synthesis of Functional Materials" [1,2].

Reproducing the O_2-binding ability of red blood cells (RBC), that is, the development of a synthetic O_2 carrier that does not need hemoglobin (Hb), was the starting point of our study. In general, central ferric iron of a heme is immediately oxidized by O_2 in water, preventing the O_2 coordination process from being observed. Therefore, the electron transfer must be prevented. We were able to detect the formation of the O_2-adduct complex, but for only several nano seconds, by utilizing the molecular atmosphere and controlling the electron density in the iron center. Based on this finding, we succeeded in 1983 with reversible and stable O_2 coordination and preparation of phospholipid vesicles embedded amphiphilic-heme, known as lipidheme/phospholipids vesicles (Fig. 1) [3–6]. This was the world's first example of reversible O_2-binding taking place under physiological conditions. For example, human blood can dissolve about 27 ml of O_2 per dl, however a 10 mM lipidheme-phospholipid vesicle solution can dissolve 29 ml of O_2 per dl. This material is suitable for O_2-Infusion.

Soon after this discovery, Professor Kobayashi of Keio University asked Professor Tsuchida for a chance to evaluate the lipidheme solution with in vivo experiments. Since then the joint research and collaboration has continued since that time. We have synthesized over one hundred types of heme, and recently synthesized new lipidheme–bearing phospholipid groups, which complete self-organization in water to form stable vesicles. In 1985 Dr. Sekiguchi at Hokkaido Red Cross Blood Center proposed that Professor Tsuchida consider the utilization of outdated red blood cells and Hbs because, while the totally synthetic system is definitely promising it appeared that it

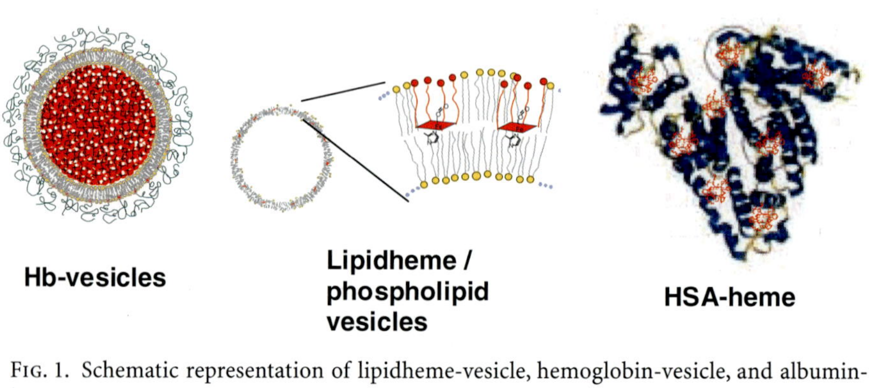

FIG. 1. Schematic representation of lipidheme-vesicle, hemoglobin-vesicle, and albumin-heme

would take considerable time to arrive at a social consensus for its use. We started to produce Hb-vesicles (HbV) using purified Hbs and molecular assembly technologies. In the late 1990's, a mass-production system for recombinant human serum albumin (rHSA) was established and we then prepared albumin-heme hybrids (rHSA-heme) using its non-specific binding ability, which is now considered to be a promising synthetic material.

Based on our effective integration of molecular science and technologies for functional materials developed by Waseda University, and the outstanding evaluation system of safety and efficacy developed by Keio University using animal experiments, we have made strong progress in our research on the O_2-Infusion Project. During this period, we have received substantial funding support from the Japanese government. In the near future, mass production and clinical tests of O_2-Infusion will be started by a certain pharmaceutical industry.

Background and the Significance of HbV

Historically, the first attempt of Hb-based O_2 carrier in this area was to simply use stroma-free Hb. However, several problems became apparent, including dissociation into dimers that have a short circulation time, renal toxicity, high oncotic pressure and high O_2 affinity. Since the 1970s, various approaches were developed to overcome these problems [7,8]. This includes intramolecular crosslinking, polymerization and polymer-conjugation. However, in some cases the significantly different structure in comparison with red blood cells resulted in side effects such as vasoconstriction [9].

Another idea is to encapsulate Hb with a lipid bilayer membrane to produce HbV that solves all the problems of molecular Hb [10]. Red blood cells have a biconcave structure with a diameter of about 8000 nm. Red blood cells can deform to a parachute-like configuration to pass through narrow capillaries. The possibility of infection and blood-type mismatching, and short shelf life are the main problems. Purified Hb does not contain blood-type antigen and pathogen, thus serves as a safe raw material for HbV.

HbV, with a diameter of 250 nm, do not have deformability but are small enough to penetrate capillaries or constrict vessels that RBC cannot penetrate. The surface of the vesicles is modified with polyethylene glycol (PEG) to ensure homogeneous dispersion when circulated in the blood and a shelf life of two years. The idea of Hb encapsulation with a polymer membrane mimicking the structure of RBC originated from Dr. Chang at McGill University [7]. After that, the encapsulation of Hb within a phospholipid vesicle was studied by Dr. Djordjevici at the University of Illinois in the 1970s [11]. However, it was not so easy to make HbV with a regulated diameter and adequate O_2 transport capacity. We made a breakthrough in routinely producing HbV by using fundamental knowledge of macromolecular and supramolecular sciences. Some of the related technologies have already been published in academic journals [12–19]. Several liters of HbV are routinely prepared in a completely sterile condition. Hb is purified from outdated red blood cells, and concentrated to 40 g/dl. Virus removal is performed using a combination of pasteurization at 60°C and filtration with a virus removal filter. The Hb encapsulation with phospholipids bilayer membrane and size regulation was performed with an extrusion method. The vesicular surface is modified with PEG chains. The suspension of Hb-vesicles is dated at the final stage.

The particle diameter of HbV is regulated to about 250 nm, therefore, the bottle of HbV is turbid, and is a suspension. One vesicle contains about 30,000 Hb molecules, and it does not show oncotic pressure. There is no chemical modification of Hb. Table 1 summarizes the physicochemical characteristics of HbV. O_2 affinity is controllable with an appropriate amount of allosteric effectors, pyridoxal 5-phosphate. Hb concentration is regulated to 10 g/dl, and the weight ratio of Hb to total lipid approaches 2.0 by using an ultra pure and concentrated Hb solution of 40 g/dl, which is covered with a thin lipid bilayer membrane. The surface is modified with 0.3 mol% of PEG-lipid. Viscosity, osmolarity, and oncotic pressure are regulated according to the physiological conditions.

HbV can be stored for over two years in a liquid state at room temperature [17]. There is little change in turbidity, diameter, and P_{50}. MetHb content decreases due to the presence of reductant inside the HbV, which reduces the

TABLE 1. Physicochemical characteristics of HbV suspended in 5% albumin (HSA)

Parameters	HbV/HSA	Human blood (RBC)	Analytical method
diameter (nm)	220–280	8000	Light scattering method
P_{50} (Torr)	27–34[1]	26–28	Hemox Analyzer
[Hb] (g/dl)	10 ± 0.5	12–17	CyanometHb method
[Lipid] (g/dl)	5.3–5.9	1.8–2.5[2]	Molibuden-blue method
[Hb]/[Lipid] (g/g)	1.6–2.0	6.7[3]	—
[PEG-lipid] (mol%)	0.3	—	^{1}H-NMR
metHb (%)	<3	<0.5	CyanometHb method
viscosity (cP)[4]	3.7	3–4	Capillary rheometer
osmolarity (mOsm)	300	ca. 300	(suspended in saline)
oncotic press. (Torr)	20	20–25	Wescor colloid osmometer
pH at 37°C	7.4	7.2–7.4	pH meter
Endotoxin (EU/mL)	<0.1	—	LAL assay
Pyrogen	Free	—	rabbit pyrogen test

[1] Adjustable, [2] Total cell membrane components, [3] Weight ratio of Hb to total cell membrane components, [4] At 230 s^{-1}.

trace amount of metHb during storage. This excellent stability is obtained by deoxygenation and PEG-modification. Deoxygenation prevents metHb formation. The surface modification of HbV, with PEG chains prevents vesicular aggregation and leakage of Hb and other reagents inside the vesicles. Liquid state storage is convenient for emergency infusion compared to freeze-dried powder or the frozen state.

In Vivo Efficacy of HbV

The efficacy of HbV has been confirmed with isovolemic hemodilution and resuscitation from hemorrhagic shock. Some of the results have already been published in academic journals in the fields of emergency medicine and physiology [20–28]. In this chapter two important facts are described. One is isovolemic hemodilution with 90% blood exchange in a rat model. The other is resuscitation from hemorrhagic shock in a hamster model.

To confirm the O_2 transporting ability of HbV, extreme hemodilution was performed with HbV suspended in human serum albumin (HSA) [21,23] (Fig. 2). The final level of blood exchange reached 90%. Needle-type O_2 electrodes were inserted into the renal cortex and skeletal muscle, and the blood flow rate in the abdominal aorta was measured with the pulsed Doppler method. Hemodilution with albumin alone resulted in significant reductions in mean

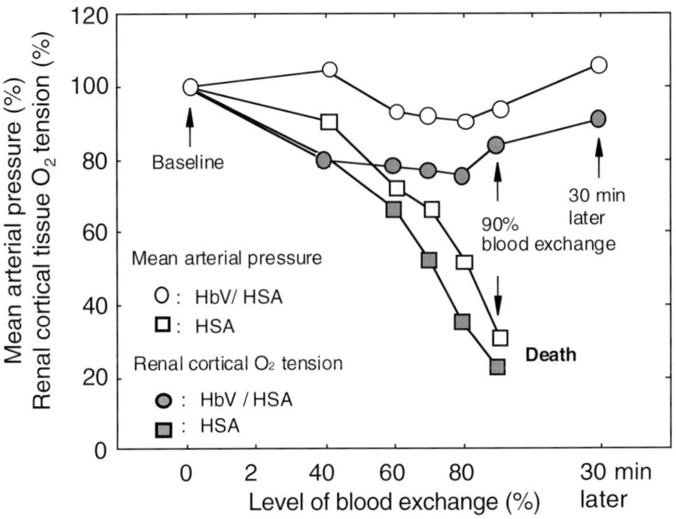

Fig. 2. 90% exchange-transfusion with HbV suspended in HSA (HbV/HSA), or HSA alone. Mean arterial pressure and renal cortical oxygen tension were monitored

arterial pressure and renal cortical O_2 tension, and finally all the rats died of anemia. On the other hand, hemodilution with HbV, suspended in HSA sustained both blood pressure and renal cortical O_2 tension, and all the rats survived. These results clearly demonstrate that HbV, has sufficient O_2 transporting capability.

To observe the microcirculatory response to the infusion of Hb products, we used the intravital microscopy equipped with all the units to measure blood flow rates, vascular diameter, O_2 tension, and so on. This system was developed by Professor Intaglietta at the University of California, San Diego. We used the hamster dorsal-skin fold preparation that allows observation of blood vessels from small arteries to capillaries. We evaluated the HbV suspension as a resuscitative fluid for hemorrhagic-shocked hamsters [26]. About 50% of the blood was withdrawn, and the blood pressure was maintained at around 40 mmHg for 1 h. The hamsters either received HbV suspended in HSA (HbV/HSA), HSA alone, or shed blood (Fig. 3). Immediately after infusion, all the groups showed increases in mean arterial pressure, however, only the albumin infusion resulted in incomplete recovery. The HbV/HSA group showed the same recovery with the shed autologous blood infusion. During the shock period, all the groups showed significant hyperventilation that was evident from the significant increase in arterial O_2 partial. Simultaneously,

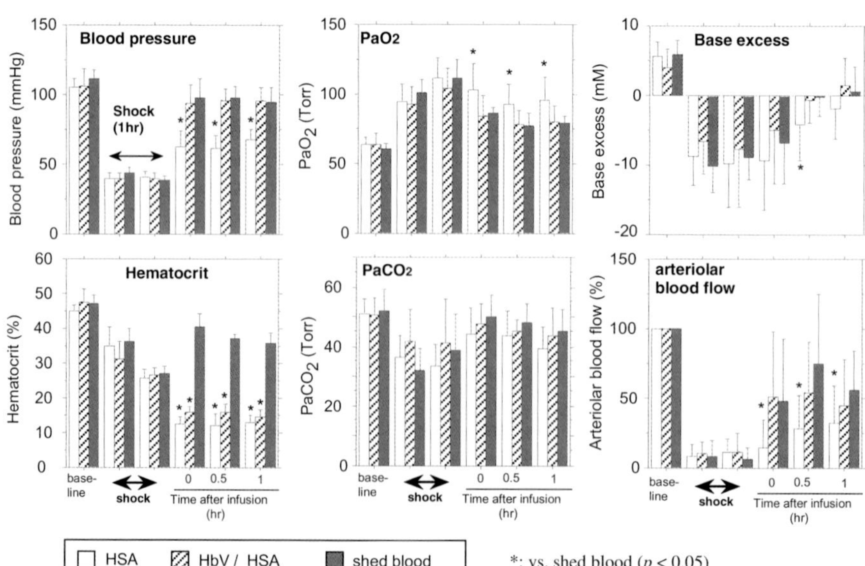

FIG. 3. Resuscitation from hemorrhagic shock with HbV suspended in HSA (HbV/HSA) in hamster dorsal skinfold model. Mean ± SD

base excess and pH decreased significantly. Immediately after resuscitation, all the groups tended to recover. However, only the HSA group showed sustained hyperventilation. Base excess for the HSA group remained at a significantly lower value one hour after resuscitation. Blood flow decreased significantly in arterioles to 11% of basal value during shock. The HbV/HSA and shed autologous blood groups immediately showed significant increases in blood flow rate after resuscitation, while the albumin group showed the lowest recovery.

In Vivo Safety of HbV

We further examined the safety profile of HbV such as cardiovascular responses, pharmacokinetics, influence on reticulo endothelial system (RES), influence on clinical measurements and daily repeated infusion [29–35].

We observed the responses to the infusion of intra-molecularly cross-linked Hb (XLHb) and HbV into conscious hamsters. XLHb (7 nm in diameter) showed a significant increase in hypertension equal to 35 mmHg, and simultaneous vasoconstriction of the resistance artery equal to 75% of the baseline levels [30] (Fig. 4). On the other hand, HbV at 250 nm, showed minimal change. The small acellular XLHb is homogeneously dispersed in the plasma, and it diffuses through the endothelium layer of the vascular wall and reaches the smooth muscle. Intra-molecular cross-linked Hb traps nitric oxide (NO) as an endothelium-derived relaxation factor, and induces vasoconstriction, and hypertension. On the other hand, the large HbV stay in the lumen and do not induce vasoconstriction. Several mechanisms are proposed for Hb-induced vasoconstriction. These include NO-binding, excess O_2 supply, reduced shear stress, or the presence of Hb recognition site on the

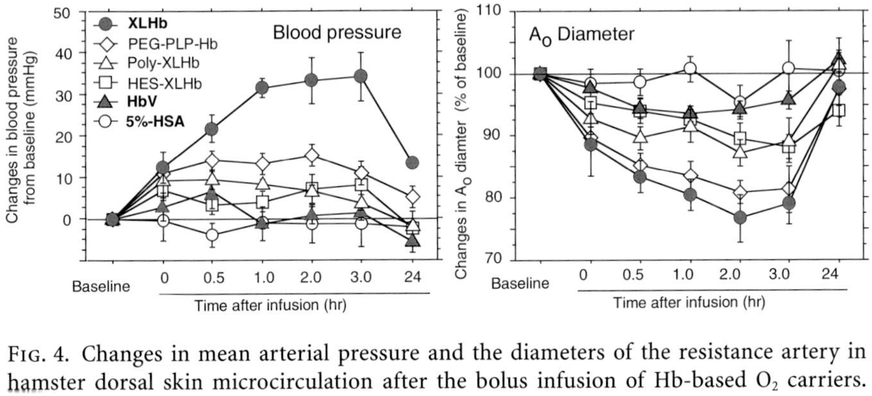

FIG. 4. Changes in mean arterial pressure and the diameters of the resistance artery in hamster dorsal skin microcirculation after the bolus infusion of Hb-based O_2 carriers. Mean ± SD

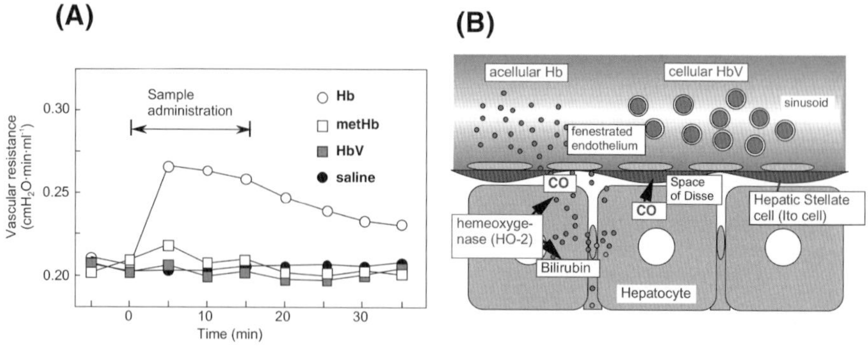

FIG. 5. **A** Changes in vascular resistance during perfusion of exteriorized rat liver with HbV, Hb, metHb, or saline. **B** Schematic representation of hepatic microcirculation: The small Hb molecule extravasate across the fenestrated endothelium to reach to the space of Disse, where heme of Hb is catabolised by hemeoxygenase-2 (HO-2) and CO is released as a vasorelaxation factor. However, the excess amount of the extravasated Hb traps CO and induces vasoconstriction and the resulting higher vascular resistance. On the other hand, the larger HbV retains in the sinusoid and there is no extravasation and vasoconstriction

endothelium. But it is clear that Hb-encapsulation shields against the side effects of acellular Hbs.

Professor Suematsu at Keio University has revealed the effects of Hb-based O_2 carriers in hepatic microcirculation [29,32] (Fig. 5). On the vascular wall of the sinusoid in hepatic microcirculation, there are many pores, called fenestration, with a diameter of about 100 nm. The small Hb molecules with a diameter of only 7 nm extravasate through the fenestrated endothelium and reach the space of Disse. On the other hand, HbV particles, which are larger than the pores, do not extravasate. Heme of extravasated Hb is excessively metabolized by hemeoxygenase-2 in hepatocyte to produce CO and bilirubin. Even though CO acts as a vasorelaxation factor in the liver, the excess amount of Hb rapidly binds CO, resulting in the vasoconstriction and an increase in vascular resistance. On the other hand, HbV (250 nm in diameter) is large enough to remain in the sinusoid, and the vascular resistance is maintained.

So, what is the optimal molecular dimension of Hb-based O_2 carriers? The upper limitation is below the capillary diameter to prevent capillary plugging, and for sterilization by membrane filters (Fig. 6). On the other hand, smaller sizes exhibit a higher rate of vascular wall permeability with side effects such as hypertension and neurological disturbances. HbV exhibits a very low level of vascular wall permeability. Therefore, the HbV appears to be appropriate from the viewpoint of hemodynamics. We have clarified the influence of HbV on the RES, because the fate of HbV is RES trapping.

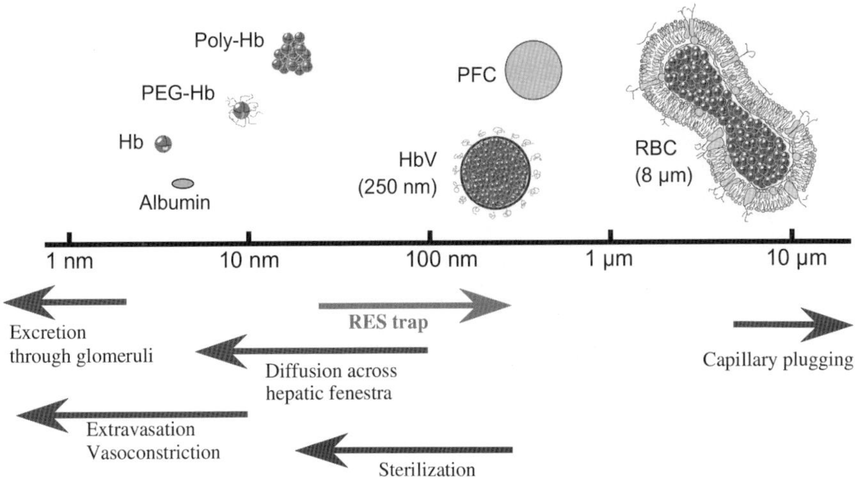

FIG. 6. Optimal diameter of Hb-based oxygen carriers from the view point of physiological response and production process

Circulation persistence was measured by monitoring the concentration of radioisotope-labeled HbV in collaboration with Dr. W.T. Phillips at the University of Texas at San Antonio. The circulation half-life is dose dependent, and when the dose rate was 14 ml/kg, the circulation half-life was 24 h. The circulation time in the case of the human body can be estimated to be twice or three times longer; or about 2 or 3 days at the same dose rate. Gamma camera images of radioisotope-labeled HbV showed the time course of biodistribution. Just after infusion, HbV remains in the blood stream so that the heart and liver that contain a lot of blood showed strong intensity. However, after it is finished playing its role in O_2 transport, a total of 35% of HbV are finally distributed mainly in the liver, spleen and bone marrow.

The time course of liver uptake was monitored with a confocal fluorescence microscope. Hb-vesicle was stained with a lipid fluorophore. The liver of an anesthetized hamster was exposed and a fluorescence-labeled-HbV was infused intravenously. Due to the motion of respiration, the picture oscillates. However, a static frame can be obtained. The individual particles of HbV cannot be recognized. When the vesicles are accumulated in phagosomes of Kupffer cells, they can be recognized with a strong fluorescence. How is HbV metabolized in macrophages? The transmission electron microscopy (TEM) of the spleen 1 day after infusion of HbV clearly demonstrated the presence of HbV particles in macrophages, where HbV particles that appear as black dots are captured by the phagosomes [34] (Fig. 7). Red blood cells and HbV contain a lot of ferric iron with a high electron density, so that they show

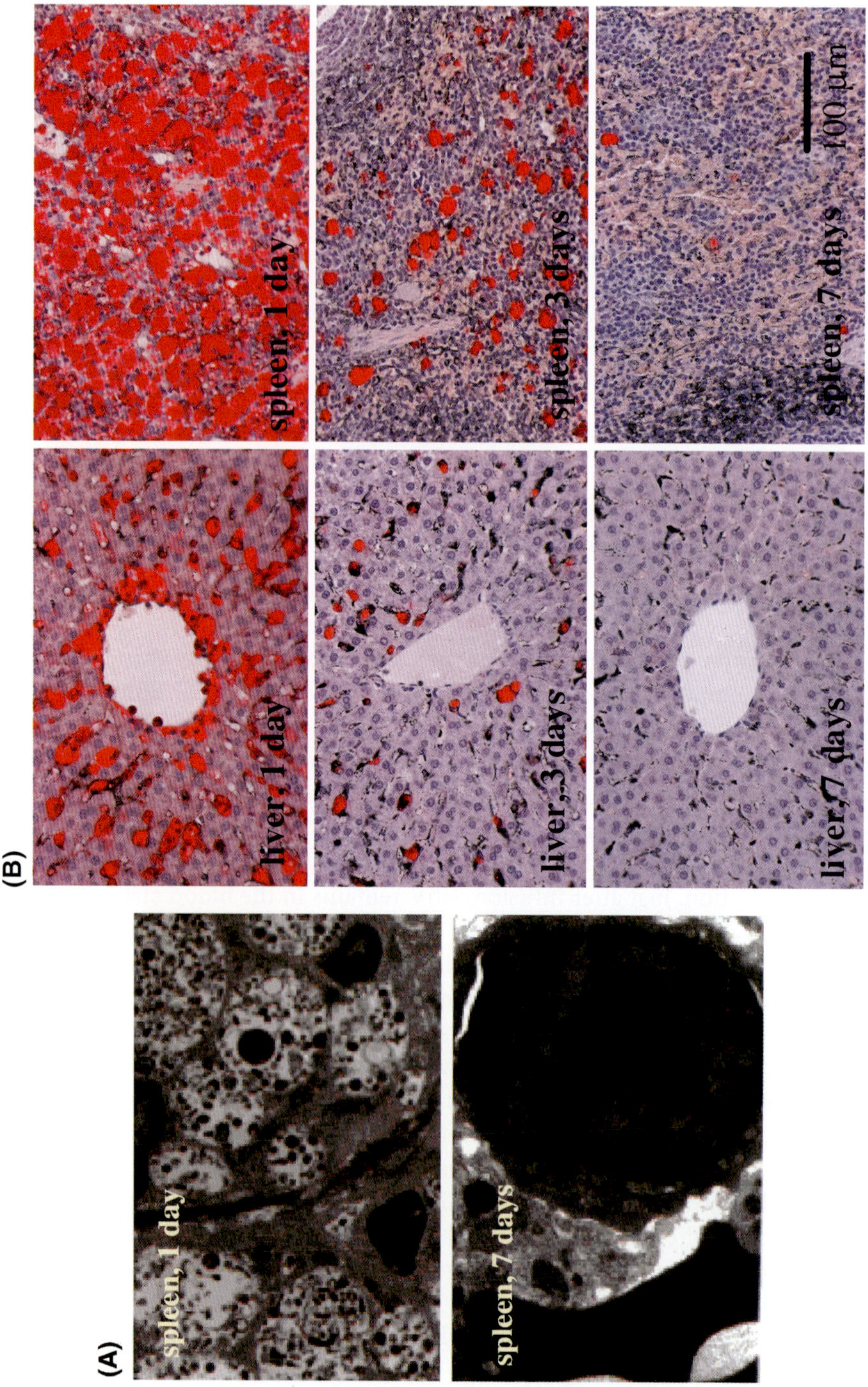
(A)
spleen, 1 day
spleen, 7 days
(B)
liver, 1 day
spleen, 1 day
liver, 3 days
spleen, 3 days
liver, 7 days
spleen, 7 days
100 μm

strong contrast in TEM. However, after 7 days, the HbV structure cannot be observed. We confirmed no abnormalities in the tissues and no irreversible damage to the organs or complete metabolism within a week. A Polyclonal anti-human Hb antibody was used as the marker of Hb in the HbV. This antibody does not recognize rat Hb. The red-colored parts indicate the presence of Hb in HbV, and almost disappear after 7 days in both the spleen and liver. This shows that HbV can be metabolized quite promptly.

One issue of the Hb-based O_2 carriers is that they have a significant influence on clinical laboratory tests. They remain in the plasma phase in hematocrit capillaries after centrifugation of blood samples, and interfere with the colorimetric and turbidimetric measurements. However, HbV can be simply removed from blood plasma either by ultracentrifugation or centrifugation in the presence of a high-molecular-weight dextran to enhance precipitation. We can obtain a very clear supernatant for accurate analyses [35]. This is one advantage of HbV in comparison with acellular Hb solutions. Accordingly we examined the influence on organ functions by serum clinical laboratory tests after the bolus infusion of HbV at a dose rate of 20 ml/kg. Albumin, alanine aminotransferase (ALT), aspartate aminotransferase (AST), and lactic dehydrogenase (LDH), which reflect the liver function, moves their values within normal range. Concentrations of bilirubin and ferric ion are maintained at a low level. The concentration of lipids transiently changed. In particular, the cholesterols increased significantly. And phospholipids slightly increased, however, they returned to the original level after 7 days. These results indicate that the membrane components of HbV, once they reappear from RES, are metabolized on the physiological pathway.

We recently tested a daily repeated infusion of HbV in Wistar rats as a safety study. The dose rate was a 10-ml/kg/day infusion for 14 days. All rats well tolerated and survived. Body weight showed a monotonous but slightly depressed increase in comparison with the saline group. However, after 2 weeks there was no significant difference with the saline control group. All the rats seemed very healthy and active. There was no piloerection. As for the hematological parameters, the numbers of white blood cells and platelets did not exhibit a significant difference from the HbV group and the saline control group. Hematocrit showed a slight reduction for the HbV group, probably due to the accumulation of the large amount of HbV in the blood. Histopathological examination one day after the final infusion of HbV showed signifi-

Fig. 7. **A** Transmission electron microscopy of rat spleen one day after the infusion of HbV (20 ml/kg) and after 7 days. Black dots are HbV particles captured in phagosomes in the spleen macrophages, and they disappeared at 7 days. **B** Staining with anti-human Hb antibody showed the presence of HbV in spleen and liver. They disappeared within 7 days. Cited from: Sakai et al (2001) Am J Pathol 159:1079–1088

cant accumulation of HbV in spleen macrophages, and liver Kupffer cells. Berlin Blue staining revealed the presence of hemosiderin indicating that the metabolism of Hb was initiated. There were no other morphological abnormalities, and the serum clinical chemistry indicated transient but reversible increases in lipid components. AST and ALT were within the normal range. From these results we are confident with the safety of HbV.

Design and Physicochemical Properties of rHSA-Heme

We have been conducting research on totally synthetic O_2 carriers, or so-called albumin-heme that does not require Hb. Human serum albumin is the most abundant plasma protein in our blood stream, but its crystal structure has not been elucidated for long time. In 1998, Dr. Stephen Curry of the Imperial College of London was the first elucidate the crystal structure of the human serum albumin complexed with seven molecules of myristic acids [36]. He found that the dynamic conformational changes of albumin take place by the binding of fatty acid.

In Japan, recombinant human serum albumin is now manufactured on a large scale by expression in the yeast Pichia pastoris, and it will appear on the market soon [37]. A large-scale plant, which can produce one million vials per year, has been already established. From the viewpoint of clinical application, O_2-carrying albumin is quite exciting and may be of extreme medical importance. With this background, we have found that synthetic heme derivative is efficiently incorporated into recombinant human serum albumin (rHSA), creating a red-colored rHSA-heme hybrid. This rHSA-heme can reversibly bind and release O_2 molecules under physiological conditions in the same manner as Hb. In other words, our rHSA-heme hybrid is a synthetic O_2-carrying hemoprotein, and we believe that its saline solution will become a new class of red blood cell substitute. We have already published these chemistry findings and technologies in international journals [38–49].

Figure 8 summarizes the structure of the albumin-heme molecule. The Maximal binding numbers of heme to one albumin are eight, and the magnitude of the binding constants ranged from 10^6 to 10^4 (M^{-1}). The isoelectric point of rHSA-heme was found to be 4.8, independent of the binding numbers of heme. This value is exactly the same as that of albumin itself. Furthermore, the viscosity and density did not change after the incorporation of heme molecules, and the obtained solution showed a long shelf life of almost two years at room temperature. The O_2-binding sites of rHSA-heme are iron-porphyrin, therefore the color of the solution changed in a similar way to Hb. Upon addition of O_2 gas through this solution, the visible absorption pattern immediately changed to that of the O_2-adduct complex. Moreover, after bub-

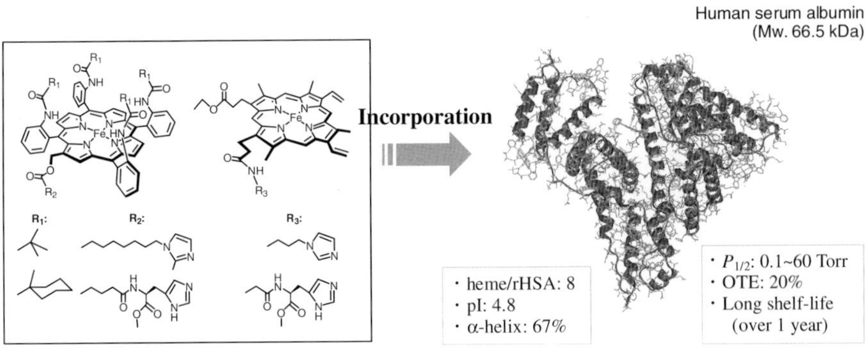

FIG. 8. Structure of the albumin-heme molecule

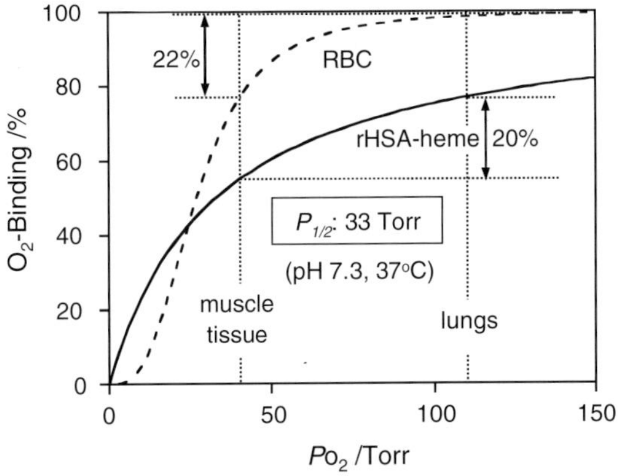

FIG. 9. O_2-binding equilibrium curve of albumin-heme

bling carbon monoxide gas, albumin-heme formed a very stable carbonyl complex.

Figure 9 shows the O_2-binding equilibrium curve of rHSA-heme. The O_2-binding affinity, of rHSA-heme is always constant, independent of the number of heme, and the O_2-binding profile does not show cooperativity. However, the O_2-transporting efficiency of albumin-heme between the lungs where PaO_2 is 110 Torr and muscle tissue where PtO_2 is 40 Torr increases to 20%, which is similar to 22% efficiency of red blood cells. The O_2-binding property of albumin-heme can be controlled by changing the chemical structure of heme derivatives incorporated. More recently, we have found that a proto-heme derivative is also incorporated into albumin and can bind and release O_2 as well [50].

In Vivo Safety and Efficacy of rHSA-Heme

Based on these findings, we can say that rHSA-heme can become an entirely synthetic O_2-carrier, and satisfy the initial clinical requirements for a red blood cell substitute. However, we have another problem to solve before we can use this material as an O_2-carrier in the circulatory system. This problem is NO scavenging. Of course, it can bind NO, and it may be anticipated that the injection of rHSA-heme also induce hypertensive action. We have evaluated the efficacy and safety of this rHSA-heme solution with animal experiments.

As described before, small Hb molecules extravasate through the vascular endothelium and react with NO, thus inducing vasoconstriction and acute increases in systemic blood pressure. Contrary to the expectations, the observation of the intestinal microcirculation after the infusion of rHSA-heme into an anesthetized rat revealed that the diameters of the venules and arterioles were not deformed at all [51]. Indeed, only a small change in the mean arterial pressure was observed after the administration of the rHSA-heme solution (Fig. 10). In contrast, the infusion of Hb elicited an acute increase in blood pressure. Why does albumin-heme not induce vasoconstriction or hypertension? The answer probably lies in the negatively charged molecular surface of albumin. One of the unique characteristics of serum albumin is its low permeability through the capillary pore, which is less than 1/100 that for Hb due to the electrostatic repulsion between the albumin surface and the glomerular basement membrane around the endothelial cells.

We are now evaluating the O_2-transporting ability of this albumin-heme molecule in the circulatory system with further animal experiments [52]. First, we determined the physiological responses to exchange transfusion with rHSA-heme solution into rats after 70% hemodilution and 40% hemorrhage

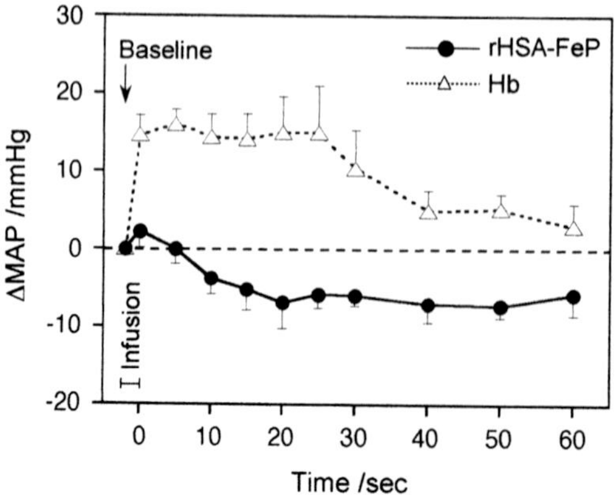

FIG. 10. Change of MAP after the administration of rHSA-heme solution in the anesthetized rats (n = 5). All data are shown as changes from the basal values (ΔMAP) just before the infusion and expressed as mean ± S.E. Basal value is 90.1 ± 3.0 mmHg

(Fig. 11). The declined mean arterial pressure and blood flow after a 70% exchange with albumin and further 40% bleeding of blood showed a significant recovery of up to 90% of the baseline values by the infusion of the rHSA-heme solution. On the other hand, all rats in the control group only injected with albumin died within 30 min. Furthermore, muscle tissue O_2-tension significantly increased. These responses indicate the in vivo O_2-delivery of the rHSA-heme solution.

More recently, we have synthesized human serum albumin dimer, which can incorporate sixteen hemes in its hydrophobic domain [53]. The human serum rHSA-heme dimer solution dissolves 1.2 times more O_2 compared to that of red blood cells and keeps its colloid osmotic pressure at the same level as the physiological value.

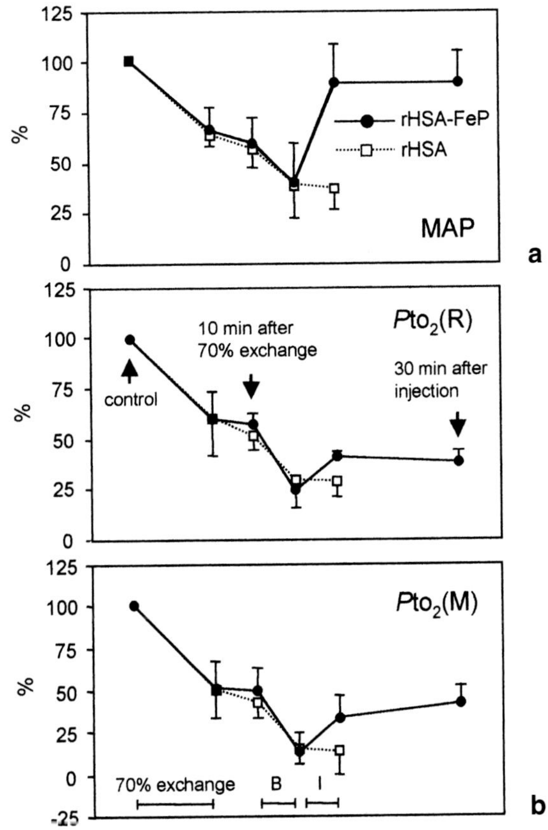

FIG. 11. Change of (a) MAP and (b) O_2-tension in renal cortex during the 70% hemodilution with 5 wt% rHSA and further 40% exchange transfusion with rHSA-heme in anesthetized rats (n = 5). All data are shown as changes from the basal values and expressed as mean ± S.E.

Potential Applications of Artificial O_2 Carriers

For almost 20 years our group at Keio University in collaboration with Dr. Tsuchida's group at Waseda University have been trying to produce artificial O_2 carriers. To date, we have produced several types of O_2 carriers and evaluated their efficacy and biocompatibility. In this chapter, we have shown what we have done to produce O_2 carriers. Below, we would like to show you the potential applications of artificial O_2 carriers, as well as a glimpse of the vast possibilities that lie ahead.

Tumor Oxygenation

Unlike vessels in normal tissues, the development of a vasculature in a tumor lacks normal course of angiogenesis and is hence, highly heterogeneous. Consequently, areas of hypoxia are quite common in tumors. In these hypoxic regions, it can be added that tumor cells acquire resistance to treatments such as chemotherapy and radiation. Our rHSA-heme was injected into the responsible artery that supplies circulation to an implanted tumor (Fig. 12) [54]. O_2 tension of the tumor rises immediately after intra-arterial infusion of albumin heme up to 2.4 times that of the baseline value. Our findings in animals indicate that tumor tissue O_2 levels can be elevated by the administration of artificial O_2 carriers due to the difference in O_2 transporting properties from red blood cells. Whether this increase in tissue O_2 can potentiate cancer treatment is currently under investigation.

Organ Preservation

One of the most important agenda in transplantation medicine is long-term organ preservation and circumvention of ischemia reperfusion injuries. We

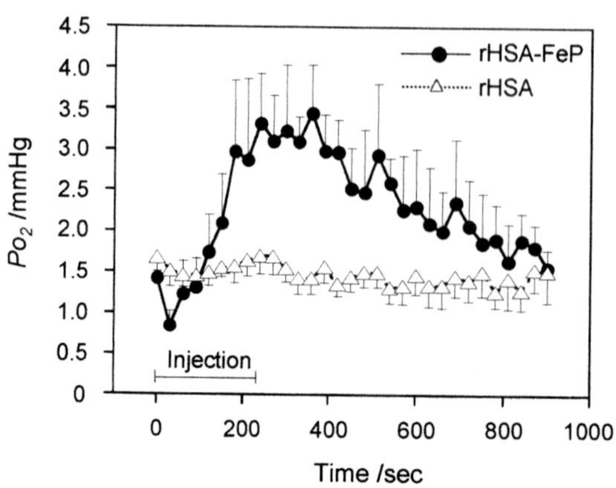

FIG. 12. Changes in the O_2 tension of the hypoxic region of the ascites hepatoma LY80 solid tumor after the administration of the O_2 saturated rHSA-heme or rHSA solutions in the anesthetized rats (n = 4 each). All data are shown as changes from the basal values (Po_2) just before the infusion and expressed as mean ± S.E.

think that artificial O_2 carriers can be applied as a perfusate for donor tissue in order to overcome these problems. In particular, its O_2 carrying capacity has the potential to significantly extend the preservation period. This will make it easier to transport organs. Also, utilizing the extra time, we may in the future be able to perform additional organ tests for better compatibility, or even perform genetic modifications during this period. We believe that through these applications, the concept of organ preservation can be expanded to organ culture, and furthermore to include the preservation of cells derived from donor tissues.

Extracorporeal Circulation

Extracorporeal circulation is quite common in cardiac surgery. Improvements are being made in the priming solutions but red cells are often still required to fill the device circuit, particularly in compromised cases and in children [55]. We believe that the use of artificial O_2 carriers in the priming solution can decrease or completely eliminate the need for a transfusion in such cases, and hence reduce the incidence of infection or GVHD.

Tissue Ischemia

Tissue ischemia can ensue from impairment of peripheral perfusion due to a variety of diseases such as arteriosclerosis obliterans, diabetes, and Burger's disease. The key event in the progression of ischemic diseases is the inability of red cells to flow through the capillaries, beyond obstruction ulceration and gangrene formation become imminent. We believe that this critical phase can be avoided or delayed by the application of artificial O_2 carriers, which can be designed to flow through these damaged capillaries or collateral circulation [27,28].

Liquid Ventilation for Acute Lung Injury

For patients who present acute lung injury or acute respiratory distress syndrome (ARDS), gas exchange in the lung exhibits severe deterioration and sometimes even the newest mechanical ventilation method fails to establish adequate oxygenation of the blood. In this type of critical case, liquid ventilation using an artificial O_2 carrier can establish optimal oxygenation of the blood and may reproduce the integrity of lung parenchyma [56]. Briefly explained, oxygenated liquid ventilation fluid is administered into the lung through trachea and O_2 molecules are transferred through diseased alveolus by diffusion and oxygenate the blood. Currently, this method is thought to be effective for patients with congenital diaphragmatic herniation. Efficacy for adult acute lung injuries is now under investigation. Perfluorochemicals are the main fluid used for clinical use, however, aqueous artificial O_2 carriers may have the potential to be used for liquid ventilation.

Epilogue

The research field of the red cell substitutes is moving forward very rapidly. Also as you have seen, the paradigm in this field is expanding from red cell substitutes to "O_2 therapeutics". The quality control and the pre-clinical test will be completed on the carriers produced at the pilot plant, after which clinical trials will proceed. We look forward to the day that our research will play an effective role in treating patients.

Acknowledgments. The authors gratefully thank Dr. H. Ikeda (Hokkaido Red Cross Blood Center), Prof. M. Suematsu (Keio University), Dr. M. Takaori (Higashitakarazuka Satoh Hospital), Prof. S. Hoka (Kitasato University), Prof. R. Ogawa (Nippon Medical College), Prof. M. Intaglietta (University of California San Diego), Prof. W.T. Phillips (University Texas San Antonio), and Prof. S. Curry (Imperial College, London), and their colleagues for the meaningful discussions and contributions to the research.

This work has been supported by The Ministry of Education, Culture, Sports, Science and Technology, The Ministry of Health, Labor and Welfare, and the Japan Science and Technology Corporation. The authors would like to express the sincere gratitude to the generous support of the Keio University Medical Science Fund founded on the basis of a donation from Dr. and Mrs. Mitsunada Sakaguchi.

References

1. Tsuchida E (ed) (1991) Macromolecular complexes, dynamic interactions and electronic processes. VCH New York
2. Ciardelli F, Tsuchida E, Wöhrle D (eds) (1996) Macromolecule-metal complexes. VCH New York
3. Matsushita Y, Hasegawa E, Eshima K, et al (1983) Synthesis of amphiphilic porphinatoiron complexes having phosphocholine groups. Chem Lett 1983:1387–1389
4. Tsuchida E (1985) Liposome-embedded iron-porphyrins as an artificial oxygen carrier. Ann New York Acad Sci 446:429–442
5. Tsuchida E, Nishide H (1986) Hemoglobin model—artificial oxygen carrier composed of porphinatoiron complexes. Top Curr Chem 132:63–99
6. Tsuchida E, Nishide H (1988) Liposome/heme as a totally synthetic oxygen transporter. In: Greoriadis G (ed) Liposomes as drug carriers, Wiley, Chichester, pp 569–582
7. Chang TMS (1997) Blood substitutes: principles, methods, products, and clinical trials. Karger, Basel
8. Riess JG (2001) Oxygen carriers (Blood Substitutes)-raison d'etre, chemistry, and some physiology. Chem Rev 101:2797–2919
9. Sloan EP, Koenigsberg M, Gens D, et al (1999) Diaspirin cross-linked hemoglobin (DCLHb) in the treatment of severe traumatic hemorrhagic shock. JAMA 282: 1857–1864

10. Tsuchida E (1998) Blood substitutes: present and future perscpectives. Elsevier, Amsterdam
11. Djordjevich L, Mayoral J, Miller IF, et al (1987) Cardiorespiratory effects of exchange transfusions with synthetic erythrocytes in rats. Crit Care Med 15:318–323
12. Takeoka S, Ohgushi T, Sakai H, et al (1993) Preparation conditions of human hemoglobin vesicles covered with lipid membrane. Artif Organs Today 3:129–136
13. Sakai H, Takeoka S, Yokohama H, et al (1993) Purufication of concentrated Hb using organic solvent and heat treatment. Protein Expression Purif 4:563–569
14. Takeoka S, Ohgushi T, Terase K, et al (1996) Layer-controlled hemoglobin vesicles by interaction of hemoglobin with a phospholipid assembly. Langmuir 12:1755–1759
15. Naito Y, Fukutomi I, Masada Y, et al (2002) Virus removal from hemoglobin solution using Planova membrane. J Artif Organs 5:141–145
16. Fukutomi I, Sakai H, Takeoka S, et al (2002) Carbonylation of oxyhemoglobin solution using a membrane oxygenator. J Artif Organs 5:102–107
17. Sou K, Endo T, Takeoka S, et al (2000) Poly(ethylene glycol)-modification of the phospholipid vesicles by using the spontaneous incorporation of poly(ethylene glycol)-lipid into the vesicles. Bioconjugate Chem 11:372–379
18. Sakai H, Tomiyama K, Sou K, et al (2000) Poly(ethyleneglycol)-conjugation and deoxygenation enable long term preservation of hemoglobin vesicles as oxygen carriers. Bioconjugate Chem 11:425–432
19. Sou K, Naito Y, Endo T, et al (2003) Effective encapsulation of proteins into size-controlled phospholipid vesicles using the freeze-thawing and extrusion. Biotechnol Prog 19
20. Izumi Y, Sakai H, Hamada K, et al (1996) Pysiologic responses to exchange transfusion with hemoglobin vesicels as an artificial oxygen carrier in anesthetized rats: changes in mean arterial pressure and renal cortical tissue oxygen tension. Crit Care Med 24:1869–1873
21. Izumi Y, Sakai H, Takeoka S, et al (1997) Evaluation of the capabilities of a hemoglobin vesicle as an artificial oxygen carrier in a rat exchange transfusion model ASAIO J. 43:289–297
22. Kobayashi K, Izumi Y, Yoshizu A, et al (1997) The oxygen carrying capability of hemoglobin vesicles evaluated in rat exchange transfusion models. Artif Cells Blood Substitues Immobilization Biotechnol 25:357–366
23. Sakai H, Park SI, Kose T, et al (1997) Surface modification of hemoglobin vesicles with poly(ethyleneglycol) and effects on aggregation, viscosity, and blood flow during 90% exchange transfusion in anesthetized rats. Bioconjugate Chem 8:23–30
24. Sakai H, Tsai AG, Kerger H, et al (1998) Subcutaneous microvascular responses to hemodilution with a red cell substitute consisting of polyethyleneglycol-modified vesicles encapsulating hemoglobin. J Biomed Materials Res 40:66–78
25. Sakai H, Tsai AG, Rohlfs RJ, et al (1999) Microvascular responses to hemodilution with Hb-vesicles as red cell substitutes: Influences of O_2 affinity. Am J Physiol 276(Heart Circ Physiol 45):H553–H562
26. Sakai H, Takeoka S, Wettstein R, et al (2002) Systemic and Microvascular responses to the hemorrhagic shock and resuscitation with Hb-vesicles. Am J Physiol Heart Circ Physiol 283:H1191–H1199
27. Erni D, Wettstein R, Schramm S, et al (2003) Normovolemic hemodilution with hemoglobin-vesicle solution attenuates hypoxia in ischemic hamster flap tissue. Am J Physiol Heart Circ Physiol 284:H1702–H1709
28. Contaldo C, Schramm S, Wettstein R, et al (2003) Improved oxygenation in ischemic hamster flap tissue is correlated with increasing hemodilution with Hb vesicles and their O_2 affinity. Am J Physiol Heart Circ Physiol 284

29. Goda N, Suzuki K, Naito S, et al (1998) Distribution of heme oxygenase isoform in rat liver: topographic basis for carbon monoxide-mediated micorvascular relaxation. J Clin Invest 101:604–612
30. Sakai H, Hara H, Yuasa M, et al (2000) Molecular dimensions of Hb-based O_2 carriers determine constriction of resistance arteries and hypertension in conscious hamster model. Am J Physiol Heart Circ Physiol 279:H908–H915
31. Wakamoto S, Fujiwara M, Abe H, et al (2001) Effects of PEG-modified hemoglobin vesicles on agonist induced platelet aggregation and RANTES release in vitro. Artif Cells Blood Substitues Immobilization Biotechnol 29:191–201
32. Kyokane T, Norimizu S, Taniai H, et al (2001) Carbon monoxide from heme catabolism protects against hepatobiliary dysfunction in endotoxin-treated rat liver. Gastroenterology 120:1227–1240
33. Ito T, Fujihara M, Abe H, et al (2001) Effects of poly (ethyleneglycol)-modified hemoglobin vesicles on N-formyl-methionyl-leucyl-phenylalanine induced respoonses of polymorphonuclear neutrophils in vitro. Artif Cells Blood Substitues Immobilization Biotechnol 29:427–438
34. Sakai H, Horinouchi H, Tomiyama K, et al (2001) Hemoglobin-vesicles as oxygen carriers: influence on phagocytic activity and histopathological changes in reticuloendothelial systems. Am J Pathol 159:1079–1088
35. Sakai H, Tomiyama K, Masada Y, et al (2003) Pretreatment of serum containing Hb-vesicels (oxygen carriers) to avoid their interference in laboratory tests. Clin Chem Lab Med 41:222–231
36. Curry S, Mandelkow H, Brick P, et al (1998) Crystal structure of human serum albumin complexes with fatty acid reveals an asymmetric distribution of binding sites. Nature Struct Biol 5:827–835
37. Sumi A, Ohtani W, Kobayashi K, et al (1993) Purification and Physicochemical Properties of Recombinant Human Serum Albumin. In: Rivat C, Stoltz J-F (eds) Biotechnology of Blood Proteins Vol. 227, John Libbey Eurotext Montrouge, pp 293–298
38. Komatsu T, Ando K, Kawai N, et al (1995) O_2-Transport Albumin: A New Hybrid-haemoprotein Incorporating Tetraphenylporphinatoiron(II) Derivative. Chem Lett 1995:813–814
39. Tsuchida E, Ando K, Maejima H, et al (1997) Properties of oxygen binding by albumin-tetraphenylporphyrynatoiron(II) derivative complexes. Bioconjugate Chem 8:534–538
40. Wu J, Komatsu T, Tsuchida E (1998) Resonance raman studies of O_2-binding to *ortho*-substituted tetraphenyl- and tetranaphthyl-porphinatoiron(II) derivatives with a covalently linked axial imidazole. J Chem Soc Dalton Trans 1998:2503–2506
41. Komatsu T, Hamamatsu K, Wu J, et al (1999) Physicochemical properties and O_2-coordination structure of human serum albumin incorporating tetrakis(*o*-pivalamido) phenylporphinatoiron(II) serivatives. Bioconjugate Chem 10:82–86
42. Tsuchida E, Komatsu T, Mastukawa Y, et al (1999) Human serum albumin incorporating tetrakis(*o*-pivalamido)phenylporphinatoiron(II) derivative as a totally synthetic O_2-carrying hemoprotein. Bioconjugate Chem 10:797–802
43. Komatsu T, Matsukawa Y, Tsuchida E (2000) Kinetics of CO and O_2 Binding to Human Serum Albumin-heme Hybrid. Bioconjugate Chem 11:772–776
44. Komatsu T, Matsukawa Y, Tsuchida E (2001) Reaction of Nitric Oxide with Synthetic Hemoprotein, Human Serum Albumin Incorporating Tetraphenylporphinatoiron(II) Derivatives. Bioconjugate Chem 12:71–75
45. Nakagawa A, Komatsu T, Tsuchida E (2001) Photoreduction of autooxidized albumin-heme hybrid in saline solution: revival of its O_2-binding ability. Bioconjugate Chem 12:648–652

46. Komatsu T, Okada T, Moritake M, et al (2001) O_2-Binding properties of double-sided porphyrinatoiron(II)s with polar substituents and their human serum albumin hybrids. Bull Chem Soc Jpn 74:1695–1702
47. Wu Y, Komatsu T, Tsuchida E (2001) Electrochemical studies of albumin-heme hybrid in aqueous media by modified electrode. Inorg Chim Acta 322:120–124
48. Komatsu T, Matsukawa Y, Tsuchida E (2002) Effect of heme structure on O_2-binding properties of human serum albumin-heme hybrids: intramolecular histidine coordination provides a stable O_2-adduct complex. Bioconjugate Chem 13:397–402
49. Tsuchida E, Komatsu T, Yanagimoto T, et al (2002) Preservation stability and in vivo administration of albumin-heme hybrid solution as an entirely synthetic O_2-carrier. Polym Adv Technol 13:845–850
50. Nakagawa A, Komatsu T, Ohmichi N, et al (2003) Synthetic dioxygen-carrying hemoprotein: human serum albumin including iron(II) complex of protoporphyrin IX with an axially coordinated histidylglycyl-propionate. Chem Lett 32:504–505
51. Tsuchida E, Komatsu T, Matsukawa Y, et al (2003) Human serum albumin incorporating synthetic heme: red blood cell substitute without hypertension by nitric oxide scavenging. J Biomed Mater Res 64A:257–261
52. Tsuchida E, Komatsu T, Hamamatsu K, et al (2000) Exchange transfusion of albumin-heme as an artificial O_2-infusion into anesthetized rats: physiological responses, O_2-delivery and reduction of the oxidized hemin sites by red blood cells. Bioconjugate Chem 11:46–50
53. Komatsu T, Hamamatsu K, Tsuchida E (1999) Cross-linked human serum albumin dimers incorporating sixteen (tetraphenylporphinato)iron(II) derivatives: synthesis, characterization, and O_2-binding property. Macromolecules 32:8388–8391
54. Kobayashi K, Komatsu T, Iwamaru A, et al (2003) Oxygenation of hypoxic region in solid tumor by administration of human serum albumin incorporating synthetic hemes. J Biomed Mater Res 64A:48–51
55. Kobayashi K, Izumi Y, Yamahata T, et al (1996) Efficacy of synthetic oxygen-carrying substances. In: Proceedings of Int. Congr. Ser. 1995. Elsevier, pp 305–310
56. Horinouchi H, Tajima A, Kobayashi K (2001) Liquid ventilation using artificial oxygen carrier. Artif Blood 9:2–5 (in Japanese)

Red Blood Cell Substitutes: Past, Present, and Future

Thomas Ming Swi Chang

Summary. Polyhemoglobin is already well into the final stages of clinical trials in humans. One has been approved for routine clinical use in South Africa. Perfluorochemicals are chemical oxygen carriers that are being actively developed with some in the advanced stages of clinical trials. Meanwhile, new generations of modified Hb are being developed that can modulate the effects of nitric oxide. Other systems are also being developed to include antioxidant properties for those clinical applications that may have potential problems related to oxygen radicals. Other products in advanced stages of animal testing are based on hemoglobin-lipid vesicles, heme-albumin and heme-lipid vesicles. A further development is the use of nanotechnology and biodegradable copolymers to prepare nano-dimension artificial red blood cells containing hemoglobin and complex enzyme systems.

Key words. Blood substitutes, Nanotechnology, Nanocapsules, Hemoglobin, Red blood cells, Polyhemoglobin

Introduction

Serious efforts to develop blood substitutes [1–5] for human use started only in the 1980s. The impetus for this was public concern about human immunodeficiency virus (HIV), hepatitis C virus and others present in donated blood. Unlike red blood cells, blood substitutes can be sterilized by pasteurization, ultrafiltration and chemical means. This inactivates the pathogens responsible for HIV, hepatitis and other infections. Furthermore, since blood substi-

---

Artificial Cells & Organs Research Centre, MSSS-FRSQ Research Group on Blood Substitutes in Transfusion Medicine, Faculty of Medicine, McGill University, 3655 Drummond Street, Montreal, Quebec, Canada H3G 1Y6

tutes do not have a cell membrane with blood group antigens, cross-matching and typing are not required before use. This saves time and facilities, allowing instant transfusions, which are especially useful in emergencies. Blood substitutes can be stored for more than one year, some at room temperature. This is compared to 40 days for donated blood stored using standard methods.

Past Approaches

The need for red blood cell substitutes is such that there have been numerous unsuccessful attempts using different approaches. One of these relates to the use of the unmodified oxygen carrying native hemoglobin extracted from red blood cells. In 1937, a hemoglobin solution obtained by lysing red blood cells was used for experimental transfusion in animals [6]. It was effective in the delivery of oxygen, but was highly toxic to the kidneys. This led to the removal of membrane stroma material from the Hb solution to develop stroma free hemoglobin that had less renal toxicity in the animals [7]. As a result, a Phase-I clinical trial was carried out in humans in 1978 [8]. The results showed that even highly purified native hemoglobin was still toxic to the kidneys. Inside the red blood cells Hb is a tetramer with two α subunits and two β subunits. When free Hb is infused into the body, the tetramer ($\alpha 1\beta 1\alpha 2\beta 2$) breaks down into toxic dimers ($\alpha 1\beta 1$ and $\alpha 2\beta 2$), which are rapidly filtered by the kidneys to enter the renal tubules where high concentration of dimers causes renal toxicity. Although this approach has not been successful, the research has produced important basic information regarding the toxicity of hemoglobin.

Present Approaches Based on Modified Hemoglobin

Since hemoglobin is too toxic to be used as a blood substitute, the challenge is to modify the hemoglobin molecule. Research on the use of encapsulated and cross-linked Hb as blood substitutes started many years ago [9–11]. However, it was only after free hemoglobin was shown to be toxic that others become interested in modified hemoglobin. The different types of modified Hb include cross-linked polyhemoglobin, cross-linked tetrameric hemoglobin, conjugated hemoglobin, recombinant hemoglobin and encapsulated hemoglobin.

Polyhemoglobin

Bifunctional agents were used to cross-link the reactive amino groups of Hb, producing polyhemoglobin (polyHb) [9–11] and preventing the breakdown of the cross-linked Hb molecules into dimers. The first reagents used to cross-link hemoglobin were sebacyl chloride [9–10] and glutaraldehyde [11]. Glutaraldehyde-cross-linked human polyHb was developed for animal testing followed by clinical trials [12–15]. Pyridoxalated glutaraldehyde-cross-linked human polyHb is in advance stages of Phase-III clinical trials [12,13]. This preparation contains less than 1% of cross-linked tetrameric Hb [12]. The clinical trials use high doses (up to 20 units or 10 litres) in randomized, controlled Phase III studies for comparing its safety and efficacy with that of allogeneic blood.

The use of glutaraldehyde cross-linked bovine polyHb is another polyhemoglobin [14,15]. Unlike human Hb, the P_{50} of bovine Hb is controlled by chloride and therefore does not require 2,3-DPG. Bovine polyHb containing less than 5% cross-linked tetrameric Hb has been extensively tested in clinical trials. It has been approved for routine clinical applications in South Africa [16].

In another approach, a 2,3-DPG-pocket modifier has been prepared using dialdehyde derived from o-raffinose [17,18]. This is now being used to form human polyHb for use in Phase III clinical trials [18]. Being a 2,3-DPG pocket modifier, this preparation has a good P_{50} without the need to add pyridoxal-phosphate [17].

Another two approaches are attempts to prepare larger polyhemoglobin. Professor Bucci discusses "non-extravasatinghemoglobin polymer" in his chapter. Barnikol and colleagues in Germany have been studying the preparation of porcine hemoglobin hyperpolymers.

Conjugated Hemoglobin

Hb has also been cross-linked to polymers to form an insoluble conjugated Hb [9,10]. This approach has been extended to produce a soluble conjugated Hb formed by cross-linking individual Hb molecules to soluble polymers such as dextran [19], polyoxyethylene [20] and polyethylene glycol (PEG) [21]. This is in ongoing clinical trials [22]. More recently, a new Maleimide PEG-hemoglobin [23] has been developed and is now in Phase II clinical trials. This will be discussed in more detail by Dr. Winslow in his chapter.

Cross-Linked Tetrameric Hb

In polyhemoglobin the Hb molecules are cross-linked both internally (intramolecular) and to one another (intermolecular). For cross-linked tetremeric Hb, cross-linker like bis(N-maleimidomethyl)ether, only cross-links the Hb intramolecularly [24] This forms cross-linked tetrameric Hb and prevents the breakdown of the Hb into dimers. Another cross-linker, bis(3,5-dibromosalicyl) fumarate, can cross-link the two α subunits of the Hb intramolecularly and modify the 2,3-DPG pocket [25]. This results in a cross-linked tetrameric Hb molecule with a high P_{50} There were substantial vasoactivities related to the use of tetrameric cross-linked hemoglobin during clinical trials.

Recombinant Human Hemoglobin

Recombinant human Hb can be produced by genetically engineered *Escherichia coli* [26] by fusing the two α subunits to prevent the breakdown of the resulting tetrameric Hb into dimmers. Furthermore, an amino acid substitution has been introduced that alters oxygen affinity resulting in a high P_{50} [26,27]. Like the above cross-linked tetrameric hemoglobin, clinical trials show substantial vasoactivities. As a result, a new recombinant hemoglobin has been developed by this group. Recombinant Hbs are prepared with mutagenesis of the distal heme pocket in order to change the reactivity of Hb for nitric oxide [28]. This has obviated the side effects related to nitric oxide removal.

Properties of Modified Hemoglobin

Vasoactivity

Nitric oxide plays an important role in controlling the vascular tone of blood vessels with a reduction in the nitric-oxide level resulting in vasoconstriction. Although Hb and albumin have approximately the same molecular weight, albumin has highly negatively charged surfaces while Hb does not. Thus, unlike the larger polyHb, tetrameric Hb (cross-linked or recombinant) can more readily cross the intercellular junctions of the endothelial-cell layer to enter the interstitial space. These tetrameric Hb molecules have high affinity for nitric oxide and thus act as a sink, binding and removing nitric oxide resulting in vasoconstriction and thus an increase in blood pressure. Lower nitric oxide levels may also affect the nerve plexus and smooth muscles resulting, for example, in esophageal spasms and other gastrointestinal effects. Premedication and general anesthesia would prevent these gastrointestinal effects. Thus, one may not see gastrointestinal effects in anesthetized patients. Polyhemoglobin solution that contains little or no tetrameric hemoglobin did not cause vasoconstriction [12,13]. Those polyhemoglobins that contain more tetrameric hemoglobin may cause varying degrees of vasoconstriction. Thus, vasoactivities of polyhemoglobin solutions are related to the amounts of tetrameric hemoglobin present in the preparation. One of the strongest indicators for the role of tetrameric hemoglobin is that the new recombinant Hb with low affinity for nitric oxide demonstrably has little or no vasoactive effects [28]. Another proposal is that the vasoactivities of some types of modified Hb may be due to an excessive delivery of oxygen to the arterioles, leading to autoregulatory vasoconstriction [2].

Immunological Properties

The initial concerns that cross-linking of macromolecules such as Hb may result in alterations of the antigenicity of the resulting modified macromolecules has not appeared with modified human Hb [5,12]. Even in the case of bovine polyHb, infusion into humans did not result in adverse local or systemic allergic or adverse reactions [14,15].

Circulation Half-Life of Modified Hemoglobin

Ongoing clinical trials using polyhemoglobin and conjugated hemoglobin show that these have several useful clinical applications especially in elective surgery. Their circulation half-life in humans averaging around 24–28h, in comparison with 40 days for donor blood. Thus, when used for the replacement of blood loss during surgery or trauma, it is effective in the first 24h. After this, if the total hemoglobin concentration is below the transfusion trigger for the particular patient, then donor blood transfusion will be required. However, the patient's own blood can be collected over a period of time before surgery (autologous donation), or collected and replaced with blood substitutes just prior to surgery. This way, blood loss during surgery can be replaced by blood substitutes and, at the completion of surgery, the autologous blood can be returned to the patients as required. If the blood loss is not excessive this would further help to reduce the need for donor blood transfusion. However, in some trauma, cancer, and major orthopedic surgery, the blood loss may be too massive to avoid the need for donor blood after 24h. Donated blood is hardly free from adverse effects [1–4], and modified Hb has the potential of avoiding some of the adverse effects of donated blood including the inactivation of infectious agents. Furthermore, modified Hb does not require cross-matching and typing before use and can be transfused immediately, making it especially useful in emergencies.

Future Modified Hemoglobin with Antioxidant Properties

Hemoglobin is a reactive molecule, especially in the generation of oxidants [29,30]. Red blood cells contain catalase and superoxide dismutase which are important in the removal of superoxide and peroxide. Many of the modified-Hb blood substitutes are prepared using ultrapure hemoglobin. The potential solution of the effects of the lack of antioxidants in the current modified-Hb blood substitutes are being investigated [30–34]. For example, studies are being carried out to cross-link catalase and superoxide dismutase to polyHb [30–33]. The resulting PolyHb-catalase-superoxide dismuatase (PolyHb-SOD-CAT) when compared to polyHb has a much lower tendency to generate free-radicals in vitro and in vivo [30–33]. In a combined hemorrhagic shock and cerebral vascular occlusion rat model, it was shown that, with sustained ischemia, reperfusion using PolyHb-SOD-CAT, unlike PolyHb, did not cause disruption of blood-brain barrier or brain edema [33]. Another group is studying the use of polynitroxylated hemoglobin with antioxidant activity [34]. This chemical modification gives rise to SOD-CAT like activities.

Encapsulated HB as Future Generation Red Blood Cell Substitute

Artificial red blood cells formed by the encapsulation of Hb and enzymes resemble red blood cells more closely and their surface properties can also be modified to increase their circulation time. In this way, Hb or specially prepared cross-linked Hb or recombinant Hb can also be encapsulated inside the artificial cells.

Microencapsulation of Hb and Enzymes

The first encapsulation of the contents of red blood cells, including Hb and enzymes, inside artificial red blood cells with artificial membranes was reported in 1957 [35] and this system has an oxygen-dissociation curve comparable to that of red blood cells [35]. Red-blood-cell enzymes such as carbonic anhydrase [9] and catalase [35] have been included in these artificial red blood cells where they continue to function. For example, artificial cells containing Hb and catalase have been used to replace the antioxidant functions in mice with an inborn defect in red-blood-cell catalase [35]. The major problem was a short circulation time resulting from rapid uptake by the reticuloendothelial system [10]. Removal of sialic acid from red-blood-cell membranes results in the rapid removal of red blood cells from the circulation [10]. This observation led to the use of membranes with different surface properties including a negative surface charge and the addition of polysaccharides such as sialic-acid analogs [9,10]. Although this resulted in a significant increase in circulation time, the problem was that the diameters of the microcapsules were relatively large (1–5 μ). This has led to the next step in artificial red blood cell development.

Hemoglobin Lipid Vesicles

In 1980, small lipid-membrane artificial red blood cells approximately 0.2 μm in diameter were prepared using lipid-membrane liposomes [36] and found to remain in the circulation for a longer period than those described above. Extensive research on bilayer-lipid membrane artificial red blood cells has been carried out [37–39]. PEG-lipid vesicles are especially effective in increasing the circulation time [38]. Hemoglobin lipid vesicles have been used successfully to replace most of the red blood cells in rats and also for the treatment of massive hemorrhage [37–39]. The Waseda-Keio(Prof Tsuchida and Kobayashi) project on "oxygen infusion" have completed detailed safety and efficacy studies and they will be describing in chapter by K. Kobayashi.

Biodegradable-Copolymer Membrane Nanocapsules Containing Hb and Red-Blood-Cell Enzymes

Polylactide and polyglycolide are degraded in the body into water and carbon dioxide. Polylactic acid encapsulated Hb and enzymes have been prepared in the micron range [40]. However, these are too large to survive for long in the circulation. More recently, polylactic acid Hb nanocapsules of 0.08–0.180 μm in diameter have been developed [41–43]. Unlike Hb lipid vesicles, the membrane material of nanocapsules is made almost entirely of biodegradable polymers and, as polymers are stronger and more porous than lipids, less membrane material is required. Superoxide dismutase catalase and methemoglobin reductase can also be included with the Hb [41,42]. Hemoglobin inside the red blood cell is being continuously converted into the non-oxygen-carrying form of methemoglobin. Red blood cells contain the methemoglobin reductase system to enzymatically convert methemoglobin to hemoglobin. Nanocapsules are permeable to glucose and other small hydrophilic molecules. This allows one to prepare Hb nanocapsules containing the methemoglobin reductase system [42,43]. Reducing agents can also diffuse into the nanocapsules to convert metHb to Hb as has been demonstrated by in vitro studies [42–45].

We have recently synthesized a number of new polylactide-polyethylene glycol copolymers. One of these, when used for the membrane of nanocapsules, can increase the circulation time of the nanodimension artificial red blood cells to double that of polyhemgolobin [44–46]. This has solved the problem of the short circulation time of the polylactide nanocapsules. As a result, we are now into safety and efficacy studies. Infusion of one-third the blood volume into rats did not result in vasoactivities. The hemodynamic remains normal. Long-term follow-up has been completed and there is no adverse effect for biochemistry, enzymes and histology. Detailed efficacy studies including exchange transfusion and resuscitation for hemorrhagic shock is ongoing.

Chemical Approach Based on Perfluorochemicals

There is another type of blood substitute based on a chemical approach using perfluorochemicals. Perfluorochemicals (PFCs) are synthetic fluids in which oxygen can dissolve [47] and that can be made into fine emulsions for use as oxygen carriers [47,48]. Their greatest advantage is that PFCs can be produced in large amounts. Furthermore, their purity can be more easily controlled. With the demonstration that this can replace most of the blood in rats [48] this approach was developed in Japan into a product called fluosol-DA (20%) [49]. This consists of a mixture of Perfluorodecalin and perfluorotripropylamine with Pluronic F-68 as the emulsifier. This has been tested extensively in clinical trials [49,50] It was approved by the F.D.A. for coronary artery balloon angioplasty (PTCA).

Improved fluorochemicals have recently allowed a higher concentration of PFC to be used, and a blood substitute based on perfluoro-octyl bromide ($C_8F_{17}Br$) with egg-yolk lecithin as the surfactant [51,52] is now well into clinical trials. The use of egg-yolk as the emulsifier [51] has solved the problem related to complement activation from Pluronic F-68. Smaller doses and smaller particle size are used to avoid flu-like symptoms caused by the infusion of large amounts of larger emulsions resulting in uptake of PFC by macrophages and the release of cytokines [52]. One of the important potential uses of PFC is for patients whose religion does not allow them to use donated blood or products prepared from it.

Synthetic Heme: Another Future RBC Substitute

Professor Tsuchida has successfully developed synthetic heme [39]. This has now reached a successful stage and has been studied extensively in animal safety and efficacy studies as part of the Waseda-Keio Joint Project on "Oxygen Infusions". These include albumin-heme consisting of recombinant human serum albumin incorporating hemes and lipidheme-vesicle consisting of phospholipid liposome embedding lipidheme. This is discussed in detail by Professor Tsuchida and Professor Kobayashi in this book.

Conclusion

Polyhemoglobin is already well into the final stages of clinical trials in humans. One of these has been approved for routine clinical use in South Africa [16]. Meanwhile, new generations of modified Hb are being developed that can modulate the effects of nitric oxide. Other systems are also being developed to include antioxidant properties for those clinical applications that may have potential problems related to oxygen radicals. A further development is the use of lipids or biodegradable polymer membranes to prepare artificial red blood cells containing Hb and complex enzyme systems. The use of synthetic heme is another exciting area. Perfluorochemicals is another area that is being actively developed.

Acknowledgments. This author gratefully acknowledges the support of the Canadian Institutes for Health Research (CIHR), the Virage Award of Centre of Excellence in Biotechnology from the Quebec Ministry of Higher Education and Science, the Bayer/Canadian Blood Agency/Hema Quebec/CIHR Research Funds, and the Quebec Ministry of Health in the form of the MSSS-FRSQ Research Group (Equipe) on Blood Substitutes in Transfusion Medicine.

References

1. Klein HG (2000) The prospects for red-cell substitutes. N Engl J Med 342(22): 1666–1668
2. Winslow RM (2000) Blood substitutes. Adv Drug Deliv Rev 40:131–142
3. Chang TMS (2002) Oxygen carriers. Current Opinion in Investigational Drugs, 3(8):1187–1190
4. Squires JE (2002) Artificial blood. Science 8:295(5557):1002–1005
5. Chang TMS (1997) Blood substitutes: principles methods, products and clinical trials. vol.1. Karger, Basel, pp 1–141
6. Amberson WR (1937) Blood substitute. Biol Rev 12:48–53
7. Rabiner SF, Helbert JR, Lopas H, and Friedman LH (1967) Evaluation of stroma-free hemoglobin solution as a plasma expander. J Exp Med 126:1127–1132
8. Savitsky JP, Doozi J, Black J, Arnold JD (1978) A clinical safety trial of stroma-free hemoglobin. Clin Pharm Ther 23:73–80
9. Chang TMS (1964) Semipermeable microcapsules. Science. 146(3643):524–525
10. Chang TMS (1972) Artificial cells. Charles C Thomas, Springfield, IL
11. Chang TMS (1971) Stabilization of enzyme by microencapsulation with a concentrated protein solution or by crosslinking with glutaraldehyde. Biochem Biophys Res Com 44:1531–1533
12. Gould SA, Sehgal LR, Sehgal HL, DeWoskin R, Moss GS (1998) The clinical development of human polymerized hemoglobin. In: Chang TMS (ed) Blood substitutes: principles, methods, products and clinical trials. vol.2. Karger, Basel, pp 12–28
13. Gould SA, Moore EE, Hoyt DB, Burch JM, Haenel JB, Garcia J, DeWoskin R, and Moss GS (1998) The first randomized trial of human polymerized hemoglobin as a blood substitute in acute trauma and emergent surgery. J Am Coll Surg 187:113–120
14. Pearce LB, Gawryl MS (1988) Overview of preclinical and clinical efficacy of Biopure's HBOCs. In: Chang TMS (ed) Blood substitutes: principles, methods, products and clinical trials. vol. 2. Karger, Basel, pp 82–98

15. Sprung J, Kindscher JD, Wahr JA, Levy JH, Monk TG, Moritz MW, O'Hara PJ (2002) The use of bovine hemoglobin glutamer-250 (Hemopure) in surgical patients: results of a multicenter, randomized, single-blinded trial. Anesth Analg 94(4):799–808
16. Lok C (2001) Blood product from cattle wins approval for use in humans. Nature 410(6831):855
17. Adamson JG, Moore C, Hemolink TM (1998) An o-Raffinose crosslinked hemoglobin-based oxygen carrier. In: Chang TMS (ed) Blood substitutes: principles, methods, products and clinical trials. vol. 2. Karger, Basel, pp 62–79
18. Carmichael FJ (2001) Recent developments in hemoglobin-based oxygen carriers—an update on clinical trials. Transfus Apheresis Sci 24(1):17–21
19. Wong JT (1988) Rightshifted dextran hemoglobin as blood substitute. Biomaterials, Artificial Cells and Artificial Organs. 16:237–245
20. Shorr RG, Viau AT, Abuchowski A (1996) Phase 1B safety evaluation of PEG hemoglobin as an adjuvant to radiation therapy in human cancer patients. Artificial Cells, Blood Substitutes and Immobolization Biotechnology, an International Journal, 24:407–412
21. Iwashita Y, Yabuki A, Yamaji K, Iwasaki K, Okami T, Hirati C, Kosaka K (1988) A new resuscitation fluid "Stabilized hemoglobin," preparation and characteristics. Biomaterials, Artificial Cells and Artificial Organs, 16:271–280
22. De Angelo J (1999) Nitric oxide scavengers in the treatment of shock associated with systemic inflammatory response syndrome. Exp Opin Pharmacother 1:19–29
23. Winslow R (2002) In: Kjellstrom T, Lowe K (eds) Abstract volume, Fourth International Symposium on Current Issues in Blood Substitute Research, June 5–8, Stockholm, Sweden
24. Bunn HF, Jandl JH (1968) The renal handling of hemoglobin. Trans Assoc Am Physicians 81:147–150
25. Nelson DJ (1998) Blood and HemAssistTM (DCLHb): potentially a complementary therapeutic team, In: Chang TMS (ed) Blood substitutes: principles, methods, products and clinical trials. vol. 2. Karger, Basel, pp 39–57
26. Hoffman SJ, Looker DL, Roehrich JM, et al (1990) Expression of fully functional tetrameric human hemoglobin in escherichia coli. Proc Natl Acad Sci USA 87:8521–8525
27. Freytag JW, Templeton D (1997) Optro TM (Recombinant Human Hemoglobin): a therapeutic for the delivery of oxygen and the restoration of blood volume in the treatment of acute blood loss in trauma and surgery. In: Rudolph AS, Rabinovici R, Feuerstein GZ (eds) Red cell substitutes; basic principles and clinical application, Marcel Dekker, New York, pp 325–334
28. Doherty DH, Doyle MP, Curry SR, Vali RJ, Fattor TJ, Olson JS, Lemon DD (1998) Rate of reaction with nitric oxide determines the hypertensive effect of cell-free hemoglobin. Nature Biotechnol 16:672–676
29. Alayash Al (1999) Hemoglobin-based blood substitutes: oxygen carriers, pressor agents, or oxidants? Nature Biotechnol 17(6):545–549
30. D'Agnillo F, Chang TMS (1998) Polyhemoglobin-superoxide dismutase catalase as a blood substitute with antioxidant properties. Nature Biotechnol 16(7):667–671
31. Chang TMS, D'Agnillo F, Razack S (1998) A second-generation hemoglobin-based blood substitute with antioxidant activities. In: Chang TMS (ed) Blood substitutes: principles, methods, products and clinical trials. vol. 2. Karger, Basel, pp 178–186
32. D'Agnillo F, Chang TMS (1997) Modified hemoglobin blood substitute from cross-linked hemoglobin-superoxide dismutase-catalase. USA patent 5,606,025
33. Powanda D, Chang TMS (2002) Cross-linked polyhemoglobin-superoxide dismutase-catalase supplies oxygen without causing blood brain barrier disruption or brain

edema in a rat model of transient global brain ischemia-reperfusion. Artificiall cells, blood substitutes and immobilization Biotechnology, an international journal 30:25–42
34. Buehler PW, Mehendale S, Wang H, Xie J, Ma L, Trimble CE, Hsia CJ, Gulati A (2000) Resuscitative effects of polynitroxylated alpha-alpha-cross-linked hemoglobin following severe hemorrhage in the rat. Free Radic Biol Med 29(8):764–774
35. Chang TMS (1988) Hemoglobin corpuscles: Report of a research project for honours physiology, Medical Library, McGill University 1957. Also reprinted as part of 30th anniversary in artificial red blood cells research, J Biomaterials, Artificial Cells & Artificial Organs 16:1–9
35. Chang TMS, Poznansky MJ (1968) Semipermeable microcapsules containing catalase for enzyme replacement in acatalsaemic mice. Nature 218(5138):242–245
36. Djordjevich L, Miller IF (1980) Synthetic erythrocytes from lipid encapsulated hemoglobin. Exp Hematol 8:584
37. Rudolph AS, Rabinovici R, Feuerstein GZ (eds) (1997) Red blood cell substitutes: basic principles and clinical applications. Marcel Dekker, New York
38. Philips WT, Klpper RW, Awasthi VD, Rudolph AS, Cliff R, Kwasiborski VV, Goins BA (1999) Polyethylene glyco-modified liposome-encapsulated hemoglobin: a long circulating red cell substitute. J Pharm Exp Ther 288:665–670
39. Tsuchida E (ed) (1998) Blood substitutes: present and future perspectives. Elsevier, Amsterdam
40. Chang TMS (1976) Biodegradable semipermeable microcapsules containing enzymes, hormones, vaccines, and other biologicals. J Bioengineer 1:25–32
41. Yu WP, Chang TMS (1996) Submicron polymer membrane hemoglobin nanocapsules as potential blood substitutes: preparation and characterization. Artificial cells, blood substitutes and Immobilization Biotechnology, an international journal 24: 169–184
42. Chang TMS, Yu WP (1997) Biodegradable polymer membrane containing hemoglobin for blood substitutes. USA Patent 1997:5670173
43. Chang TMS, Yu WP (1998) Nanoencapsulation of hemoglobin and rbc enzymes based on nanotechnology and biodegradable polymer. In: Chang TMS (ed) Blood substitutes: principles, methods, products and clinical trials. vol. 2. Karger, Basel, pp 216–231
44. Chang TMS, Yu WP (2001) Biodegradable polymeric nanocapsules and uses thereof. US provisional patent No 60/316,001
45. Chang TMS, Powanda D, Yu WP (2002) Biodegradable polymeric nanocapsules and uses thereof. PCT 2002
46. Chang TMS, Powanda D, Yu WP (2003) Ultrathin polyethylene-glycol-polylactide copolymer membrane nanocapsules containing polymerized hemoglobin and enzymes as nano-dimension red blood cell substitutes. Artificial Cells, Blood Substitutes & Biotechnology, an international journal 31(3):231–247
47. Clark LC Jr, Gollan F (1966) Survival of mammals breathing organic liquids equilibrated with oxygen at atmospheric pressure. Science 152:1755
48. Geyer RP, Monroe RG, Taylor K (1968) Survival of rats totally perfused with a fluorocarbon-detergent preparation. In: Norman JC, Folkman J, Hardison WG, Rudolf LE, Veith FJ (eds) Organ perfusion and preservation. Appleton Century Crofts, New York, pp 85–96
49. Naito R, Yokoyama K (1978) An improved perfluorodecalin emulsion. In: Jamieson GA, Greenwalt TJ (eds) Blood substitutes and plasma expanders. Alan R Liss, New York, p 81

50. Mitsuno T, Ohyanagi (1985) Present status of clinical studies of fluosol-DA (20%) in Japan. In: Tremper KK (ed) Perfluorochemical oxygen transport. Little Brown, Boston, pp 169–184
51. Riess JG (2001) Oxygen carriers ("blood substitutes"). Chem Rev 101:2797–2919
52. Keipert PE (1998) Perfluorochemical emulsions. In: Chang TMS (ed) Blood substitutes: principles, methods, products and clinical trials. vol. 2. Karger, Basel, pp 127–156

Inhaled Nitric Oxide: Update 2003

W.M. Zapol

Summary. Use of the novel biological mediator nitric oxide is described as a selective pulmonary vasodilator when inhaled in low concentrations.

Key words. Selective pulmonary vasodilator, Inhalation therapy

We hypothesized that inhaled Nitric Oxide (NO) would diffuse into the pulmonary vasculature of ventilated lung regions and cause relaxation of the pulmonary vascular smooth muscle. Since the NO is inhaled, the gas should be distributed predominantly to well-ventilated alveoli and not to collapsed or fluid-filled regions of the lung. In the presence of increased vasomotor tone, the selective vasodilatation of well-ventilated lung regions by inhaled NO should cause a "steal" or diversion of pulmonary artery blood flow towards well-ventilated alveoli, and improve the matching of ventilation to perfusion, thereby enhancing arterial oxygenation (PaO_2). Such an effect would be in marked contrast to the increased mismatch of ventilation and perfusion caused by intravenously administered vasodilators such as nitroprusside, nitroglycerin, and prostacyclin. Although these intravenous agents decrease pulmonary artery pressure, they increase intrapulmonary shunting of deoxygenated blood, by non-selectively dilating hypoventilated lung segments, and reduce the systemic PaO_2. Also, inhaled NO should not produce systemic vasodilatation because, unlike available intravenous vasodilators, it is avidly bound to hemoglobin and rapidly inactivated [1].

Rossaint et al. [2] compared the effects of inhaling 18 and 36 parts per million by volume (ppm) NO to intravenously infused prostacyclin in nine patients with acute respiratory distress syndrome (ARDS). Inhaled NO selectively reduced mean pulmonary artery pressure from 37 ± 3 to 30 ± 2 mmHg

---

Massachusetts General Hospital, Boston, MA, USA

(mean ± SE) and improved oxygenation by decreasing venous admixture (Q_{VA}/Q_t). The improved efficiency in oxygen exchange during NO inhalation was reflected in an increase of the PaO_2/FIO_2 ratio from 152 ± 15 mmHg to 199 ± 23 mmHg. While the intravenous infusion of prostacyclin also reduced pulmonary artery pressure, mean arterial pressure and PaO_2 decreased as Q_{VA}/Q_t increased. Subsequent reports have documented that inhalation of lower concentrations of NO (less than 20 ppm) also decreases pulmonary artery pressure and improves PaO_2 levels [3]. Even very small inhaled concentrations of NO (as low as 250 parts per billion) may be effective in some patients [3]. Right ventricular ejection fraction increases in some patients breathing inhaled NO, suggesting that decreasing pulmonary artery pressure may unload the right heart and be hemodynamically beneficial [3,4].

A marked variation has been reported for the hemodynamic and respiratory effects of clinical NO inhalation in ARDS, both among patients and within the same patient at different times in their illness. It is possible that pre-existing pulmonary disease as well as the concomitant administration of other vasoactive drugs and the effects of septic mediators may contribute to the observed variability. In general, the level of elevation of pulmonary vascular resistance predicts the degree of pulmonary vasodilation that is possible by NO inhalation. Those with the greatest degree of pulmonary hypertension appear to respond best to NO inhalation. Several recent trials have shown no effects on outcome (survival weaning from ventilation, etc.) of NO breathing in acute lung injury (ALI) [5].

NO Inhalation in Neonatal Respiratory Failure

In the fetus, intense pulmonary vasoconstriction causes oxygenated blood returning from the placenta to shunt right-to-left across the patent foramen ovale and ductus arteriosus to bypass the collapsed lungs. At birth, the lungs are distended with air and there is a sustained decrease in pulmonary vascular resistance and an increased pulmonary blood flow. In some babies, pulmonary blood flow does not increase after birth. Persistent pulmonary hypertension of the newborn (PPHN) is characterized by an increased pulmonary vascular resistance, right-to-left shunting of deoxygenated blood across the ductus arteriosus and foramen ovale, and severe systemic hypoxemia. Although breathing high levels of oxygen and induced alkalosis decreases pulmonary hypertension in some patients with PPHN, these therapies are often unsuccessful. The use of intravenous vasodilator therapy is limited by severe systemic hypotension, which may further reduce the PaO_2 by increasing right-to-left shunting in patients with PPHN. Extracorporeal membrane oxygenation (ECMO) is often used to support babies who remain hypoxemic despite maximal ventilator and medical therapies. Endogenous production of NO by the pulmonary vasculature is likely to be decreased in PPHN. Therefore, a therapeutic strategy that selectively increases NO activity in the lung may be beneficial to many infants with pulmonary hypertension.

Several clinical studies of NO inhalation have been performed in neonates [6,7], and infants and children with pulmonary hypertension [8]. Each demonstrates that inhalation of NO selectively decreases pulmonary hypertension and increases PaO_2. In three prospective randomized trials in term gestation newborns with hypoxic respiratory failure breathing NO acutely increases systemic oxygen levels and decreases the need for ECMO [9–11]. The Federal Drug Administration (FDA) approved the clinical use of inhaled NO for the treatment of hypoxic newborn respiratory failure in December 1999. Additionally, in children with many forms of congenital heart disease inhaled NO decreases pulmonary hypertension [8].

In pediatric as well as adult patients the pulmonary vasodilator response to NO inhalation is variable. In the neonatal lung, the degree of improvement of arterial oxygenation with NO depends on the initial degree of pulmonary vasoconstriction and hypoxemia [9] and recruitment of an adequate lung volume.

References

1. Steudel W, Hurford WE, Zapol WM (1999) Inhaled nitric oxide: basic biology and clinical applications. Anesthesiology 91:1090–1121
2. Rossaint R, Falke KJ, Lopez F, et al (1993) Inhaled nitric oxide for the adult respiratory distress syndrome. N Engl J Med 328:399–405
3. Gerlach H, Pappert D, Lewandowski K, et al (1993) Long-term inhalation with evaluated low doses of nitric oxide for selective improvement of oxygenation in patients with adult respiratory distress syndrome. Intensive Care Med 19:443–449
4. Wysocki M, Vignon P, Roupie E, et al (1993) Improvement in right ventricular function with inhaled nitric oxide in patients with the adult respiratory distress syndrome (ARDS) and permissive hypercapnia. Am Rev Respir Dis 147:A350
5. Lundin S, Mang H, Smithies M, et al (for the European Study Group of Inhaled Nitric Oxide) (1999) Inhalation of nitric oxide in acute lung injury: results of a European multicentre study. Intensive Care Med 25:911–919
6. Roberts JD, Polaner DM, Lang P, et al (1992) Inhaled nitric oxide in persistent pulmonary hypertension of the newborn. Lancet 340:818–819
7. Kinsella JP, Shaffer E, Neish SR, et al (1992) Low-dose inhalational nitric oxide in persistent pulmonary hypertension of the newborn. Lancet 340:8819–8820
8. Roberts JD, Jr., Lang P, Bigatello L, et al (1993) Inhaled nitric oxide in congenital heart disease. Circulation 87:447–453
9. Roberts JD, Fineman JR, Morin FC, et al (1997) Inhaled nitric oxide and persistent pulmonary hypertension of the newborn: results of a randomized controlled trial. N Engl J Med 336:605–610

10. Neonatal Inhaled Nitric Oxide Study Group (1997) Inhaled nitric oxide in full-term and nearly full-term infants with hypoxic respiratory failure. N Engl J Med 336(9): 597–604
11. Clark RH, Kueser TJ, Walker MW, et al (for the Clinical Inhaled Nitric Oxide Research Group) (2000) Low-dose nitric oxide therapy for persistent pulmonary hypertension of the newborn. N Engl J Med 342:469–474

The Role of p50 in Tissue Oxygen Delivery by Cell-Free Oxygen Carriers

Robert M. Winslow

Summary. The concept that the p50 of a cell-free O_2 carrier ("blood substitute") should approximate that of human blood is rooted in the assumption that the p50 is an important determinant of O_2 delivery. This assumption is based on antiquated measurements in subjects exposed to hypoxia, for whom a theory was developed that an increase in red cell 2,3-DPG shifts the oxygen equilibrium curve to the right (high p50, low O_2 affinity), thereby providing "adaptation" to hypoxia. This concept has been carried over to efforts to pharmacologically raise the p50 of human red cells and to preserve 2,3-DPG concentration in banked blood. More recent measurements in high altitude natives demonstrate that such a right-shift is not critical to adaptation; in fact, a left shift is probably essential to maintain arterial saturation at extreme altitude. Furthermore, evidence of therapeutic benefit from increasing p50 in humans is scant. In the case of cell-free hemoglobin, the mechanisms of O_2 transfer to tissue are completely different, such that unless p50 is significantly reduced, O_2 oversupply will result, engaging autoregulatory mechanisms that leads to vasoconstriction. A second generation of O_2 carriers has been designed with increased O_2 affinity, and the suggestion is made that the optimal p50 for cell-free hemoglobin should be approximately that of the target tissue for oxygenation. In the case of highly metabolic tissue such as the myocardium or exercising skeletal muscle, this is in the range of 3–5 mmHg.

Key words. p50, PEG, O_2 transport, Blood substitute, Hemoglobin

Sangart Inc., 11189 Sorrento Valley Road, Suite 104, San Diego, CA 92121, USA
Department of Bioengineering, University of California, San Diego, CA, USA

Introduction

p50 is the pO_2 at which hemoglobin is half saturated with oxygen, a number that appears to be fairly constant in nature. In humans, the p50 of blood is approximately 28 mmHg [1]. The tetrameric structure of hemoglobin ($\alpha_2\beta_2$) and a switch between 2 conformations of the subunits (oxy and deoxy) gives rise to the familiar sigmoid oxygen equilibrium curve (OEC, see Fig. 1) [2]. Oxygen affinity is determined by the structure of the hemoglobin molecule and it is influenced primarily by temperature, H^+, CO_2 and, within the red blood cell, by various salts, including Cl^-, ATP and 2,3-DPG. The structure of hemoglobin is conserved to a high degree throughout vertebrates, and similar O_2 transport molecules are found even in nonvertebrates and plants. Myoglobin, similar to a single subunit of hemoglobin, is abundant in muscle, and its function has been ascribed to O_2 storage: diving animals have a very large amount of this protein. Simple animals, such as protozoans, can obtain O_2 from their environment by diffusion, because the distance between the environment and metabolic sites is short. However, in order to achieve greater complexity, higher animals are faced with the problem of moving O_2 from the environment (lung) to remote metabolic sites (mitochondria). Although this problem is solved in different ways in animals, nowhere is it more dramatic than in mammals. In order to successfully oxygenate tissue in complex organisms such as mammals, at least 4 requirements must be fulfilled:

1. A transport molecule is needed. The solubility of O_2 in aqueous solutions is very low: only 2.3 mL of O_2 can dissolve in 100 mL of plasma at one atmosphere of O_2. Since at sea level the earth's atmosphere provides an oxygen partial pressure of approximately 150 mm Hg in air and 100 mmHg in the alveolus, arterial blood plasma contains only $2.3 \times 100/760$ or 0.3 mL/dL of O_2. With a cardiac output of 5 L/min and a basal O_2 requirement of 5 ml/kg/min, a 70 kg human requires a minimum of 7 mL O_2/dL. If all O_2 were transported as dissolved in plasma, a 70 kg human would require a minimum cardiac output of 350 L/min! Clearly, an O_2 carrier is essential to life for humans.
2. The O_2 transport molecule (hemoglobin) must be protected from degradation by a cell membrane. Since a large amount of the carrier is needed, and its degradation in the plasma would be rapid, it must be protected by inclusion in the red cell. By doing this, the useful O_2-carrying life of hemoglobin is prolonged from a few hours to more than 100 days. Without such protection, the body could scarcely produce enough hemoglobin to support itself under basal conditions.
3. Tissue must be protected from the toxic effects of iron-containing heme. Oxygen transporters throughout nature are heme proteins. Protective mechanisms must be in place to prevent direct tissue damage by iron oxidation.

This is achieved, again, but inclusion of the protein within the red cell, which not only prevents degradation, but protects it from oxidation by enzymatic reducing systems.

4. The release of O_2 from the circulation prior to entering capillaries must be minimized. All movement of O_2 is by concentration gradients. The low solubility of O_2 in plasma serves to "insulate" against the loss of O_2 as red cells move from the lung to tissue. Once reaching capillaries, where red cells are in close contact with endothelium, the distance for diffusion is minimal, and O_2 can most readily be released from red cells to plasma then to tissue.

5. A regulatory system must sense impending O_2 deficiency well before supply is critical. The O_2 delivery system needs to be flexible, to accommodate bursts of very high consumption (flight or fight) or survival in nutritional deficiencies or disease. A mechanism that detects insufficient O_2 at the site of metabolism (mitochondria) would be unacceptable, since there are no striking metabolic changes until O_2 supply is critically low, in the range of tissue pO_2 of 2–3 mmHg, where tissue death would be imminent. This is accomplished through the sigmoid shape of the OEC (Fig. 1), where the change of O_2 delivery in respect to the change in pO_2 (slope) is maximal at a pO_2 of approximately 30–40 mmHg. Arterioles, which regulate blood flow to specific capillary networks, are sensitive to pO_2 changes in this region [4].

Traditional thinking has been that the p50 of cell-free O_2 carriers should be the same as the p50 of normal human blood in order to deliver oxygen ade-

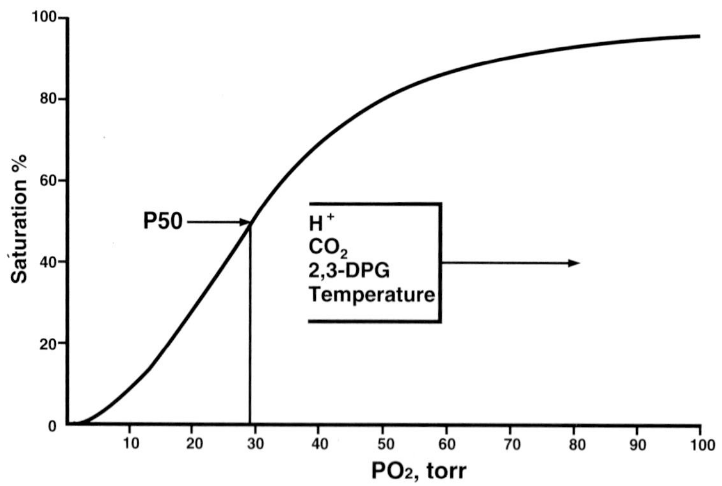

Fig. 1. The normal whole blood oxygen equilibrium curve (OEC). p50 is the pO_2 at which hemoglobin is half-saturated with O_2. The principal effectors that alter the position and shape of the curve under physiological conditions are indicated. From [3]

quately to tissue. This assumption is based upon the idea that oxygen is delivered in the same way by cell-free hemoglobin as it would be by red blood cells. From the discussion above, it should be clear that these assumptions need to be examined closely. This brief review will examine some of the key historical points and assumptions underlying the p50 concept, particularly as applied to oxygen carriers. The discussion will touch briefly on hypoxia, high affinity hemoglobin mutants, stored blood, and cell-free hemoglobin.

Hypoxia: Mountains as Natural Laboratory

Red cell p50 has been considered to be critical to adaptation to hypoxia. Polycythemia was first observed in high altitude residents in the Peruvian Andes [5], and the connection between hematocrit and hypoxia seemed obvious. The prominent Cambridge physiologist, Joseph Barcroft, conducted studies at Cerro de Pasco (4250 m) and 1921 where he observed that at a given pO_2 blood saturation in high altitude natives was higher than the saturation at the same pO_2 in sea level natives (Fig. 2) [7]. Barcroft concluded that blood increases its affinity for oxygen in order to become saturated in the lung. These studies led to the concept of acclimatization to high altitude, and were readily

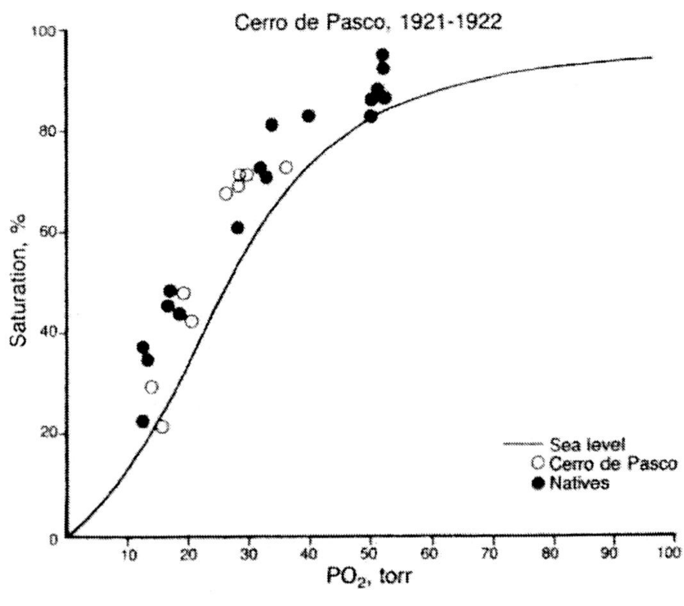

Fig. 2. Hemoglobin saturation from Cerro de Pasco, Barcroft expedition of 1921–22. The solid line is the normal OEC of sea level natives [6]. The circles are measurements made on acclimatized sea level residents (*open*) and natives (*closed*). From [7]

embraced by governments and private companies eager to attract workers to the mines at very high altitudes. Furthermore, the studies were thought to be immediately relevant to understanding performance of pilots in WWII.

Research supported by the U.S. Army in this context was extended in the Peruvian Andes by an academic group led by Alberto Hurtado, who reported data opposite to those of Barcroft (Fig. 3) [8]: at Morococha (4550 m), Hurtado found that at a given pO_2 blood of high altitude natives had reduced O_2 saturation. According to Hurtado's interpretation, this right shift of the oxygen dissociation curve (lower affinity, higher p50) increased the efficiency of oxygen unloading in tissues. These results must have been reassuring to military commanders whose pilots were exposed to hypoxic conditions on every combat mission.

We re-evaluated this historical discrepancy in the same Peruvian locations using modern methods to measure oxygen equilibrium curves (Fig. 4). The earlier Hurtado work had been hampered by the need to transport blood samples to sea level laboratories, during which red cell metabolites (such as 2,3-DPG) would be degraded. Modern equipment allowed us to measure arterial and venous blood gases and saturation, with continuously recorded oxygenation curves using fresh blood on-site [6]. In agreement with Hurtado, we found that the oxygen equilibrium curve is slightly right-shifted due to increased 2,3-DPG under standard conditions (pH 7.4, pCO_2 40). However high-altitude natives are alkalotic due to hyperventilation; reduced pCO_2 and

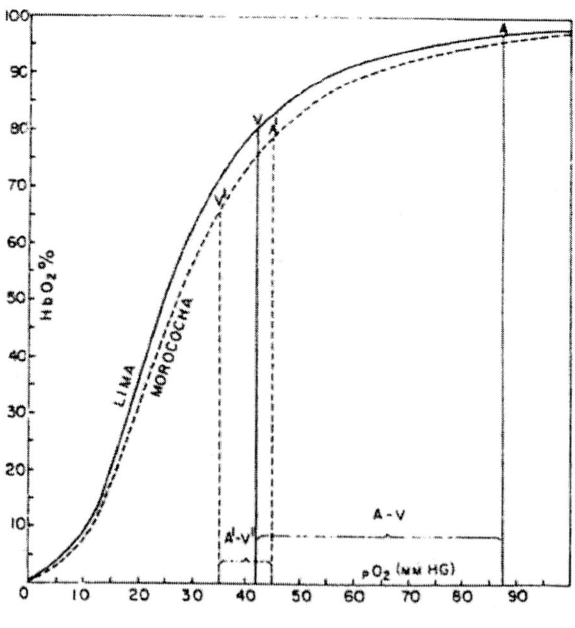

Fig. 3. Hurtado's blood saturation data from Morococha. In contrast to the Barcroft data, Hurtado claimed that high-altitude natives had slightly reduced O_2 saturation at a given pO_2. From [8]

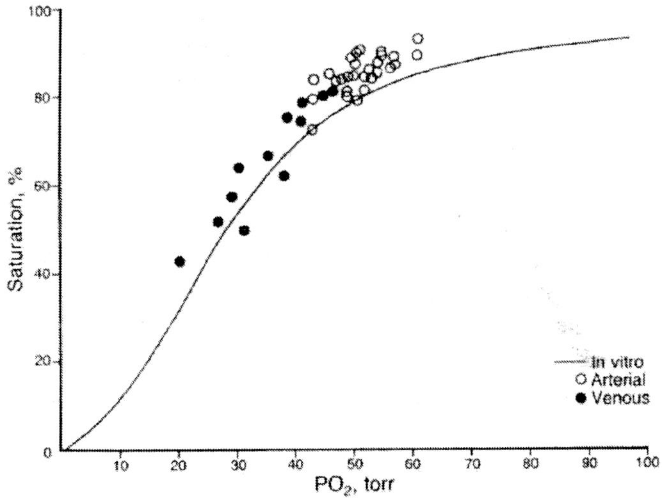

FIG. 4. Modern measurements of O_2 saturation at Morococha. The *solid line* is the normal OEC of sea level natives [9]. The *circles* are measurements made on natives in either arterial (*open*) or venous (*closed*) blood. From [5]

increased pH both offset the 2,3-DPG effect, with a net result that the p50 in high-altitude natives was not distinguishable from sea level values [10].

We also found a considerable variability in p50, not only in high altitude residents, but also at sea level, with "normal" in vivo p50's ranging from 26 to 34 mmHg at both locations. There were no differences in general health of individuals at either end of this range. We concluded that while p50 appears to be under precise biochemical regulation, the physiological determinants of oxygen transport are redundant and numerous, so that within limits, changes in p50 are easily compensated by other mechanisms, including blood flow (cardiac output), ventilation and acid-base status. To confirm the broad basis for O_2 transport, we demonstrated that reduction of hematocrit from 64% to 40% in a single high altitude resident improved exercise performance, cardiac output and pulmonary function [11].

Further studies in extreme hypoxia were carried out on Mount Everest in 1981, where blood gases and the oxygen equilibrium curves were measured in climbers at stages from sea level to the summit [12]. We found that as altitude increases, rising red cell 2,3-DPG shifts the dissociation curve to the right but increasingly severe alkalosis opposes the effect at altitudes above 6000 m. Beyond that point, pH and pCO_2 reach extreme levels (7.78 and 7.5 mmHg respectively, at the summit) with an in vivo p50 of 19.4 mmHg on the summit. We concluded that reduced p50 is critical to maintenance of arterial O_2 saturation, in agreement with Barcroft's initial hypothesis.

Our lesson from these studies in high altitude natives and sojourners was clear: physiological mechanisms for oxygen transport are many and redundant. p50, if maintained within limits, is not a major determinant of O_2 delivery in humans. The studies did not provide data to define what the limits may be, and other data would be needed to provide this information.

Hemoglobinopathies

Some definition of the lower limits of acceptable p50 for human blood can be obtained from another experiment of nature, genetically abnormal hemoglobins with high oxygen affinity. The first of these to be described was hemoglobin Chesapeake an α chain mutant whose abnormal O_2 affinity leads to polycythemia in affected family members [13]. The mechanism for the rise in hematocrit is reduced oxygenation of the kidney, which stimulates erythropoietin production. Another example with even higher oxygen affinity, identified by our group, was hemoglobin McKees Rocks, named for the residence of the affected family [14]. This is an interesting termination mutant, the first to be reported in humans, in which two amino acids are deleted from the carboxyl terminus of the β chain. The carriers of this mutation have a blood p50 of approximately 16 mmHg and elevated hematocrit (Fig. 5).

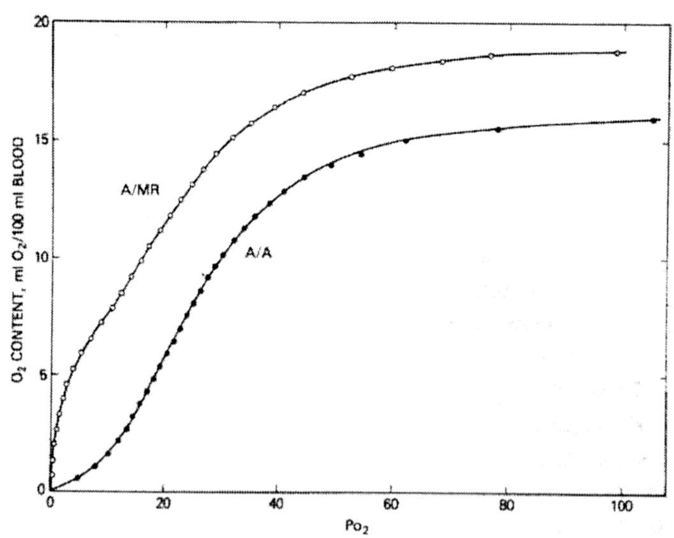

FIG. 5. Blood OEC in a patient with hemoglobin McKees Rocks (*A/MR*) compared with normal blood (*A/A*). Note the abnormal curve is biphasic: a component is present which oxygenates rapidly at low pO_2. From [14]

Studies in human subjects with high affinity mutations have sought to confirm the physiological consequences of low p50. In spite of almost four decades of observation in these families, no significant abnormality, other than plethora, has been found. Infant mortality is not increased [15], even in α-chain mutations which would also affect fetal hemoglobin. Also, there is no increased incidence of cardiovascular disease or stroke. In fact, some studies have shown that lower p50 confers adaptive advantage in altitude hypoxia in rats [16] and humans [17]. Furthermore, animals native to high altitudes have reduced, rather than increased blood p50 [18] which casts doubt on the importance of the right shift in the delivery of oxygen to tissues.

Once again we were impressed that while the molecular biology of hemoglobin confers exquisite biochemical control over p50, physiological mechanisms of oxygen transport are so redundant that any change in a molecular property such as p50 is easily compensated by other changes such as cardiac output, ventilation and acid-base balance.

Altered Red Cells

In the 1970s and 1980s there as a wave of research to attempt to pharmacologically shift the oxygen dissociation curve to the right in order to facilitate the unloading of oxygen in tissues [19–21]. The theoretical driving force was the classical physiological literature on high-altitude natives mentioned above from Hurtado and his group. Some studies seemed to confirm that decreased O_2 affinity (higher p50) can increase tissue pO_2 [22,23]. Studies continue with pharmacological manipulation of the p50 [24,25] and final conclusions are not yet possible. It appears that increasing the p50 of red blood cells, if sufficient oxygen is supplied, can increase tissue oxygenation in some clinical circumstances.

Stored Red Cells

The discovery that 2,3-diphosphoglycerate (2,3-DPG), a normal glycolytic metabolite, can influence the red cell p50 [26,27] had a major impact on concepts about the regulation of oxygen delivery. Later studies showed that the level of 2,3-DPG was regulated by intracellular pH [28], thereby linking hypoxia, hyperventilation, alkalosis, 2,3-DPG upregulation and lowered red cell oxygen affinity. Studies at moderately high altitude confirmed the increase in 2,3-DPG with moderate altitude [29].

Studies with banked blood showed a decrease of 2,3-DPG with storage, particularly at acid pH, but that it was slowly regenerated after infusion into a recipient [28]. In the context of the high altitude research, this was widely interpreted as compromised O_2 delivery capacity by stored blood. Efforts to demonstrate physiological consequences of 2,3-DPG depletion have been more complicated, however [30]. Although the question remains open, it is widely accepted that stored red blood cells have inadequate O_2 delivery capacity because of reduced 2,3-DPG.

Our research group was skeptical of this theory, having shown that p50 had little relevance even at high altitude. The problem with the story was the lack of good experimental evidence to link p50 with tissue oxygen supply. Nevertheless, 2,3-DPG became a surrogate for oxygen transport, which led to efforts to increase its concentration in stored red blood cells by additives.

Cell-Free Oxygen Carriers

As early as 1927, Hartridge and Roughton [31] showed that O_2 uptake by red blood cells was approximately 40 times slower than by a comparable cell-free hemoglobin solution. This observation, and the greater rate of release of O_2 from cell-free hemoglobin compared to red cells, has subsequently been confirmed by more recent studies [32,33]. The theory has been advanced [34,35] that the major barrier to uptake and release of O_2 from red cells is the low solubility of O_2 in the surrounding medium.

Some developers of hemoglobin-based O_2 carriers have proposed that this increased diffusive O_2 delivery from cell-free hemoglobin would be beneficial to tissue oxygenation. However, we proposed the opposite in a theoretical paper [36]: if O_2 is too available in precapillary vessels, potent autoregulatory vasoconstrictive mechanisms could be engaged. Support for this concept came from observations in the microcirculation in which functional capillary density in the rabbit tenuismus muscle was found to be inversely proportional to pO_2 [37]. This has been recently confirmed in the hamster skinfold window model [38]. Subsequently [39] we expanded on this idea and presented a mathematical model, based on pO_2 measurements in the microcirculation.

Clearly, O_2 transfer by cell-free hemoglobin is subject to different rules and constraints than transfer from red blood cells. Given this conclusion, the question then is, how to design a cell-free hemoglobin molecule that does not engage autoregulatory mechanisms, yet is able to deliver O_2 to capillary networks. For this, some understanding of the mechanism of increased O_2 transfer by cell-free hemoglobin must be formulated. A considerable literature exists on the concept of "facilitated diffusion", based on pioneering work by Wittenberg on myoglobin [40] and Scholander on hemoglobin [41]. Accord-

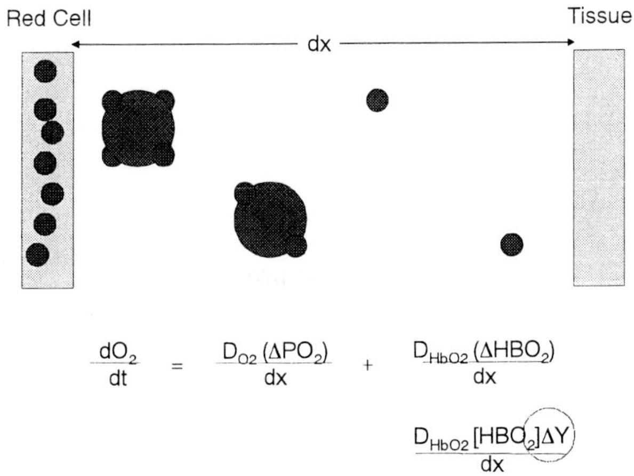

FIG. 6. Facilitated diffusion. Oxygen moves from left (red cell) to right (tissue) through plasma of distance dx, both as simple diffusion, and bound to hemoglobin (facilitated diffusion). The formulas show that the rate of O_2 transfer by the latter mechanism is dependent on a saturation gradient, determined by p50

ing to the concept of facilitated diffusion (Fig. 6), O_2 moves through plasma not only as dissolved molecules in the plasma but as oxyhemoglobin which itself can diffuse along its concentration gradient. This can be a significant increase in plasma O_2 content: as little as 1 g/dL of cell-free hemoglobin can double the amount of plasma O_2 under arterial conditions. In turn, this would double the O_2 gradient between plasma and tissue.

The key to understanding the role of facilitated diffusion in regard to cell-free hemoglobin lies in the fact that in order to transport O_2, the cell-free hemoglobin must itself diffuse; if it does not, O_2 released at the vessel wall will not be replaced by new HbO_2. The diffusive movement of hemoglobin in the plasma is expressed by Fick's diffusion equation:

$$\frac{d[HbO_2]}{dt} = D_{HbO_2} \frac{[HbO_{2rbc}] - [HbO_{2wall}]}{\Delta x} \tag{1}$$

Where $[HbO_{2rbc}]$ is the HbO_2 concentration at the red cell membrane, $[HbO_{2wall}]$ is the HbO_2 concentration at the vessel wall, Δx is the distance between these 2 points, and D_{HbO2} is the diffusion constant for HbO_2. In order for the HbO_2 concentration to be different at these 2 points, the O_2 saturation must decrease over the distance, Δx. Equation 1 can be simplified to

$$\frac{d[HbO_2]}{dt} = D_{HbO_2} \frac{\Delta Y[HbO_{2plasma}]}{\Delta x} \tag{2}$$

Where ΔY is the hemoglobin saturation gradient from the red cell to the vessel wall, which is a function, in turn, of p50. Also critical to facilitated diffusion, is the diffusion constant for HbO_2, D_{HbO2}, which is a function of molecular radius and viscosity, as represented by the Stokes-Einstein equation

$$D_{HbO_2} = \frac{kT}{6\pi\eta r} \quad (3)$$

In this equation, k is the Boltzman constant, T is absolute temperature, η is viscosity, and r is the radius of the HbO_2 molecule. Thus, diffusion of HbO_2 can be controlled through manipulation of molecular radius, viscosity and p50.

To test this approach to O_2 carrier design, we studied the hamster dorsal skinfold model, which allows direct measurement of O_2 transfer at various levels of the microcirculation. After hemodilution to hematocrit of 11%, arteriolar pO_2 is about 35 mmHg (42). Our model would predict that maximal O_2 delivery via the facilitated diffusion mechanism would occur with a cell-free hemoglobin whose p50 is about 35 mmHg and which has significant cooperativity such that the OEC is steepest in its mid-portion. In fact, a cell-free hemoglobin, designed to have the same p50 and cooperativity (Hill coefficient) as human red cells would have just these properties, and we would predict would be maximally vasoconstrictive. In contrast, a molecule that is still substantially saturated at 35 mmHg (ie, p50 much lower) and without cooperativity, would not be expected to delivery any O_2 by the facilitated mechanism in arterioles. These concepts were shown by direct measurement in the hamster microcirculation [42].

Our theory of O_2 transport by cell-free hemoglobin was tested in a simple artificial capillary system [43] (Fig. 7). The gas-permeable capillary was suspended in an atmosphere of N_2, and oxygenated solutions were then perfused through it at different rates. It would be expected that at high perfusion rates, the solutions would be only partially deoxygenated, while at lower rates, the degree of deoxygenation would be greater. Since the oxygen equilibrium curves for all solutions were known exactly, as well as the dimensions and diffusion characteristics of the capillary itself, the only unknown in modeling the release of O_2 was diffusion. The diffusion constant for molecular O_2 is also known, so it only remained to model the diffusion constants for oxyhemoglobin. The results of this experiment show surprisingly that a modified hemoglobin molecule can be designed which releases O_2 in a fashion similar to that of red blood cells, if the p50 is 12 mmHg, as is the case with PEG-Hb, a large molecule surface modified with polyethylene glycol.

Interestingly, the experiment showed that 2 hemoglobins, hemoglobin A_0, and hemoglobin crosslinked between the α chains ($\alpha\alpha$Hb) have similar O_2

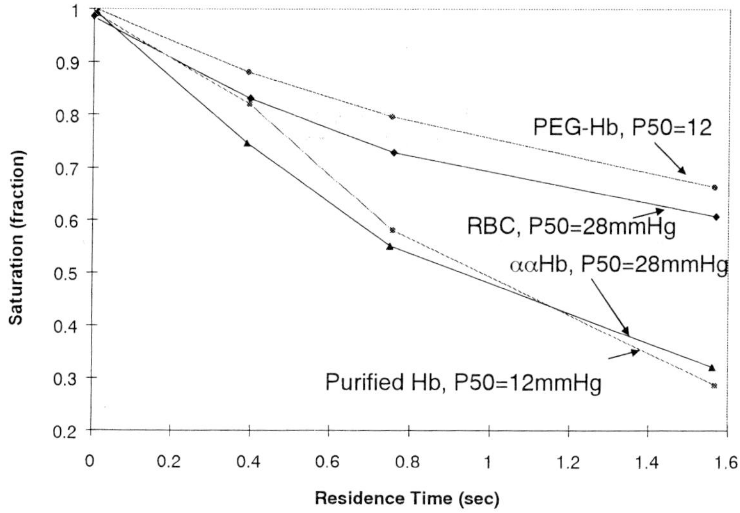

FIG. 7. Hemoglobin saturation as a function of residence time in a flowing capillary suspended in an N_2 atmosphere. The release of O_2 from PEG-Hb is similar to that of red blood cells in spite of high O_2 affinity (p50 12 mmHg). Two hemoglobins with very different p50 values have similar O_2 delivery. These data emphasize that both p50 and molecular size are critically important in determination of facilitated diffusion. Data from [43]

release characteristics, in spite of very different p50 values. Also, ααHb and PEG-Hb have very different O_2 release profiles but with similar p50.

This research is ongoing, and much more work remains to be done, but our current working hypothesis is that for cell-free hemoglobin, the optimal p50 should be in the range of the tissue targeted for oxygenation. If the value is too high, O_2 will be oversupplied to arterioles resulting in reflexive vasoconstriction.

In summary, our hypothesis is that in order to efficiently transfer O_2 to capillaries by cell-free hemoglobin, the critical properties appear to be molecular size, p50 and viscosity, so as to avoid engaging reflexive autoregulatory vasoconstriction. Work remains to determine the relative importance of each of these properties. A molecule that appears to satisfy these requirements is MalPEG-hemoglobin, which is currently in clinical trials.

Acknowledgments. Dr. Winslow is President and CEO of Sangart Inc., a company involved in the research and development of O_2 carriers. This work was supported, in part, by grants RO1 HL64579, R43 HL64996, R44 HL62818, R24 64395, R01 40696, R01 62354, R01 62318 from the NHLBI, NIH, to Sangart, Inc.

References

1. Winslow RM, Swenberg M, Berger R, et al (1977) Oxygen equilibrium curve of normal human blood and its evaluation by Adair's equation. J Biol Chem 252: 2331–2337
2. Bolton W, Perutz M (1970) Three dimensional fourier synthesis of horse deoxyhemoglobin at 2 Angstrom units resolution. Nature 228:551–552
3. Winslow R (1992) Hemoglobin-based red cell substitutes. Johns Hopkins University Press, Baltimore
4. Intaglietta M, Johnson P, Winslow R (1996) Microvascular and tissue oxygen distribution. Cardiovasc Res 32:632–643
5. Winslow RM, Monge CC (1987) Hypoxia, polycythemia and chronic mountain sickness. Johns Hopkins University Press, Baltimore
6. Winslow R, Morrissey J, Berger R (1978) Variability of oxygen affinity or normal blood: an automated method of measurement. J Appl Physiol 45:289–297
7. Barcroft J, Binger C, Bock A, et al (1923) Observations upon the effect of high altitude on the physiological processes of the human body carried out in the Peruvian Andes chiefly at Cerro de Pasco. Philos Trans R Soc Lond S Biol Sci 211:351–480
8. Hurtado A (1964) Animals in high altitudes: resident man, Sect. 4, Ch. 54. Washington, D.C.: Am Physiol Soc
9. Winslow RM, Morrissey JM, Berger RL, et al (1978) Variability of oxygen affinity or normal blood: an automated method of measurement. J Appl Physiol 45:289–297
10. Winslow R, Monge C, Statham N, et al (1981) Variability of oxygen affinity of blood: human subjects native to high altitude. J Appl Physiol 51:1411–1416
11. Winslow R, Monge C, Brown E, et al (1985) The effects of hemodilution on O_2 transport in high altitude polycythemia. J Appl Physiol 59:1495–1502
12. Winslow R, Samaja M, West J (1984) Red cell function at extreme altitude on Mount Everest. J Appl Physiol 56(1):109–116
13. Charache S, Weatherall D, Clegg J (1966) Polycythemia associated with a hemoglobinopathy. J Clin Invest 45:813
14. Winslow RM, Swenberg M-L, Gross E, et al (1976) Hemoglobin McKees Rocks ($\alpha_2\beta_2$145Tyr->Term). A human "nonsense" mutation leading to a shortened b-chain. J Clin Invest 57:772–781
15. Charache S, Jacobson R, Brimhall B, et al (1978) Hb Potomac (101 Glu replaced by Asp): speculations on placental oxygen transport in carriers of high-affinity hemoglobins. Blood 51:331–338
16. Eaton J, Skelton T, Berger E (1974) Survival at extreme altitude: protective effect of increased hemoglobin-oxygen affinity. Science 185:743–744
17. Hebbel R, Eaton J, Kronenberg R, et al (1978) Human llamas. Adaptation to altitude in subjects with high hemoglobin oxygen affinity. J Clin Invest 62:593–600
18. Monge CC, Leon-Velarde F (1991) Physiological adatation to high altitude: oxygen transport in mammals and birds. Physiol Rev 71:1135–1172
19. Gersonde K, Nicolau C (1980) Modification of the oxygen affinity of intracellular haemoglobin by incorporation of polyphosphates into intact red blood cell enhanced O_2 release in the capillary system. Biblthca Haemat 46:81–92
20. Kunert M, Liard J, Lombard J, et al (1995) Low affinity hemoglobin increases tissue PO_2 and decreases arteriolar diameter and flow in the rat cremaster muscle. Microcirculation 23 (Abstract)

21. Lalezari I, Lalezari P, Poyart C (1990) New effectors of human hemoglobin: structure and function. Biochemistry 29:1515–1523
22. Malmberg P, Hlastala M, Woodson R (1979) Effect of increased blood-oxygen affinity on oxygen transport in hemorrhagic shock. J Appl Physiol 47:889–895
23. Woodson R, Wranne B, Detter J (1973) Effect of increased blood oxygen affinity on work performance of rats. J Clin Invest 52:2717–2724
24. Randad R, Mahran M, Mehanna A, et al (1991) Allosteric modifiers of hemoglobin. 1. Design, synthesis, testing, and structure-allosteric activity relationship of novel affin decreasing agents. J Med Chem 34:752–757
25. Wireko F, Kellogg G, Abraham D (1991) Allosteric modifiers of hemoglobin. 2. Crystallographically determined binding sites and hydrophobic binding/interaction analysis of novel hemoglobin oxygen effectors. J Med Chem 34:758–767
26. Benesch R, Benesch R (1967) The effect of organic phosphates from the human erythrocyte on the allosteric properties of hemoglobin. BBRC 26:162–167
27. Chanutin A, Curnish RR (1967) Effect of organic and inorganic phosphates on the oxygen equilibrium curve of human erythrocyte. Arch Biochem Biophys 121:96–102
28. Beutler E, Wood L (1969) The in vivo regeneration of red cell 2,3-diohosphoglyceric acit (DPG) after transfusion of stored blood. J Lab Clin Med 74(2):300–304
29. Lenfant C, Sullivan K (1971) Adaptation to high altitude. N Engl J Med 284(23): 1298–1309
30. Collins J, Stechenberg L (1973) The effects of the concentration and function ofhemoglobin on the survival of rats after hemorrhage. Surgery 85(4):412–418
31. Hartridge H, Roughton F (1927) The rate of distribution of dissolved gases between the red blood corpuscle and its fluid environment. J Physiol (Lond) 62:232–242
32. Kavdia M, Pittman R, Popel A (2002) Theoretical analysis of effects of blood substitute affinity and cooperativity on organ oxygen transport. J Appl Physiol 93: 2122–2128
33. Page TC, Light WR, McKay CB, et al (1998) Oxygen transport by erythrocyte/ hemoglobin solution mixtures in an in vitro capillary as a model of hemoglobin-based oxygen carrier performance. Microvasc Res 55:54–64
34. Federspiel WJ, Popel AS (1986) A theoretical analysis of the effect of the particulate nature of blood on oxygen release in capillaries. Microvascular Research 32:164–189
35. Homer L, Weathersby P, Kiesow L (1981) Oxygen gradients between red blood cells in the microcirculation. Microvasc Res 22:308–323
36. Vandegriff K, Winslow R (1995) A theoretical analysis of oxygen transport: a new strategy for the design of hemoglobin-based red cell substitutes. In: Intaglietta M (ed) Blood substitutes. Physiological basis of efficacy. Birkhäuser, New York, pp 143–154
37. Lindbom L, Tuma R, Arfors K (1980) Influence of oxygen on perfused capillary density and capillary red cell velocity in rabbit skeletal muscle. Microvasc Res 19:197–208
38. Tsai A, Cabrales P, Winslow R, et al (2003) Microvascular oxygen distribution in the awake hamster window chamber model during hyperoxia. Am J Physiol 285:H1537–H1545
39. Winslow RM, Vandegriff KD (1997) Hemoglobin oxygen affinity and the design of red cell substitutes. In: Winslow RM, Vandegriff KD, Intaglietta M (eds) Advances in blood substitutes. Industrial opportunities and medical challenges. Birkhäuser, Boston, pp 167–188
40. Wittenberg J (1970) Myoglobin-facilitated oxygen diffusion: role of myoglobin in oxygen entry into muscle. Physiol Rev 50(4):559–636

41. Scholander P (1960) Oxygen transport through hemoglobin solutions. Science 131: 585–590
42. Tsai A, Vandegriff KD, Intaglietta M, et al (2003) Targeted O_2 delivery by cell-free hemoglobin: a new basis for oxygen therapeutics. Am J Physiol Heart Circ Physiol 285: H1411–H1419
43. McCarthy MR, Vandegriff KD, Winslow RM (2001) The role of facilitated diffusion in oxygen transport by cell-free hemoglobin: implications for the design of hemoglobin-based oxygen carriers. Biophys Chem 92:103–117

Repetitive Administration of Hemoglobin Raffimer in Experimental Models and Clinical Applications

Hae Won Kim[1], George Biro[2], and A. Gerson Greenburg[1]

Summary. Hemoglobin (Hb)-raffimer (Hemolink) is an oxygen therapeutic based on human Hb that is intramolecularly and intermolecularly crosslinked with o-raffinose. Hb-raffimer appears to be free of severe toxicity, as shown in a variety of topload/repeat dose preclinical animal studies. In addition, Hb-raffimer does not appear to be immunogenic. Limited information is available on the acute and chronic effects of high volume infusion in animals and on responses to repeated dosing in human subjects. Hb-based oxygen therapeutics have not been tested in a wide variety of possible indications. In conclusion, Hb-raffimer and other oxygen therapeutics could be potentially life saving in certain clinical situations. Current and future clinical trials will evaluate expanded indications and dosing regimens.

Key words. Hemoglobin (Hb), Hb-raffimer, Oxygen therapeutic, Repeat dose, Clinical trial

Introduction

Oxygen therapeutics are therapeutic agents designed to deliver oxygen (O_2) to tissues where normal O_2 supply is impaired or compromised due to hemorrhage or impaired blood flow. Current candidate oxygen therapeutics are mainly based on hemoglobin (Hb) or synthetic perfluorochemicals. Hemoglobin-based oxygen therapeutics are chemically modified human- or animal-derived Hbs or genetically "engineered" Hbs designed to improve on properties of unmodified stroma free hemoglobin solution obtained from

[1] Brown University and The Miriam Hospital, 164 Summit Avenue, Providence, RI 02906, USA
[2] Hemosol, Inc., Missisauga, Ontario, Canada

lysed red cells. Improving intravascular circulation time is another element of the design criteria.

Hb-raffimer (Hemolink) is an oxygen therapeutic based on human Hb that is intramolecularly and intermolecularly crosslinked with oxidized raffinose (o-raffinose) [1]. Hb-raffimer has a lower O_2 affinity (higher P50) and viscosity than native red cells, a physicochemical characteristic considered desirable in an oxygen therapeutic. Hb-raffimer has been extensively tested in preclinical animal studies without evidence of significant toxicities. In Phase I and II clinical trials with Hb-raffimer, no serious adverse effects have been revealed [2,3] although some mild undesired effects (e.g., transient hypertension, dysphagia and abdominal discomfort) have been observed in some patients [4,5]. In a Phase III trial in 148 subjects in a number of Canadian centers, the safety and efficacy of Hb-raffimer was evaluated in patients undergoing coronary artery bypass grafting (CABG) operations.

Characteristics of Hb-raffimer

Hb-raffimer is a highly purified, pasteurized, solution of human HbA_0 stabilized and covalently crosslinked with o-raffinose. Hb-raffimer is formulated as an iso-oncotic solution in Ringer's Lactate for Injection United States Pharmacopeia (USP) (Table 1). The o-raffinose crosslinking method consistently yields a distribution of molecular weight species in the range of 64–500 kDa. Hb-raffimer contains 10 g Hb/dl; >90% in ferrous deoxy state.

Mechanism of Action of Hb-raffimer

The goal of oxygen therapeutics in an acute anemic condition is normalization of tissue perfusion and improved oxygen kinetics. Optimal tissue perfu-

Table 1. Characteristics of Hb-raffimer solution (Hemolink)

Modification	Crosslinking with o-raffinose
Hb Source	Outdated human red cells
Hb concentration	10 g/dl (<7% metHb)
Colloidal osmotic pressure	25 mmHg
Hb molecular weight distribution	<64 kD: <5% 64–500 kD: >90% >500 kD: <3%
Electrolyte base	Ringer's lactate
pH	7.5
P50	52 mmHg
Hill Coefficient (n)	1.0
Sterilility (USP XXII)	Pass
Endotoxin	<0.006 EU/ml
Viscosity	1.14 (cP)

sion is the end result of complex interactions of many physiologic regulatory systems. An adequate supply of oxygen is required for normal tissue metabolism and to maintain homeostasis. How does this oxygen therapeutic work? There are many elements to consider including oxygen carrying capacity, oxygen delivery kinetics, colloids and electrolytes in solution, viscosity, effects on hemodynamics and the vascular system, leukocyte activation/deactivation and erythrocyte clumping. Three important characteristics of Hb-raffimer are: acellularity, oxygen delivery capacity, and the shape of the oxyhemoglobin dissociation curve (OHDC) (Fig. 1). The acellular nature of Hb-raffimer allows improved perfusion of capillary beds blocked by leukocytes or erythrocyte thrombi that impede blood flow. Reduced viscosity lowers blood flow resistance and oxygen in the plasma phase enhances the diffusing surface to tissue cells. An increased oxygen carrying capacity of blood enhances oxygen delivery generally and the rightshifted OHDC enables nearly as much oxygen offloading across the standard arterio-venous oxygen gradient as whole blood of similar Hb concentration. All of these factors work synergistically to effect improved tissue perfusion and acellular oxygen supply. The improved delivery of oxygen to tissues is an important mechanism of action of this oxygen therapeutic.

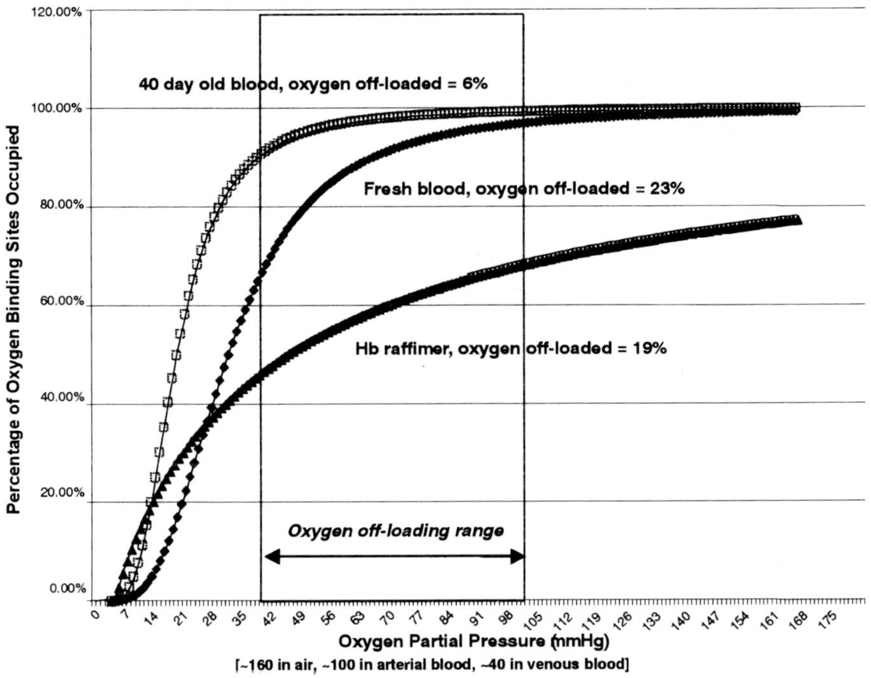

FIG. 1. Oxyhemoglobin dissociation curves for blood and Hb-raffimer

Preclinical Topload/Repeat Dose Studies

Certain clinical conditions may require multiple administrations of Hb-based oxygen therapeutics to the same subject. Repeated dosing regimens render a greater potential for toxicity than a single dose treatment because they usually result in higher blood concentration and more protracted exposure. They may also stress or overwhelm the normal clearance/metabolic mechanisms (liver, spleen, kidneys, etc.), causing accumulation of potentially toxic Hb breakdown products. Lastly, they are more likely to reveal toxic reactions that occur rarely when administered in "normal" or single doses. To test safety of repeated doses, rats and dogs were subjected to topload repeated intravenous infusions of Hb-raffimer [6].

In rats with single 5% topload, Hb-raffimer did not cause any deaths or toxic effects on the major body organs or systems. All animals showed normal activity and positive body weight gain. There were no significant detrimental effects on hematology, biochemistry, or histology. No significant immune response was noted at this dose. In studies of 14 day daily repeated dosing (iv infusion) of 5, 10, 15, or 30 ml/kg/day, dose related slowing of weight gain was observed. In addition, histopathology revealed foamy histiocytes, foamy sinusoidal cells with pigment in the liver, and pigment accumulation in the renal cortical tubular epithelia cells. Gross pathology revealed carcass discoloration and dark pigmentation of the kidneys. The carcass discoloration was no longer apparent after day 29, i.e., after 14 days of treatment free recovery. There were no deaths in any of these studies.

A similar 14-day toploading repeat dose study in dogs with 10 ml/kg/day resulted in no deaths [6]. Increased aspartate aminotransferase (AST), creatine phophokinase, amylase, total bilirubin, dark yellow/amber coloration of the urine and "bilirubin" stained cells in the urine were observed. The histopathological effects were largely reversed during the 14-day recovery period. In studies with 20 and 30 ml/kg/day, on each of fourteen consecutive days, reduction in the rate of body weight gain and feed intake was noted. There was increased pigmentation in the skin, eyes, and mucous membranes. Red cell counts and hematocrit decreased slightly but plasma hemoglobin concentration increased. Phagocytic leukocyte count was increased and bilirubin was significantly elevated. Discoloration and increased liver and kidney weights were reversed during the 14 day treatment free recovery period. At the end of recovery, there was an elevated plasma iron level with reduced iron binding capacity. No deaths resulted in any of these studies.

The repeated dosing subjected the animals to prolonged exposure to unphysiologically high concentrations of Hb-raffimer in the blood. The cumulative total doses were many times those anticipated in the clinical use of this oxygen therapeutic, and amounted to several times the animals' total red cell and Hb mass. Nevertheless, the treatment was tolerated well in these models. The biochemical and histological findings were consistent with serious loads on Hb catabolic mechanisms. Yet, no evidence of serious organ toxicity was observed in these studies.

Preclinical developmental studies are designed to fulfill two primary objectives. First, preclinical studies produce data that support and validate the effectiveness of a therapeutic candidate for its intended clinical use. Second, preclinical studies are also conducted to test potential toxicity (safety) of a therapeutic candidate. Toxicity is generally assessed in terms of changes in physiologic parameters, blood and urine chemistries, and organ/tissue function, histopathology and other relevant indicators. Because many, and often unknown, differences in genetics and physiology between animal models and human patients, results from preclinical efficacy and safety studies do not always translate into efficacy and safety in actual human patients although they are generally good predictors.

To be clinically useful, oxygen therapeutics must be free of serious toxic side effects. Therefore, one key question for the pre-clinical programs is: can preclinical studies predict serious adverse effects in the human subjects? Results of the completed preclinical studies indicate that Hb-raffimer appears to be safe in a variety of models. Using the laboratory to identify the underlying mechanisms of clinical observations is an interesting exercise in uncovering physiologic processes that may be involved in human response. In retrospect some of the issues may be addressed but animals cannot tell us about their clinical conditions such as abdominal pain, discomfort, etc. However, they provide clues by not eating or slowed rate of weight gain which could indicate some gastrointestinal and other organ functional impairment. Did we find it looking backwards? There were hints and suggestions, but not conclusive data.

Clinical Studies

The primary purpose of clinical studies are to demonstrate that oxygen therapeutics are safe and effective as described in the U.S. Food and Drug Administration Points-to-Consider guidelines [7,8]. Results from preclinical and clinical studies conducted over the last 20 years have enhanced our understanding of various safety issues such as renal toxicity, immunogenicity, and hypertensive and other effects of oxygen therapeutics. Demonstration of clinical efficacy, however, turned out to be more difficult since clinical endpoints have not been well defined [9]. Some proposed endpoints include mortality, transfusion avoidance and various laboratory and clinical indicators of organ function. Currently, transfusion avoidance appears to be a popular efficacy endpoint adopted in most oxygen therapeutics clinical trials regardless of indicated use. However, demonstration of clinical efficacy is contingent upon an indicated use. Therefore, clinical endpoints of oxygen therapeutics should be defined as distinctively as possible depending on indicated use (e.g., hemorrhagic shock resuscitation, ischemic rescue, transfusion alternative, pre/peri-operative hemodilution, adjuvant to cancer therapy, etc). More work needs to be done in this area.

To date, Hb-raffimer has been tested in over 500 human subjects in various clinical protocols including normal subjects and coronary artery bypass grafting (CABG), orthopedic surgery, and chronic renal failure patients.

Safety in Healthy Volunteers (Phase I Clinical Trial)

Safety of Hb-raffimer was evaluated in a Phase I clinical trial of 42 normal healthy volunteers, of which 33 received Hb-raffimer [2]. Hb-raffimer was administered intravenously in doses ranging from 0.025 to 0.6 g/kg or an equivalent volume of Ringer's lactate. The subjects were monitored for 3 days and followed for up to 6 weeks. Pre- and post-infusion cardiovascular, pulmonary and other major organ functions were assessed along with clinical laboratory measurements. Hb-raffimer administration was well tolerated in healthy volunteers with no evidence of serious organ dysfunction. At doses >0.4 g/kg, some subjects complained of moderate to severe abdominal pain which was relieved by smooth muscle relaxants. Hb-raffimer elicited a moderate dose-dependent transient elevation of mean arterial blood pressure which, at a 0.1 g/kg dose, plateaued approximately 14% above the pretreatment value. In these subjects, there was a concomitant bradycardia without ECG abnormalities. Dose dependent elevations of serum bilirubin and LDH values were noted. In some subjects, elevated AST, ALT, creatine kinase and serum amylase were noted. All other clinical chemistry and hematologic parameters were within the normal range. In these subjects, plasma $T_{1/2}$ of Hb-raffimer ranged from 1.6 h at 0.25 ml/kg to 15.6 hours at 5 ml/kg [10]. After 1.0 ml/kg dose, $T_{1/2}$ was 6.3 hours for the oligomeric fraction (>64 kD) and 2.6 hours for tetrameric (64 kD) fraction. At 5.0 ml/kg, T1/2 was 18.6 h for oligomers, 7.1 h for the tetrameric fraction and 2.6 h for the fraction which appeared as dimer on SDS-PAGE.

Phase II and III Clinical Trials

Hb-raffimer has been tested in patients undergoing routine coronary artery bypass grafting (CABG) operation and orthopedic surgery, or in patients with certain other conditions (Table 2). In Phase II and III clinical trials of patients undergoing elective CABG operations, Hb-raffimer was well tolerated and appears to reduce allogeneic blood transfusion in this group as median

TABLE 2. Hb-raffimer completed clinical trials

Clinical setting	Total no. subjects	Dose ranges
Phase I safety	42	0.25–6.0 ml/kg
Orthopedic surgery	16	1.5–6.0 ml/kg
Orthopedic surgery	40	25–125 g
Primary CABG	60	25–100 g
Primary CABG	60	25–75 g
Chronic renal failure	29	5–10 g
Primary CABG	299	75 g

CABG, coronary artery bypass graft.

volume of allogeneic red cells transfused was significantly lower than patients treated with control (6% hetastarch) [11,12].

In a similar study of randomized double blind study of post-operative cardiac patients, polymerized bovine hemoglobin (HBOC-201) has been shown to moderately but significantly reduce the need for red cell transfusion [13]. HBOC-201 group required a mean of 1.7 units of red cells while blood transfusion group received a mean of 2.2 units of red cell units.

Anti-Hb-raffimer antibodies were detected in 16%–20% of subjects treated with Hb-raffimer compared to 1.4% in control subjects (G. Adamson, 2002, Personal communication). There was no apparent correlation of antibody development to clinical response or adverse events. In in vitro studies, antibodies from subjects receiving Hb-raffimer did not bind to normal RBCs and did not cause red cell disruption. The potential for pathological effects is unknown.

Compassionate Use Cases

As of December 2002, 21 subjects were approved by regulatory authorities for treatment with Hb-raffimer for compassionate use. Of these, 16 subjects received Hb-raffimer (Table 3). In these subjects, nadir RBC Hb ranged from 1.1 to 5.1 g/dl and Hb-raffimer was administered in doses from 500 to 5000 ml. Of those treated, 8 of 16 subjects survived. In compassionate use cases, treatments were largely uncontrolled, thus, determination of adverse events is difficult. Elevated enzymes (amylase, lipase, bilirubin) were noted in these cases. There were incidences of transient elevation of blood pressure, abdominal pain and jaundice in some patients.

Other Potential Indications/Benefits and Issues

Solid hypoxic tumors are often resistant to radiation and chemotherapy. Because Hb-raffimer and other acellular oxygen therapeutics have low viscosity, they may provide conditions for improved perfusion in solid tumors,

TABLE 3. Compassionate use cases

Sex	Age	Indication	Nadir Hb g/dl	Hb-raffimer dose (ml)	Outcome
F	57	Burns	5.1	4500	Survived
F	54	SLE	3.7	2750	Died
M	61	UGI bleed	2.7	2750	Survived
F	75	UGI bleed	3.9	2500	Survived
M	19	GI bleed	2.7	4500	Died
F	31	Hemolytic anemia	2.7	2250	Died
F	14	ITP with bleeding	2.6	500	Survived
F	29	Blood loss	2.9	1250	Survived
M	43	Aortic dissection	1.1	3000	Died
M	39	Multiple trauma	3.0	3500	Died
F	53	Post-op bleeding	3.2	5000	Survived
F	51	Pancreatitis	3.2	500	Died
F	67	Uterine CA	3.2	1000	Died
F	67	Ruptured esophagus	2.4	2750	Died
F	20	Menstrual bleeding	3.1	1250	Survived
M	54	GI bleed	2.8	750	Survived

SLE, systemic lupus erythematosus; UGI, upper gastro-intestinal; GI, gastro-intestinal; ITP, idiopathic thrombocytopenic purpura; CA, cancer.

thereby resulting in higher tumor oxygen tension. Therefore, administration of Hb-raffimer and certain other oxygen therapeutics prior to radiation/chemotherapy may increase tumor sensitivity to these therapeutic modalities [14]. It appears that in some in-vitro systems exogenous Hb may accelerate erythropoiesis [15]. In addition, acelluar Hb based oxygen therapeutics may also be useful in treating malaria since it slowed P. falciparium growth in murine malaria [16].

Of note, it has been shown that Hb based oxygen therapeutics appear to interfere with certain, predominantly colorometric, clinical laboratory tests (e.g., serum creatinine) [17]. Therefore, when interpreting clinical laboratory test results of patients following administration of Hb based oxygen therapeutics, caution should be exercised.

Conclusion

Hb-raffimer appears to be free of severe toxicity in a variety of topload and repeat dose preclinical animal studies. In addition, Hb-raffimer does not appear to be immunogenic in animals although antibodies have been detected, and repeated dosing with heterogeneic crosslinked Hb can result in anaphylaxis in some animals. Limited information is available on acute and chronic effects of high volume infusion in animals. In addition, Hb based oxygen therapeutics have not been tested in a wide variety of possible indications. In conclusion, Hb-raffimer and other oxygen therapeutics could be potentially life saving in certain clinical situations. Current and future clinical trials will evaluate expanded indications and dosing regimens.

References

1. Jones RT, Head C, Wong LT, et al (1993) Characterization of o-raffinose crosslinked hemoglobin tetramer. Proceedings of the International Symposium on Blood Substitutes, p H7 (Abstract)
2. Carmichael FJL, Ali ACY, Campbell JA, et al (2000) A Phase I study of o-raffinose cross-linked human hemoglobin: Hemolink in Phase I. Crit Care Med 28:2283–2292
3. Mazer CD, Cheng MA, Dai B, et al (1998) Safety and efficacy of Hemolink during cardiopulmonary bypass. Anesthesiology 89(3A):A652 (Abstract)
4. Reid TJ (2003) Hb-based oxygen carriers: are we there yet? Transfusion 43:280–287
5. Xue S, Paterson W, Valdez D, et al (1999) Effect of an o-raffinose cross-linked haemoglobin product on oesophageal and lower oesophageal sphincter motor function. Neurogastroent Motil 11(6):421–430
6. Biro GP (1999) Safety toxicology evaluation of o-raffinose cross linked hemoglobin solution by daily repeated infusions in rats and dogs. Crit Care Med 27(1):A173 (Abstract)
7. Center for Biologics Evaluation and Research (1991) Points to consider in the safety evaluation of hemoglobin-based oxygen carriers. Transfusion 31:369–371
8. Center for Biologics Evaluation and Research (1994) Points to consider on efficacy evaluation of hemoglobin- and perfluorocarbon-based oxygen carriers. Transfusion 34:712–713
9. Frantantoni JC (1997) Red cell substitutes: evolution of approaches to demonstrating efficacy. Proceedings of the 7th International Symposium on Blood Substitutes, p 55 (Abstract)
10. Wicks DG, Nakao S, Champagne P, et al (1996) The pharmacokinetics of Hemolink in human volunteers determined by cyanomet-Hb and size exclusion chromatography assays. Art Cells Blood Sub Immobil Biotechnol 24(4):460 (Abstract)
11. Hill S, Gottschalk LI, Grichnik K (2002) Safety and preliminary efficacy of hemoglobin raffimer for patients udergoing coronary artery bypass surgery. J Cardiothoracic and Vascular Anesthesia 16:695–702
12. Cheng DC (2001) Safety and efficacy of o-raffinose crosslinked human hemoglobin (Hemolink) in cardiac surgery. Can J Anesth 48:S41–S48
13. Levy JH, Goodnough LT, Grelich PE, et al (2002) Polymerized bovine hemoglobin solution as a replacement for allogeneic red blood cell transfusion after cardiac surgery: results of a randomized, double-blind trial J Thoracic Cardiovas Surgery 124:35–42
14. Sun AY, Kavanagh MC, Hill RP (1995) Increasing tumor oxygenation with a human hemoglobin blood substitute (Hemolink). Proceedings of the 64th Annual Meeting of the Royal College of Physicians and Surgeons (Abstract)
15. Mueller S, Stuart SE, Masuta KK, et al (1997) The enhancement of erythropoiesis by hemoglobin. Proceedings of the 29th Annual Meeting of the American Society of Hematology (Abstract)
16. Freilich D, Branda R, Hacker M, et al (1999) Decreased lactic acidosis and anemia after transfusion of o-raffinose cross-linked and polymerized hemoglobin in severe murine malaria. Am J Trop Med Hyg 60(2):322–328
17. Ali AC, Campbell JA (1997) Interference of o-raffinose cross-linked hemoglobin with routine Hitachi 717 assays. Clin Chem 43(9):1794–1796

Oxygen Gradients In Vivo Seen by a High Oxygen Affinity HB Polymer

Enrico Bucci[1] and Raymond C. Koehler[2]

Summary. Cell-free hemoglobin based oxygen carriers (HBOC) wet the endothelial surfaces and deliver oxygen directly to tissues, bypassing plasma. Simulations show that carriers with oxygen affinity higher than blood would best deliver oxygen to tissues, although good delivery is produced within a large range of affinities. We tested this hypothesis using a solution of either a high oxygen affinity polymer (ZL-HbBv, P50 = 4 mmHg) or of sebacoyl crosslinked hemoglobin, DECA, with P50 = 30 mmHg. The polymer does not extravasate and does not produce a pressor response in infused animals. ZL-HbBv decreased the volume of cerebral infarct by 40% in mice, while in the cat the lower affinity DECA failed to reduce the infarct volume. At reduced plasma viscosity ZL-HbBv produced a cerebral vasoconstriction due to excessive oxygen delivery, while at high plasma viscosity it produced a compensating vasodilation. In rabbit jejunum membranes, superfused under hypoxic conditions, the presence of the DECA allowed metabolites transport across the mucosa. Equivalent suspensions of red cells failed to allow transport. It is suggested that non-extravasating HBOC with high oxygen affinity can still deliver oxygen to ischemic tissues. Under nonischemic conditions with reduced blood viscosity cerebral vasoconstriction appears to occur in response to hyperoxygenation of tissues.

Key words. Blood substitutes, Oxygen gradients, Stroke, Microcirculation, Zero-link polymers

[1] Department of Biochemistry and Molecular Biology, University of Maryland, Baltimore Medical School, 108 N. Greene St., Baltimore, MD 21201, USA

[2] Department of Anesthesiology and Critical Care, Johns Hopkins Medical Institutions, 600 N. Wolfe St., Baltimore, MD 21205, USA

Introduction

The design of hemoglobin based blood substitutes should satisfy two main parameters: oxygen affinity and size. The prevailing opinion is that the ideal cell-free oxygen carrier should have oxygen affinity, and binding cooperativity similar to those of blood, namely P50 = 27 mmHg and a binding cooperativity with the index "n" near 2.7.

This opinion has been challenged by Vandegriff and Winslow [1], who claim that the oxygen carriers should have affinities higher than that of blood. Regarding size, the old concept that stabilized tetramers were big enough to prevent extravasation because they did not appear in the urine of infused animal, was incorrect. In fact extravasation still was detectable in the lymphatics [2], and was associated with large increase of mean arterial pressure.

Recently we obtained data using a high affinity, nonextravasating polymer of bovine hemoglobin and a crosslinked hemoglobin with affinity similar to that of blood. Data on brain microcirculation and focal ischemia were consistent with numerical simulations anticipating oxygen delivery as function of oxygen affinity in vivo.

Gradients of Oxygen Pressure

As shown in Fig. 1, blood plasma is an interface which regulates the transport of oxygen from the lungs to the tissues. A gradient is formed from a partial pressure of oxygen near 100 mmHg at the lungs, to the partial pressure at the mitochondrial level, where oxygen pressure is very low. In the absence of a carrier, the dissolved oxygen would be gradually released in amounts paral-

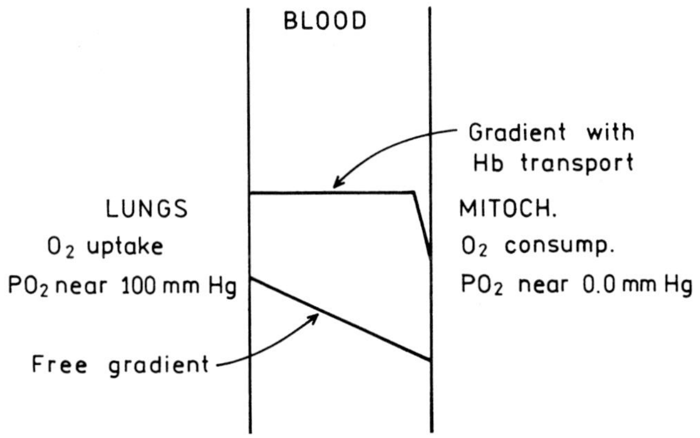

FIG. 1. Blood as an interface between lungs and mitochondria

lel to the decreasing partial pressure gradient and not much is left when it reaches the tissues. Instead when oxygen is transported by a carrier, the transported amount is released only when the gradient becomes compatible with its oxygen affinity, assuring a large amount of oxygen even at low partial pressure of oxygen.

There is a fundamental difference between the transport produced by a cell free carrier and a carrier segregated inside a membrane as in the red cells. A stringent regulation is provided by the poor solubility of oxygen in plasma. Oxygen released by the red cells cannot exceed oxygen solubility, therefore it is allowed only as replacement of consumption. The result is that red cells are an excellent buffer of plasma's oxygen tension. The end point of oxygen delivery by the red cells is plasma, not the tissues. Instead, as anticipated by the facilitated diffusion across liquid interfaces described by Wittenberg et al. [3], cell-free carriers chelate oxygen molecules at one end of the interface (in the lungs) and physically transport them to the other end (the endothelial walls of the capillaries) bypassing the fluid (plasma) and delivering oxygen directly across the interface (to tissues).

It is instructive to simulate, using the classical Hill equation, the fractional release of oxygen by cell free carrier as function of their P50 and binding cooperativity, when exposed to these gradients. For simulation purposes we assumed a partial pressure of oxygen at the mitochondria of 2.0 and

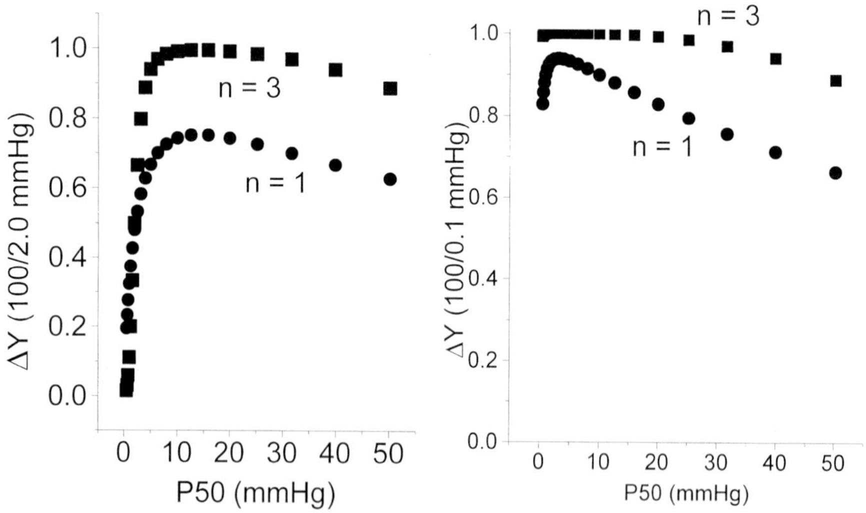

FIG. 2. Dependence of fractional delivery of oxygen (ΔY) on the P50 values of oxygen carriers exposed to the gradients of partial pressure shown in parenthesis. *Square* and *circle* are for cooperativity with n = 3 and n = 1 respectively

0.1 mmHg respectively. As shown in Fig. 2, for a gradient between 100 and 2 mmHg, with a cooperativity index n = 3 the delivery is practically the same for P50 values between 4 and 50 mmHg, where the delivery is more than 90% of the oxygen content. When the cooperativity decreases to n = 1.0. The delivery is still near 60 % between P50 of 4 and 50 mmHg. More dramatic are simulations assuming a gradient between 100 and 0.1 mmHg, For n = 3 the delivery is close to 100% at P50's between 1.0 and 20.0 mmHg, declining only slightly to 90% at higher P50 values. When n = 1 the delivery is still 90% at P50 between 2 and 5 mmHg, declining to about 60 % at higher P50 values. In essence the simulations suggest that best delivery is obtained with low, or very low P50 values. Also, the curves are flat, suggesting an ample tolerance of oxygen affinities. Cooperativity increases the delivery.

Brain Focal Ischemia and Microcirculation Evidences

We used a polymer of bovine hemoglobin (ZL-HbBv) [4], and hemoglobin A intramolecularly crosslinked with sebacic acid (DECA) [5]. Suffice here to say that ZL-HbBv is a large molecule with hydrodynamic radius Rh = 240 nm, P50 = 4.0 mmHg and no oxygen binding cooperativity. It does not extravasate and does not produce a "pressor response" in infused animals. DECA is a stabilized tetramer which does not dissociate into dimers [5]. It has P50 = 30 mmHg and binding cooperativity with n = 2.0.

Stroke Response to Infusions of ZL-HbBv

Cerebral infarct in mice was produced by occlusion of the middle cerebral artery [6]. Infusion of ZL-HbBv, with P50 near 4 mmHg, decreased by 40% the volume of the infarct, probably because of the oxygen delivered to ischemic tissues by the carrier (Fig. 3). Instead in the cat the size of cerebral stroke was not reduced by infusions of DECA [7] (Fig. 3). These data suggest that the high affinity with no binding cooperativity ZL-HbBv was more efficient than the lower affinity, high cooperativity DECA.

Microvascular Response to Infusions of ZL-HbBv

In the cat, when the viscosity of circulating blood was decreased by anemia, as produced by exchange transfusions, the oxygen carried by ZL-HbBv produced a moderate decrease in the diameter of the pial arteries, as opposed to the vasodilation produced by albumin infusion. In the absence of a pressor response, the reduced arterioles diameter was interpreted as a regulation to prevent excessive oxygen delivery [4,8]. Conversely, when plasma viscosity was increased 2.7 times by infusion of PVP, and the vasodilation produced by

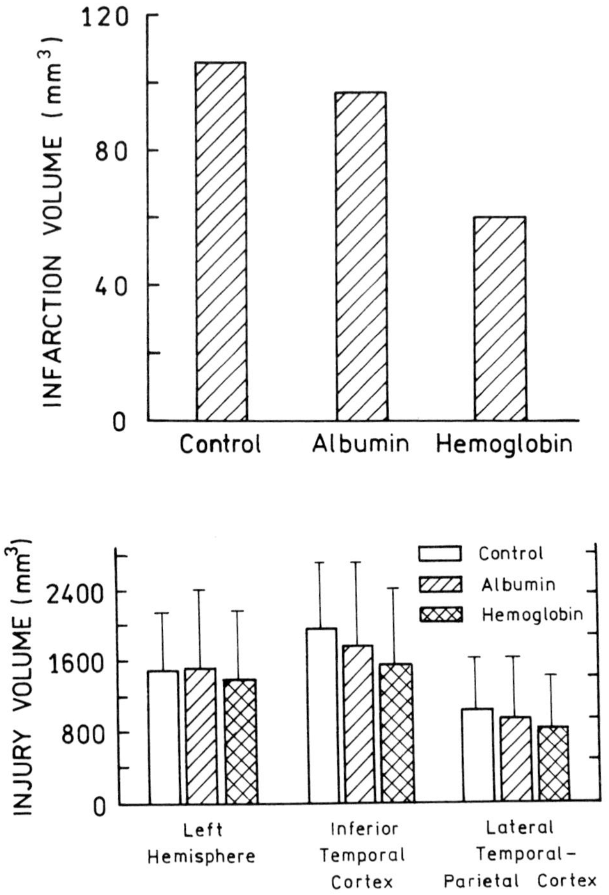

FIG. 3. **Upper panel,** A 40% exchange transfusion with ZL-HbBv polymer reduces the infarct size of mice brain, 1 day after a 2h period of middle cerebral occlusion. **Lower panel,** In the cat a 40% exhange transfusion of DECA failed to reduce the size of the infarct after 6h of middle cerebral artery occlusion

albumin solutions was not sufficient to maintain a normal oxygen supply, the oxygen carried by ZL-HbBv produced an extra vasodilation probably as if to further compensate for the diminished oxygen supply [8] (Fig. 4). These observations are consistent with simulations showing that carriers with high oxygen affinity and no oxygen binding cooperativity still transport and deliver oxygen in vivo. Actually, the oxygen delivery by ZL-HbBv elicited a regulatory response of either vasoconstriction or vasodilation to compensate for change in viscosity.

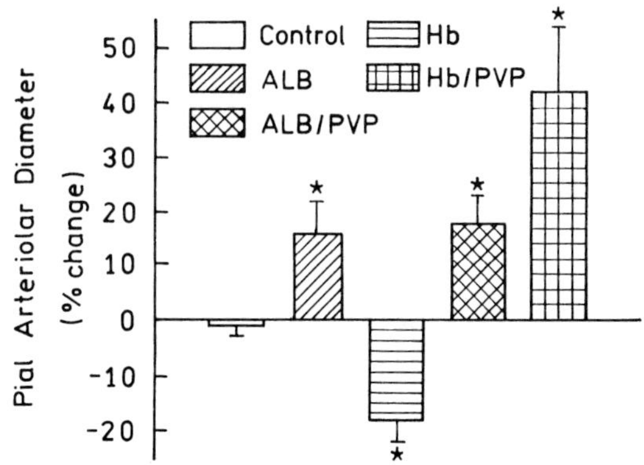

FIG. 4. Percent change in diameter of pial cerebral arteries (<50 μm) in anesthetized cats in a time control group, and 1 h after exchange transfusion with solutions of either albumin, albumin + PVP, ZL-HbBv, and Zl-HbBv + PVP. (n = 5 in all groups) (Adapted from Rebel et al. [8])

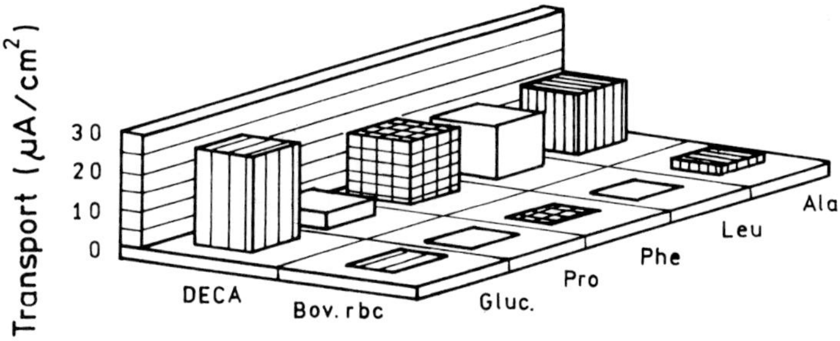

FIG. 5. Comparison of metabolite transport across rabbit jejunum membranes superfused in Ussin chambers with equivalent 3% hemoglobin in perfusates containing either cell-free DECA or bovine red cells. (Adapted from Bucci et al. [10]). Transport is proportional to the μA of the short circuit current elicited by the transport

Red Cells Deliver Oxygen only to Surrounding Fluid

Superfusion in Ussin Chambers

Rabbit jejunum membranes transport glucose and amino acids from the mucosa to the serosa side when superfused with salines in Ussin chambers [9]. The transport is oxygen sensitive. Ringer perfusates must be equilibrated with 95% oxygen and 5% CO_2. We have shown that with 3% w/v DECA in Ringer it was possible to equilibrate the perfusate with only 30% oxygen. Under these conditions Ringer alone would not allow transport. When we compared the transport obtained with equivalent 3% hemoglobin content in either DECA solutions or in bovine red cells suspensions, no transport was produced by the red cells [10] (Fig. 5). It should be stressed that the oxygen affinity of DECA and bovine red cells are very similar with P50 of 30 and 27 mmHg and a cooperativity index of 2.0 and 2.5, respectively [5,11].

As anticipated by the model, the red cells could not deliver oxygen above the amount dissolved in perfusates equilibrated with 30% oxygen. They only buffered a partial pressure of oxygen insufficient to allow metabolite transport. Instead the cell-free carrier, with a similar oxygen affinity, bypassed the Ringer and directly delivered sufficient amounts of oxygen.

Discussion

Although the proposed model is only a gross oversimplification, it is still consistent with the experimental data. The main difference between the delivery of oxygen by red cells and by cell-free HBOC's is that, due to the facilitated diffusion where oxygen molecules are physically transported by the carriers through the blood interface, cell-free hemoglobins "bypass" plasma.

These considerations strongly suggest that the oxygen affinity characteristics of cell free carriers are not a limiting factor for their physiologic competence. Our data on cerebral infarcts would suggest that high oxygen affinity carriers are more efficient than the low affinity ones in reducing the injury size. Also, at reduced viscosity ZL-HbBv seemed to deliver an excessive amount of oxygen which elicited vasoconstriction of cerebral pial arterioles. Conversely at high plasma viscosity it produced a compensatory vasodilation. These opposite effects confirm that both the vasoconstriction and vasodilation were regulatory phenomena stimulated by oxygen delivery.

It should be stressed that the effects of ZL-HbBv on brain arterioles, and in particular the vasodilation, could be interpreted as due to oxygen delivery only because ZL-HbBv did not elicit a pressor response. Also, it is very important to recognize the potentially excessive delivery of oxygen of a high affinity carrier. This property of cell free oxygen carriers should be investigated, so as either to avoid the risk of hyperoxygenation, or to take advantage of it, according to needs.

References

1. Vandegriff KD, Winslow RM (1995) A theoretical analysis of oxygen transport; a new strategy for the design of hemoglobin-based red cell substitutes. In: Winslow RM, Vandegriff KD, Intaglietta M (eds) Blood substitute, physiological basis of efficacy. Birkhauser, Boston, pp 143–155
2. Matheson B, Razynska A, Kwansa HE, et al (2000) Appearance of dissociable and crosslinked hemoglobins in renal hilar lymph. J Lab Clin Inv 135:459–464
3. Wittemberg J (1966) The molecular mechanism of hemoglobin facilitated oxygen diffusion. J Biol Chem 241:104–114
4. Matheson B, Kwansa HE, Rebel A, et al (2002) Vascular response to infusions of a non extravasating hemoglobin polymer. J Appl Physiol 93:1479–1486

5. Bucci E, Razynska A, Kwansa HE, et al (1996) Production and characterization of an infusible oxygen-carrying fluid based on hemoglobin intramolecularly crosslinked with sebacic acid. J Lab Clin Med 128:146–153
6. Bucci E, Watts TL, Kwansa HE, et al (2001) Cell-free hemoglobin, oxygen off-load and vasoconstriction. Anasthesiol Intensivmed Notfallmed Schmerzther Nov; 36 Suppl 2:S123–S124
7. Rebel A, Ulatowski JA, Joung K, et al (2002) Regional cerebral blood flow in cats with crosslinked hemoglobin transfusion during focal cerebral ischemia. Am J Physiol Heart Circ Physiol 282:H832–H841
8. Rebel A, Ulatowski JA, Kwansa H, et al (2003) Cerebrovascular response to decreased hematocrit: effect of cell-free hemoglobin, plasma viscosity and CO2. Am J Physiol Heart Circ Physiol H1600–H1608
9. Field M, Fromm d, McColl I (1971) Ion transport in rabbit elieal mucosa: I Na and Cl fluxes and short circuit current. Am J Physiol 2220:1388–1396
10. Bucci E, Watts TL, Kwansa HE, et al (2003) Different efficacy in vitro of hemoglobin based oxygen carriers and red cells. In: Wilson D (Ed) Oxygen transport to tissue, vol. XXIII: Oxygen measurements in the 21st century. Kluwer Plenum, New York, pp 89–92
11. Bucci E, Fronticelli C (1992) Hemoglobin as oxygen carriers in cell-free fluids. Maryland Med J 41:527–531

Oxygen Partition Between Microvessels and Tissue: Significance for the Design of Blood Substitutes

Amy G. Tsai[1], Barbara Friesenecker[2], and Marcos Intaglietta[1]

Summary. Correction of blood losses with blood substitutes alter the pO_2 distribution in the microcirculation, with outcomes depending on the final viscosity of the circulating blood and the vasoactivity induced to the restore normal distribution of pO_2. Vasoactivity has an oxygen cost shown by the oxygen consumption of the arteriolar microcirculation. Vasodilators lower arteriolar oxygen consumption delivering more oxygen to the tissues, and vice versa. Increased oxygen delivery to the arterioles by right shifted oxygen dissociation causes autoregulatory vasoconstriction, a problem aggravated by low blood and plasma viscosity that lowers NO endothelial NO production. Restoration of tissue function is achieved when no portion of the tissue falls below the threshold of anaerobic metabolism. This goal is attained by using high affinity modified hemoglobins that act as a reservoir of oxygen only deployed when the circulating blood arrives at tissue regions where pO_2 is very low. Given these premises, restoration of tissue function after severe blood losses requires the re-establishment of oxygen delivery capacity and pO_2 distribution. This is attained by tailoring blood and plasma viscosity and oxygen dissociation properties to insure that no portion of the tissue lacks oxygen delivery, even though overall tissue pO_2 may be abnormally low.

Key words. Vessel wall oxygen consumption, Tissue oxygenation, Oxygen delivery

[1] Department of Bioengineering, 0412, University of California, San Diego, 9500 Gilman Dr., La Jolla, CA 92093-0412, USA
[2] Division of General and Surgical Intensive Care Medicine, Department of Anesthesia and Critical Care Medicine, The Leopold-Franzens-University of Innsbruck, Austria

Introduction

The classical scheme for tissue oxygenation assumes that oxygen gathered by the lung capillaries from the atmosphere is distributed by the systemic circulation to the tissue capillaries, which yield their oxygen by being in close proximity with virtually every cell of the organism. In this process the lung capillaries receive oxygen that diffuses through a high oxygen concentration gradient, while tissue capillaries deliver oxygen by means of a low concentration gradient, a situation rendered possible because of the large surface area disparity between tissue and lung capillaries, which is about a factor of 10×.

While the capillaries are in virtual equilibrium with tissue, there is also a large disparity between arterial and tissue pO_2, which indicates that there is a significant oxygen loss from blood as it transits from the lungs to the tissue.

This oxygen loss determines a longitudinal oxygen gradient mostly developed in the microcirculation, leading to a specific distribution of intravascular oxygen tension. There is substantial evidence that the circulation is adapted to this distribution and that the organism strives to maintain this specific pattern by the process of autoregulation [1,2].

Local autoregulation is based on arteriolar vasoactivity, a process that engages the smooth muscle of the arteriolar wall leading to vasodilation and vasoconstriction, and the control of blood flow which regulates oxygen delivery to counteract the changes in intravascular oxygen distribution.

The Oxygen Cost of Blood Flow Regulation

Arterioles yield a significant amount of the oxygen that they carry directly to the tissue, instead of delivering this to the capillary system (leading to the presence of an intraluminal, longitudinal oxygen gradient), therefore in principle these microvessels should be a major source of oxygen for the tissue. Mass balance analysis of the rate of exit of oxygen from arteriolar segments showed that it was much greater than that solely accounted by the process of diffusion, leading to the proposal that the diffusion constant of the arteriolar wall was of the order of 10× of that of normal tissue [3], a process for which there is no physical evidence.

An alternative explanation is that the vessels wall is a large oxygen sink due to the high metabolic activity of the endothelium and possibly smooth muscle in vivo and in situ. The presence of such an oxygen sink was demonstrated by the measurements of Tsai et al. [4], who found large pO_2 gradients in the region of the vessel wall, a finding that was recently confirmed by Shibata et al. [5]. In this situation large oxygen gradients can also be due to a large resistance to oxygen exit, however this alternative is not compatible with the measured large rates of oxygen exit measured from arterioles.

Arteriolar wall oxygen consumption is not a static, fixed rate, and it varies in accordance to microvessels tone or level of vasoconstriction. Under normal conditions 50 μm diameter arterioles of the unanesthetized hamster window chamber preparation consume about 25% of the oxygen convected by the blood stream, a rate that is evidenced by the these vessels exhibiting a vessel wall gradient, i.e., difference between in pO_2 across the vessel wall, of 18.5 mmHg. The continuous infusion of PGE_1 (2.5 mg/kg min, i.v.) was found to increase flow by a factor of 2.18x and lower the vessel wall oxygen gradient to 15.5 mmHg. Geometrical considerations indicate that the oxygen gradient in 50 μm arterioles is 12 mmHg, the excess pO_2 difference being attributed to vessels wall oxygen consumption. The same analysis shows that the oxygen gradient of the vessels wall [6] is linearly related to its rate of oxygen consumption, thus the decrease due to PGE_1 halves vessel wall oxygen consumption. Not unexpectedly, the increased flow and lowered vessels wall oxygen consumption causes tissue pO_2 to be 31.9 mmHg, vs. 24.5 mmHg found for normal conditions. The infusion of Vasopressin (0.001 IU/kg min i.v.) a vasoconstrictor, caused flow to decrease to 0.60 of control, increased the vessel wall oxygen gradient to 31.2 mmHg, and lowered tissue pO_2 to 9.5 mmHg. Similar findings have been reported by Ye et al. [7], who measured oxygen extraction from various tissues under different levels of tone.

The Significance of Tissue pO_2

Tissue pO_2 is controlled simultaneously by the rate at which oxygen is delivered by convection to the microcirculation and the rate that it is consumed by the vessels walls, however the actual level of tissue pO_2 is only indicative of tissue oxygen supply, a factor that is significantly influenced by the shape of the oxygen dissociation curve of hemoglobin, and therefore the intraluminal distribution of oxygen in the microcirculation. In the normal hamster window chamber model large arterioles and venules have respectively 56 and 33 mmHg blood oxygen partial pressure which corresponds to an arteriolar/venular difference in oxygen saturation of 34%, leading to a tissue pO_2 of 24.5 ± 5.0 mmHg (mean $\pm$ SD) according to Intaglietta et al. [8]. By comparison, if tissue were regulated at the verge of the transition of tissue hypoxia, or about 2 mmHg, the threshold for anaerobic metabolism, and all intravascular pO_2 values were decreased by 22.5 mmHg the arteriolar/venular saturation difference would by 45%, thus if blood flow were the same, the tissue would receive more oxygen.

Normal tissue pO_2 is regulated at a level that is significantly higher than that associated with anaerobic metabolism, which commences at pO_2s lower than about 2 mmHg [9]. The disparity between level of regulation and limit of oxidative metabolism can be explained by considering a hypothetical situation in which the tissue is regulated at 7 mmHg pO_2, under otherwise identical anatomical and microhemodynamic conditions. In this form of regulation, if the pO_2 variability remains the same, 16% of the tissue would be beyond the anaerobic threshold, i.e., beyond one standard deviation or 1σ. It is apparent that regulating tissue at 24.5 mmHg places 99.98% of the tissue within the aerobic metabolism, the anaerobic portion being beyond 4σ.

Oxygen Distribution in the Design of Blood Substitutes

To the present, blood substitutes have been mostly formulated using hemoglobin as the oxygen carrier. Formulations based on human hemoglobin must in principle provide a material that is as plentiful an efficacious as the natural blood, namely should be the result of a process that increase, or at least is equal to the amount of human blood utilized. In other words a practical product should yield an equivalent unit of blood utilizing at most a unit of natural blood. Formulations that use non-human hemoglobin or recombinant hemoglobin are not exempt from considerations of economy of oxygen carrier, since they are costly to produce.

An economic product can in principle be formulated if the material is vasoinactive and is utilized in minimal concentrations. However, overall hemoglobin concentrations (red blood hemoglobin plus product hemoglobin) that are significantly lower than that of natural blood will correspondingly significantly lower tissue pO_2 placing substantial portions of the tissue in conditions of anaerobic metabolism, as shown in our previous example.

The statistical nature of oxygen distribution, however, indicates that even at low tissue pO_2 conditions there are parts of the tissue whose pO_2 is higher than the tissue average, therefore a solution of this problem is to introduce an oxygen reservoir that is only deployed for tissue regions at very low pO_2s. This is readily accomplished by utilizing an oxygen carrier whose equivalent p50 is very low, i.e., a material that releases oxygen only in anoxic regions. This analysis also shows that this approach is only possible if the material is vasoinactive, otherwise the comparatively small amounts of oxygen transported by the low concentration formulation is utilized by the energy requirements of vasoconstriction. Parenthetically and additional advantage of oxygenating the tissue at low pO_2 is that vessel wall oxygen consumption is proportional to blood pO_2 [6], thus less oxygen would be consumed by the arteriolar walls.

These concepts have been validated by the experiments of Sakai et al., 1999 [10], who tested tissue oxygenation by hemoglobin vesicles formulated at varying p50s in a hemodilution protocol in hamster and determined that for this type of oxygen carrier optimal performance was attained at p50 = 16 mmHg vs. p50 = 36 mmHg for hamster blood. A material incorporating these features, namely vasoinactivity, low p50, i.e., 5 mmHg, and formulated at 4% hemoglobin concentration (MalPEG-hemoglobin, Hemospan) is presently produced by Sangart Inc, San Diego, has shown to be highly efficacious in experimental studies [11] and is presently in clinical trials.

Acknowledgments. This work was supported by Bioengineering Research Partnership grant R24-HL 64395 and the grants R01-HL 62318 and R01-HL 62354.

References

1. Johnson PC (1986) Brief Review: Autoregulation of blood flow, Circ Res 59:483–495
2. Duling BR, Berne RM (1970) Longitudinal gradients in periarteriolar oxygen tension. A possible mechanism for the participation of oxygen in the local regulation of blood flow. Circ Res 27:669–678
3. Popel AS, Pittman RN, Ellsworth ML (1988) Rate of oxygen loss from arterioles is an order of magnitude than expected. Am J Physiol Heart Circ Physiol 256:H921–H924
4. Tsai AG, Friesenecker B, Mazzoni MC, Kerger H, Buerk DG, Johnson PC, Intaglietta M (1998) Microvascular and tissue oxygen gradients in the rat mesentery. Proc Nat Acad Sci USA 95:6590–6595
5. Shibata M, Ichioka S, Ando J, Kamiya A (2001) Microvascular and interstitial pO_2 measurements in rat skeletal muscle by phosphorescence quenching J Appl Physiol 91:321–327
6. Tsai AG, Johnson PC, Intaglietta M (2003) Oxygen gradients in the microcirculation. Physiol Rev 83:933–963
7. Ye JM, Colquhoun EQ, Clark MG (1990) A comparison of vasopressin and noradrenaline on oxygen uptake by perfused rat hind limb, intestine, and mesenteric arcade suggests that it is part due to contractile work by blood vessels. Gen Pharmacol 21:805–810
8. Intaglietta M, Johnson PC, Winslow RM (1996) Microvascular and tissue oxygen distribution. Cardiovasc Res 32:632–643
9. Richmond KN, Shonat RD, Lynch RM, Johnson PC (1999) Critical pO_2 of skeletal muscle in vivo. Am J Physiol Heart Circ Physiol 277:H1831–H1840
10. Sakai H, Tsai AG, Rohlfs RJ, Hara H, Takeoka S, Tsuchida E, Intaglietta M (1999) Microvascular responses to hemodilution with Hb vesicles as red blood cell substitutes: influence of O_2 affinity. Am J Physiol Heart Circ Physiol 276:H553–H562
11. Winslow RM, Gonzales A, Gonzales ML, Magde M, McCarthy M, Rohlfs RJ, Vandegriff KD (1998) Vascular resistance and the efficacy of red cell substitutes in a rat hemorrhage model. J Appl Physiol 85:993–1003

Endothelial Cell Response to Hemoglobin Based Oxygen Carriers. Is the Attenuation of Pathological Reactions Possible?*

Jan Simoni

Summary. There is no doubt that in order to design an effective free hemoglobin (Hb)-based oxygen carrier, a full understanding of the mechanism of Hb toxicity is required. The current knowledge of Hb's overall toxicity however, is very limited. Hb is such an intriguing molecule that even after many decades of researching its physical, biochemical, physiological and pathological profile, many aspects of its intrinsic toxicity are yet to be uncovered [1]. This is probably the main reason for not having a viable substitute of human blood on the market. In fact, no product has yet been approved in the U.S. for any indication [2]. The currently tested, Hb-based oxygen carriers trigger a complex array of reactions as a result of Hb's natural features [3]. A number of unwanted effects have been observed in human clinical trials. Regardless of the type of Hb chemical modification procedure, all the first generation Hb-based oxygen carriers are vasoactive [1–6]. Some products have also been linked with oxidative and inflammatory reactions, often described as "flu like" symptoms, gastrointestinal side effects and myocardial lesions [1,3,7,8].

The products currently in various phases of clinical trials were developed before the recognition of Hb's intrinsic toxicity problems. These products seem only to address the problems of Hb purity, high oxygen affinity and short circulatory half-life; which were uncovered in the 1970s and had been resolved in various ways. There are, however, newly discovered problems that need resolution. These are vasoactivity, pro-oxidant and pro-inflammatory properties of Hb [1–8]. Therefore, it was not surprising that the commercial

Department of Surgery, Texas Tech University Health Sciences Center School of Medicine, Lubbock, TX 79430, USA

* This paper is based on the plenary lecture delivered at the 13th Keio University International Symposium for Life Sciences and Medicine; Research and Development of Artificial Oxygen Carrier—Its Frontline 2003, Keio University, Tokyo, Japan.

development of HemAssist, a diaspirin αα-cross-linked human Hb, (Baxter Healthcare, Round Lake, IL, USA) was halted, and the development of Hemolink, a *o*-raffinose polymerized human Hb, (Hemosol, Mississauga, Canada) was paused because of the high mortality rate or increase of myocardial infarctions in humans [9,10]. Earlier, the commercial development of Optro, a recombinant Hb, (Somatogen, Boulder, CO, USA) was canceled because of the serious side effects observed in the patients tested [11]. The only product under FDA review for a Biological License Application (BLA) is Biopure's (Cambridge, MA, USA) Hemopure, a glutaraldehyde polymerized bovine Hb, intended to be used in elective surgery patients [2]. Recently, the FDA asked for more information on the product and cited "safety concerns" had halted further clinical trials of Hemopure. In 2002, Northfield Laboratories, (Evanston, IL, USA) failed to get U.S. regulatory approval for its PolyHeme, a pyridoxylated and glutaraldehyde polymerized human Hb solution, used in elective surgery patients. Now, Northfield is taking a second stab at an approval, this time via a study in which PolyHeme will be used on trauma patients [12]. This is an important approach because the first indication for a successful Hb-based oxygen carrier would be hemorrhage and trauma [2,3].

It is reasonable to expect, that the products presently under clinical trials, will represent the "first family" of Hb-based oxygen carriers, with efforts now directed towards a "new generation" of blood substitutes which addresses all of the Hb intrinsic toxicity problems. It is believed that the second-generation products will be used for all clinical indication, including treatment of hemorrhagic shock and trauma.

Endothelial cells are among the first exposed to injected Hb-based oxygen carrier [13]. Several clinical and in vitro points of evidence have been presented, that the currently tested Hb-based oxygen carriers can interfere with the many basic functions of the endothelium [1,3–6,8,13–21]. The effects of Hb on the endothelium have become a central focus for research because of the vasoconstriction seen during the clinical trials [1–4,7,8].

Key words. Hemoglobin-based oxygen carrier, Endothelial cell, Toxicity, Radicals, Cell signaling

Consequences of Endothelial Cells Exposed to Hemoglobin

Normal endothelium maintains a balance in vasculature between vasoconstriction and vasodilation, blood cell adherence and non-adherence, anticoagulation and pro-coagulation, and growth promotion and inhibition. In these ways, the endothelial cells control vasomotor tone, regulate vascular structure, maintain blood fluidity, and mediate both inflammatory and immunologic responses. Endothelial cells respond to various biologic signals and are involved in the synthesis and release of an immense number of factors [22–24]. Hb-based oxygen carriers could mediate many endothelial responses including: up- or down-regulation of secretory activity, change in the functional and morphological status, aggravation of endothelial oxidative stress and affect in redox balance, augmentation of endothelial pro-inflammatory responses, and many other reactions based on signaling/transcriptional events.

Role of Vascular Endothelium in Hemoglobin Catabolism

In healthy subjects, the only condition in which free Hb appears in circulation is the hemolysis of aged red blood cells. Characteristically, Hb-haptoglobin (Hp) complexes, formed during intravascular hemolysis, are taken up by the liver parenchyma cells, followed by the bone marrow and spleen, whereas phagocytic and endothelial cells appear to be held in reserve in terms of Hb accumulation [13,25–29]. The kidneys normally play a minor role in the overall catabolism of Hb and only account for 2% of the total normal daily Hb turnover. The threshold of tubular reabsorption is less than 100 mg of Hb per dl of plasma [30,31]. Heme oxygenase (HO) activities, which catalyze the degradation of heme to carbon monoxide (CO) and biliverdin (then converted to bilirubin by biliverdin reductase) are an important part of the catabolic fate of Hb [32]. The heme molecule is the most effective pro-oxidant, thus its degradation to bilirubin (a potent antioxidant) effectively prevents cellular damage. While HO activity appears to be physiologically present in high concentrations in the liver, spleen, bone marrow and phagocytic cells, its basal activity in endothelial cells is much lower. Some of the intact heme derived from the catabolism of Hb-Hp may be incorporated into apoheme proteins in the microsomes, and function as the prosthetic group of hemoprotein [33]. Free hemin, however, that can be released from Hb during autoxidation can be detoxified by hemopexin proteins and plasma albumin [34,35]. The hemopexin bound hemin is completely inactive as an oxidant, whereas the albumin-hemin complex serves as a temporary hemin reservoir that possesses peroxidase-like activity. These Hb catabolic processes will be effective to some extent, and are related to extracellular Hp and hemopexin concentrations, HO activities, and the ferritin and apoheme intracellular pool.

In pathological conditions, such as incompatible transfusions, traumatic injury, malaria and etc., intravascular hemolysis can exceed the capacity of the detoxifying system, and plasma free Hb becomes toxic. In hemodialysis patients as often observed, a large amount of free Hb in plasma is now being considered as a progressive factor of end stage renal disease [36,37]. Also, free

Hb is linked to neuronal injury during head trauma and hemorrhagic stroke [38–42]. Most importantly, however, a massive amount of free Hb will appear in the plasma as a consequence of the transfusion of Hb-based oxygen carriers. In such situations, the natural Hb detoxification system will not be effective. Moreover, certain chemical modification procedures used in the preparation of the first generation Hb-based oxygen carriers can completely eliminate or decrease the binding properties of Hb to Hp [43–45]. These chemical modification procedures, by altering Hb autoxidation kinetics and other related redox characteristics, may destabilize the heme-globin binding force and increase the release of hemin [46,47].

The failure of Hb's natural catabolism causes enhanced Hb absorption by phagocytic [26–28] and endothelial cells [29,48,49]. Both monocytes and macrophages phagocytize Hb under suitable conditions, and the iron released from the heme rapidly accumulates in ferritin, which can then be released from the cells [50,51]. Endothelial cells, however, have a less sophisticated Hb detoxification system that is solely based on the availability of HO-1 and ferritin [29,35,52,53]. The availability of ferritin in the endothelium is very important since HO is the enzyme that opens the porphyrin ring, producing not only biliverdin and CO, but also a very dangerous product free redox-active iron that can only be sequestrated with this multimeric protein [54]. It was demonstrated that the free heme released from ferrous-Hb during autoxidation primes the endothelium for oxidative damage [29]. In this study, exposure of the endothelial cells to a low concentration of ferric-Hb increased their heme oxygenase mRNA and enzyme activity, thereby supporting, to a certain extent, heme uptake. The ferritin production has also increased after such exposure, thus attesting eventual incorporation of iron [29]. This protective mechanism, however, will not be fully effective after a massive transfusion of Hb-based oxygen carriers that can greatly enhance endothelial susceptibility to oxidant-mediated injury [13,15–17,21,49,54,55]. In a similar study, acellular ferrous-Hb solutions were also found to augment to some extent the endothelial HO activity [16]. This effect, however, did not protect the endothelial cells against Hb-mediated oxidative damage. In this study, a marked reduction in endothelial injury was achieved with deferoxamine, whereas dimethylthiourea provided only partial protection [16]. It seems that the excess of Hb and subsequent deficiency in heme-catabolizing enzyme and ferritin will be the leading causes of endothelial damage. In fact, heme oxygenase deficiency patients exhibit extensive endothelial dysfunction [56].

Hitherto, no strategy has been developed to overcome the toxic consequences of endothelial Hb catabolism after a massive transfusion of Hb-based oxygen carriers. Experimental studies from the Mayo Clinic and Rockefeller University suggest that complete endothelial protection against heme and hemoglobin toxicity can only be achieved by transfection of the endothelial cells with the human heme oxygenase gene [56,57]. Endothelial cells transfected with the human HO, acquired substantial resistance to the toxicity produced by exposure to Hb solutions and heme as compared to non-transfected cells. This finding, however, sounds impractical for the Hb-based oxygen carriers. It seems that a much simpler strategy is to better stabilize the heme-globin binding force, and design a Hb molecule that will mimic the Hb.Hp complex and would not be subjected for endocytosis.

Hemoglobin Extravasation Endocytosis and Transcytosis

Extravasation

The luminal surface of the endothelial cells and the outer membranes of phagocytic cells have a net negative charge. This negative charge is attributed primarily to the carboxyl groups of sialic acid in the membrane [58]. The distribution and movement of charge on the cell membrane surface influences various membrane-associated processes and may affect the barrier function of the endothelial cell layer. There is evidence that the negative surface charge is of importance for the permeability to macromolecules of various vascular beds and for restraining cell to cell interaction [58]. There is mounting evidence that the permeability of systemic microvessel to macromolecules is influenced by the net electric charge as well as the molecular size and shape of the permeating molecules [59–64]. Large and not dissociated macromolecules, with electronegative charge, would not extravasate. The other factors that may increase vascular permeability to macromolecules include: hypertension, shear stress, oxidants, adenosine-5′-triphosphate (ATP) and reduced glutathione (GSH) depletion, hyperglycemia, inflammation and etc. [65–69]. The factors that are known to decrease endothelial permeability to macromolecules include adenosine, glutathione, nitric oxide and etc. [70–72].

Molecular Mass vs. Isoelectric Point

It is well known that the cationization of serum albumin [61] and ferritin [62] results in their higher transcapillary movement. This is the best example for how anionic macromolecules, such as most plasma proteins, may be restricted from movement across the vascular endothelium. The fixed anionic charges of the endothelium act much like a cation exchange gel to rapidly take up electropositive proteins and retard anionic molecules of the same size. The native Hb, however, with an isoelectric point (pI) of 6.8–7.0 should be considered as a moderately, or in some circumstances slightly electropositive, cationic molecule [25]. Since the transcapillary exchange of macromolecules is only minimally affected by molecular masses of up to 300 kDa [73], the native Hb [31,74–78] as well as the modified Hb solutions without an altered pI, might extravasate [76].

The elegant study done at the University of Tokyo showed that the endothelial permeability of unmodified Hb was almost twice that of serum albumin and that the intramolecular cross-linking only slightly reduced Hb's transendothelial passage [76]. In this study, the conjugation of Hb with polyethylene glycol (PEG) or Hp further reduced, but not eliminated, the Hb transendothelial flux. The study done at the University of Arizona, showed that cross-linked αα-Hb, PEG-Hb and glutaraldehyde polymerized Hb induced venular leakage in the mesentery by mechanisms similar to those previously observed after treatment with histamine or nitric oxide inhibitors [77,78]. Hb-induced microvascular leakage was accompanied by changes in the endothelial actin cytoskeleton and by an increased number of endothelial gaps [77]. The recent study at Texas Tech University, further explored the effect of Hb on endothelial cell permeability to anionic macromolecules [42]. The human brain capillary endothelial cells exposed to tetrameric Hb, showed a higher permeability rate to human albumin. This effect was greatly potentiated in GSH depleted cells [42].

For almost two decades, it was speculated that an apparently higher rate of glomerular filtration and extravasation of native Hb over albumin reflects the dissociation of Hb tetramers into dimers, which pass with greater ease through the endothelial barrier [79–81]. It was thought that the dimers, having a molecular mass of ca. 32 kDa traversed the pores of the glomeruli. At that time, no theoretical connection between the modification type of Hb and its pI had been made, and the proposed dissociability of the Hb tetramers was the only explanation for its extravasation and glomerular filtration [81,82]. The study done at Texas Tech University, however, successfully challenged previous reports attributing Hb extravasation to the tendency of the Hb tetramer to dissociate into dimers [31]. It was found that the 64 kDa Hb tetramer is able to extravasate. The earlier suggested presence of Hb dimers in the urine was not confirmed in this study. Moreover, Hb tetramers by binding to the glomerulus during filtration and decrease in the number of anionic groups, increased glomerular permeability to anionic macromolecules such as plasma proteins [31]. In contrast, the alteration of the surface charge of Hb polymers and tetramers to the pI of 6.1–6.2 has completely blocked their transglomerular passage. This data suggests that the extravasation of Hb could not be related to the ability of Hb to dissociate into dimers, but rather to the Hb net surface electric charge.

Ignoring the fact that in addition to molecular size, the electric charge of macromolecules plays an important role in preventing their glomerular filtration and transcapillary exchange, the developers of the first generation products have solely focused on the prevention of Hb dimerization by cross-linking and/or increasing Hb molecular weight by conjugation or polymerization [1–3,7,83]. For this purpose, the following five types of Hb modification have been developed so far: (1) intermolecular cross-linking-polymerizations, (2) intramolecular cross-linking of alpha or beta chains, (3) conjugation of Hb with other molecules, (4) various combinations of the above methods, and (5) recombinant Hb in which two alpha-globin polypeptides are genetically joined, resulting in a stable tetramer [1,83]. The currently used Hb chemical modification methods that stabilize the Hb tetramer and/or increase its molecular weight can only produce non uniform, partial changes to the Hb surface charge. Such a Hb solution often possesses diverse physicochemical properties from its constituents, with an isoelectric point varied from positive to moderate [1,81,84]. It is noteworthy that the macromolecules with such an electric potential are able to pass the negatively charged endothelial barrier. Thus, the presently used chemical modification techniques can only partially decrease transcapillary Hb passage [83]. Since, the extravasation of Hb and its presence in the subendothelial space is required to interfere with endothelial dependent vasorelaxation, the observed changes in the hemodynamics of the currently tested products can be related to the ability of these products to pass the transendothelial barrier [1–7,83]. It seems that the clever strategy to avoid extravasation of Hb, (besides increasing its molecular mass), is to reduce the Hb molecules isoelectric potential.

Endocytosis and Transcytosis

Recently, a group of scientists form Universite Henri Poincare-Nancy demonstrated that Hb could penetrate into the endothelial cells [48]. In this study, despite the large molecular size of Hb-based oxygen carriers to prevent Hb extravascular leakage, Hb was detectable inside the endothelial cells. The authors concluded that the vascular endothelium could uptake Hb by an endocytosis mechanism. They also suggested that the vascular endothelial cells could help Hb to cross the endothelial barrier toward the media by a transcytosis mechanism. This new finding is very important in the better understanding of the mechanism of the pressor effect of modified Hb solutions. The independent study conducted at Texas Tech University confirmed the above finding [21]. During the fluorometric measurement of cytostolic calcium in human coronary artery endothelial cells exposed to different Hb solutions, it was found that the endocyted tetrameric Hb interfered with an emission wavelength of 505 nm. The immunohistochemical staining confirmed the intracellular localization of Hb. In this study, the electronegatively charged Hb molecules were not up-taken by the endothelial cells. This was not a great surprise, because it was already known that incubation of the endothelium with Hb could provide the cells with heme [29]. In situ hybridization study for heme oxygenase reveals accumulation of this enzyme in the microvascular endothelium, implying the incorporation of heme into endothelial cells.

Endothelial Participation in Hemoglobin Mediated Vasoconstriction

Numerous laboratories have demonstrated a clear vasoconstrictive effect, particularly in pulmonary, coronary, cerebral and renal vascular beds, after the administration of different Hb solutions. Although the pathophysiology of Hb-induced hemodynamic changes is still unclear, recent scientific reviews suggest that the modulation of vascular tone could be the result of Hb stimulatory-inhibitory activity under control of mediators released by the vascular endothelial cells [1–7,13,14,18–21]. Many factors that are in control of the vascular tone can be influenced by free-Hb. The factors that modify arterial diameter, include: physical factors (pressure, flow, viscosity); metabolic factors from cells surrounding the arteries (pH, potassium ions, adenosine); hormonal factors (angiotensin II, adrenaline); neuronal-sympathetic factors (noradrenaline, ATP); neuronal-parasympathetic factors (Ach, VIP); neuronal-sensory factors (CGRP); and endothelial factors (e.g., nitric oxide, endothelin, prostaglandins (eicosanoids), isoprostanes) [22–24,85,86].

The vascular endothelium may vary in its response to pathophysiologic stimuli. Endothelial cells are not homogeneous instead they are heterogeneous [87]. The structure and function of endothelial cells are differently regulated in space and time [87]. Since the 1960s, it has been reported that there are striking differences between large and small coronary arteries in their responsiveness to catecholamines, nitroglycerin, and adenosine [88–91]. While nitroglycerin has been shown to affect preferentially large coronary arteries, the adenosine affects preferentially small coronary arteries [89–91]. A more recent study has shown that the endothelium produces at least three diffusible molecules (NO, EDHF and prostacyclin) that relax smooth muscle cells; but not all endothelial cells release all of the factors [22,24,92]. In humans, large arteries appear to rely on NO for relaxation, and smaller ones rely more on EDHF or prostanoids [92].

The published research related to endothelial participation in Hb-mediated vasoconstriction was almost exclusively done on the endothelial cells from human umbilical vein, bovine aorta, and human coronary artery. Omission in these studies of endothelial cells from other vessels is perhaps, the main reason for our lack of a full understanding of the mechanism of Hb-mediated vasoconstriction, seen after the administration of Hb solutions. Presently, several mechanisms could explain the vasoconstrictive effects observed after the administration of Hb-based oxygen carriers. The most popular explanation is based on the high affinity of Hb for endothelial NO [1,8,19,24,93–97].

Nitric Oxide

Endothelium mediated relaxation of vascular smooth muscle is dependent in part on the endothelial production of NO from L-arginine, through the action of nitric oxide synthase (NOS). NO stimulates soluble guanylate cyclase (sGS) by the formation of a nitrosyl-heme complex at the activator site of the enzyme. Activated sGC subsequently converts intracellular guanosine triphosphate (GTP) to 3′,5′-cyclic guanosine monophosphate (cGMP). This lowers the free intracellular ionized Ca^{2+} concentration to promote vasodilation and depression of the tone of the underlying vascular smooth muscle cells; and is accomplished via the action of cGMP-dependent protein kinases and/or a direct effect of the nucleotide on sarcoplasmic reticulum or plasma membrane Ca^{2+}-activated ATP-ases. Intracellular calcium triggers smooth muscle contraction via a calcium-dependent enzyme cascade. In smooth muscle, actin and myosin cannot interact unless the myosin regulatory light chain is phosphorylated on Ser19. Phosphorylation of myosin is catalyzed by calcium-calmodulin-dependent activation of the myosin light chain kinase (MLCK). Myosin phosphorylation depends on the balance of activities of MLCK and MLC phosphatase. It has recently become clear that the activity of MLC phosphatase is regulated and has important consequences or force generation in arterial smooth muscle [24,97].

Most blood substitute investigators believe that extravasated Hb to the subendothelial environment, is able to remove NO before it interacts with sGC, thus promoting vasoconstriction [24,93–97]. This is based on the evidence that ferrous-Hb reacts with NO to yield nitrate (NO_3^-) and ferric-Hb [94,96,98]. By these investigators, this reaction is considered to be a major pathway of NO elimination from the endothelial cell environment. Some recent reports, however, have suggested that NO binds to Hb cooperatively [99–101]. In other words it was postulated that Hb might be involved in the systemic transport and delivery of NO to tissues and in the facilitation of O_2 release. This is based on the observation that NO can preferentially bind to the minor population of Hb's vacant hemes, nitrosilates Hb thiols, and subsequently forms S-nitrosoHb. Some researchers, however, question this new hypothesis [102]. Recently they reported that NO is consumed, rather than conserved, by reaction with ferrous-Hb under physiological condition [103].

The NO-Hb hypotheses have both strength and weaknesses and many questions remaining. The scientists from University of California, San Diego, believe that vasoconstriction observed upon exchange transfusion with Hb solutions can not be the result of NO scavenging reactions at the heme, but rather must be due to alternative physiologic mechanisms [104]. They proposed that the "autregulation theory" that increased diffusive O_2 delivery, paradoxically decreased O_2 uptake by tissues because of vasoconstriction [7]. Yet, the researchers from Johns Hopkins University suggest that the ensuing pressor response could only be caused by high NO reactivity with Hb in the vascular lumen and/or the extravasation of the Hb molecules [105]. It has also been reported that L-arginine (a substrate for NO synthesis) and nitroglycerin (a NO donor) do not fully eliminate the vasoconstrictive effects associated with the injection of ferrous Hb [20]. Therefore, it is still unclear as to which extent the heme scavenging effect on the endothelial NO contributes to the vasoconstrictive episodes seen after the administration of Hb-based oxygen carriers.

Intracellular Ionized Calcium

In the current literature, there is some indication that Hb causes an increase in $[Ca^{2+}]_i$ in cultured endothelial and vascular smooth muscle cells [18,106]. Scientists at Texas Tech University have also investigated this possibility [21]. The results of these studies suggest that the increase in endothelial $[Ca^{2+}]_i$ may be triggered by Hb-mediated generation of oxygen free radicals. It has been demonstrated that oxygen free radicals and lipid radicals are potent activators of phospholipase C, thus generating inositol 1,4,5-triphosphate and 1,2-diacylglycerol, which cause an increase in $[Ca^{2+}]_i$, and an activation of protein kinase C (PKC), respectively [107,108]. It is also likely that $[Ca^{2+}]_i$ accumulation in the endothelial cells arises from the inhibition of $[Ca^{2+}]_i$ extrusion. This is possible, because Hb in high concentrations alters the activity of the Na^+/K^+ ATPase and Ca^{2+}-ATPase [18,109].

The consequences of higher endothelial $[Ca^{2+}]_i$ accumulation are broad, starting from Ca^{2+} dependent actin/myosin based contraction of the capillary endothelium with subsequent interendothelial gap formation, to the activation of Ca^{2+} dependent protease and protein kinase C (PKC), which are known mediators of many endothelial and vascular smooth muscle cellular responses [110,111]. The novel research conducted at Texas Tech University revealed that unmodified Hb is able to initiate shrinkage and increase of the interendothelial gap junction formation in the human brain capillary endothelial cells [112].

Protein Kinases

Although it is universally accepted that smooth muscle contraction involves Ca^{2+}-dependent phosphorylation of MLCK, additional mechanisms are also believed to be involved in the Hb-induced vasoconstriction. In 1998, a group of scientists from the University of Alberta presented a novel mechanism of Hb-mediated vasoconstriction [113]. They suggested that Hb could have a direct vasoconstrictive effect on cerebrovascular smooth muscle cells. In this study, ferrous-Hb produced a contraction of basilar artery preparation, which was reversed by an inhibitor of tyrosine kinase and an inhibitor of mitogen-activated protein kinase (MAP kinase). These investigators have also shown that Hb can induce PKC and Rho/Rho kinase, that are known to be the contributory factors in the non-endothelium-mediated vessel contraction [114,115]. In vascular smooth muscle PKC plays a role in the regulation of myogenic tone by the sensitization of myofilaments to Ca^{2+} [111,116]. PKC is known to phosphorylate voltage-dependent Ca^{2+} channels and inhibit K^+ channels, which both lead to vasoconstriction [116]. Activated PKC interacts with other signaling pathways such as MLCK, NO, intracellular Ca^{2+}, protein tyrosine kinase, and its substrates such as MAP kinases, ERK1 and ERK2 [116]. PKC activity also contributes to the endothelial hyper-permeability [117]. These results show, for the first time that Hb-mediated signaling utilizes the protein kinase-based mechanism in sustained smooth muscle contraction.

Nonetheless, the investigators from Brown University still believe that the only mechanism for Hb mediated vascular contraction is ferrous heme-iron scavenging of endothelium derived basal NO [19,118]. In a recent study, however, they reported that while pretreatment of isolated rat aorta with a calmodulin agonist and protein kinase inhibitors had no effect on Hb mediated contraction, pretreatment with a intercellular gap junction inhibitor prevented these unwanted events [118]. Based on this study, they concluded that the agonist-induced contraction appears to upregulate endothelial NO release that is mediated by Ca^{2+}-calmodulin independent mechanism.

Endothelin

In addition, several different factors could mediate the vasoconstrictive effects associated with Hb injection. In the early 1990s, it was postulated that Hb might enhance the synthesis or activity of endothelin-1 (ET-1). In fact, it has been reported that ferrous-Hb and ferric-Hb caused a significant increase in the production of ET-1 from the endothelial cells in culture [119,120]. ET-1, identified as a product of vascular EC, is a potent vasoconstrictor as well as exhibitor of vascular smooth muscle cell proliferative action [121]. It potently constricts various blood vessels via a Ca^{2+} dependent mechanism [122,123]. Elevated levels of this peptide have been reported in patients with severe hypertension [124]. Therefore, it has been suggested that ET-1 may play a role in vasoconstrictive events after Hb administration. ET is formed by the conversion of big-ET to ET-1 by the endothelin-converting enzyme (ECE). The action of ET-1 is modulated by NO and thrombin [125]. NO released during stimulation with thrombin inhibits the production of ET-1 via a cGMP-dependent pathway in aortic endothelial cells [125]. The in vivo study with diaspirin-cross-linked Hb produced evidence that the vasoconstrictive effect is only in part mediated by ET-1, because the pretreatment with phosphoramidon, an inhibitor of proendothelin to ET, does not fully eliminate Hb-mediated vasoconstriction [20]. Based on these preliminary studies, the investigators from the University of Illinois exclusively focused their research on the role of ET-1 in the pressor response of Hb solutions. They concluded that ET-1 is the factor responsible for the cardiovascular effects of Hb solutions [126,127]. Infusion of diaspirin cross-linked Hb in patients with acute ischemic stroke was associated with a dose-dependent increase in the plasma ET-1 concentration [128].

Doubt regarding the direct role of Hb in ET-1 production arose in 1992, after it was suggested that Hb might interfere with the detection of ET-1 [129]. In that study, free Hb significantly increased measurable plasma "endothelin like immunoreactivity," possibly because of a cross-reaction of the polyclonal anti-ET-1 antibody with the heme portion of Hb. Moreover, the Hb cross-reacted almost to an equal extent as the heme portion of cytochrome C, at comparable molar concentrations. The authors emphasized that to avoid such an interaction; liquid chromatography purification of the hemolytic samples must be performed. Using this precaution, the investigators at Texas Tech University were able to measure the actual Hb contribution to ET-1 production by human umbilical vein endothelial cells [130]. The results of this study did not support the role of Hb in ET-1 production. To the contrary, while ferrous- and ferric-Hb did not significantly alter ET-1 synthesis, ferryl-Hb greatly reduced ET-1 production. Based on these findings, it can be suggested that the degree of attenuation of ET-1 production by endothelial cells depends on Hb's prooxidant potential. Because ECE is a membrane bound metalloprotase, Hb induced oxidative damage to the endothelium might deactivate the enzyme required for the conversion of big ET to the biologically active mature ET-1. The scientists at Brown University reached a similar conclusion [131]. They provided evidence that the ET-1 pathway is not involved in the Hb mediated vasoconstriction.

It seems that Hb is not directly involved in the endothelial production of ET-1. Since NO suppresses ET-1 synthesis [125], it is conceivable that the scavenging of NO by Hb produces the metabolic disturbances that raise cytostolic ionized Ca^{2+} and, consequently, induce ET gene activation [123]. In fact, Hb was found to increase ET-1 production in endothelial cells by binding nitric oxide [132]. The reported diaspirin-crosslinked Hb that greatly increased the production of ET-1 has also the greatest NO scavenging potential [20,126–128]. Therefore, we cannot rule out the possibility that ferrous-Hb inhibitory activity toward the endothelial NO may enhance the production of ET-1.

Eicosanoids

Another possibility exists that Hb catalyzes the formation of other vasoconstrictive agents derived from the phospholipids in the plasma membranes. Earlier suggestions that thromboxane A_2 plays a minor role in the observed hemodynamic changes have not been substantiated in recent studies [13,133]. Although Hb was found to be an activator of cyclo-oxygenase (COX) [134] and phospholipase A_2 [135], it was also reported that an injection of Hb solution did not increase the concentration of thromboxane A_2 in plasma [136].

Isoprostanes

In the late 1980s, the investigators at Texas Tech University demonstrated that improperly purified Hb solutions might contain the vasoconstrictive factors derived from erythrocytes [13,137,138]. Early Hb solutions, contaminated with aminophospholipids, have demonstrated strong vasoconstrictive effects and have toxic effects on human endothelial cells. At that time, they speculated that amino-phospholipids themselves are vasoactive and toxic; however, their more current research provides a different answer. They found that the human coronary and human brain capillary endothelial cells incubated with tetrameric, Hb significantly increase the production of a newly described prostaglandin like compound 8-iso prostaglandin $F_{2\alpha}$ [21,112,139]. 8-iso $PGF_{2\alpha}$ is an F_2-isoprostane formed via a non-cyclooxygenase pathway under the condition of oxidative stress through free radical action on arachidonic acid on endothelial membrane [140]. 8-iso $PGF_{2\alpha}$ is a potent vasoconstrictor, particularly in pulmonary and renal arteries, acting via the thromboxane receptor [141,142]. Activation of the thromboxane receptor by 8-iso $PGF_{2\alpha}$ increases MLC kinase phosphorylation, and activates MAP kinase, while promoting the contraction of vascular smooth muscle [143]. In addition, the sub-threshold concentrations of 8-iso $PGF_{2\alpha}$ enhanced vasoconstriction by angiotensin II [144]. More recently, it was found that NO conceivably contributed to the action of 8-iso $PGF_{2\alpha}$, suggesting that a lack of NO may accelerate its vasoconstrictor activity [145]. Texas Tech University studies have shown that Hb may play a dual role in the contractile action of 8-iso $PGF_{2\alpha}$. In this study, Hb was involved in the effective removal of endothelial NO and in the production of endothelial 8-iso $PGF_{2\alpha}$ [21]. Based on this observation, the Texas Tech University investigators formulated a hypothesis that 8-iso $PGF_{2\alpha}$ could be the missing factor in the yet not fully understood Hb-mediated vasoconstriction.

Peroxynitrite

Other hypotheses imply that oxygen free radicals, perhaps produced during Hb autoxidation, can inactivate NO, and thereby promote vasoconstriction [146]. It was reported that superoxide anion can react with NO to form a toxic peroxynitrite (ONO_2^-), and it also has been shown that oxygen free radical scavengers may reduce to a certain extent, the hypertension associated with oxidative stress [146].

Summary of Hemoglobin Mediated Vasoconstriction

Despite the large number of scientific papers published, our understanding of how Hb mediates vasoconstriction is not well defined. Many hypotheses remain controversial. Nonetheless, the observed increase in blood pressure after injection of the first generation Hb-based blood substitutes is most likely caused by an increase in peripheral vascular resistance resulting from vasoconstriction [3–7]. The investigators from the University of California at Davis, reported that Oxyglobin (Biopure), a veterinary product approved by the FDA for treatment of anemia, used in hypovolemic dogs, failed to restore back to pre-hemorrhagic values the cardiac output, oxygen delivery index and systemic venous resistance [147,148].

Taken together, Hb is a pressor agent and the presently used chemical modification techniques did not correct this problem. It seems that all of the currently tested Hb-based oxygen carriers caused vascular constriction—a side effect that has been the main nemesis of blood substitute developers [1–7]. Since the full mechanism of Hb-mediated vasoconstriction is not well defined, a "single bullet" strategy for the correction of Hb's vasoactivity problems could be a highly ineffective proposition. For instance, scientists at Baxter developed a new recombinant Hb molecule with decreased affinity to NO [149]. Despite the lower hypertensive potential of this product seen in laboratory animals, some blood substitute experts are asking for more evidence that the observed reduction in blood pressure is a result of reduced vasoconstriction [7]. Several aspects of Hb-mediated vasoconstriction should be emphasized for future investigation.

At present the best strategy to counteract Hb's vasoconstrictive effects will be to: (1) make a NO resistant molecule by blocking the access of NO to heme (Hb with NO preservation shield or recombinant Hb), and (2) decrease Hb's pro-oxidative potential, particularly its ability to produce vasoconstrictive 8-isoprostane.

Endothelial Consequences of Hemoglobin Oxidation

The vascular endothelium is a major target of oxidant stress [150]. Particularly, oxidant stress augments vascular endothelial permeability and increases endothelial adhesion for leukocytes [150]. All processes are mediated by signaling mechanisms, through redox sensitive transcription factors, and can influence other basic functions of the endothelium including; vasomotor, inflammatory and immunologic responses [22,23,150].

For years, concern has been expressed about the suitability of Hb solutions as blood substitutes. This has been based on the fact that Hb might aggravate oxidant stress [151,152]. Despite the large number of scientific papers published to date on this subject, the fundamental question raised during the III International Symposium on Blood Substitutes *Hemoglobin: A lifesaver and an oxidant. How to tip the balance?* still awaits full elucidation [151].

Reactive Oxygen and Nitrogen Species

Despite the indirect involvement of Hb in the production of toxic oxygen intermediates through a respiratory burst of inflammatory cells, Hb under physiological conditions is a direct source of free radicals. The spontaneous autoxidation of extracellular Hb produces the superoxide anion ($O_2^{\cdot-}$) [153]. The dissociation of $O_2^{\cdot-}$ is accompanied by the removal of an electron from the heme iron; hence the iron is oxidized to the Fe^{3+} state. Protons increase the rate of dissociation of $O_2^{\cdot-}$ from the iron atom in a catabolic fashion, with protonation of the distal histidine. In addition, $O_2^{\cdot-}$ can serve as a catalyst to promote further Hb autoxidation [154]. In aqueous solutions, $O_2^{\cdot-}$ is extensively hydrated, much less reactive, and undergoes a dismutation reaction in the presence of superoxide dismutase (SOD) enzymes [155]. Despite the moderate chemical reactivity of $O_2^{\cdot-}$, the aqueous $O_2^{\cdot-}$ generating system has been observed doing a considerable degree of biological damage [155].

It was proposed that activated phagocytic and endothelial cells, by simultaneous production of NO and $O_2^{\cdot-}$, may form ONO_2^- [156]. Under physiological conditions, peroxynitrite may diffuse away from its site of formation before reacting with target molecules, such as membrane lipids and protein sulfhydryl groups [157]. It has also been shown that NO inactivation may cause vasoconstriction [146,158]. The ONO_2^- anion has a pKa of 6.8, so that 20% of these anions will be protonated at the physiological pH. When protonated, ONO_2^- gives rise to hydroxyl ($^{\cdot}OH$) and nitrogen dioxide ($NO_2^{\cdot-}$) radicals, which are capable of inducing tissue damage. Thus, ONO_2^- is a powerful oxidant that can be involved in many pathological processes, including oxidative damage of the endothelial cells [159]. It was reported that the presence of Hb in close proximity to the ONO_2^- production site in vasculature could contribute to possible in vivo toxicity by a mechanism involving direct oxidation of heme iron and nitration of Hb's tyrosine residues, leading to the instability of heme [160].

The endothelial cell damage accompanying Hb autoxidation arises from a complex chemistry that can also involve other toxic oxygen/Hb intermediates. Pure H_2O_2 has limited reactivity, but can freely cross biological membranes. The charged $O_2^{\cdot-}$ species crosses the membrane at a much slower rate, unless there is an anion channel, such as that in the endothelial cells [161]. The toxicity of H_2O_2 to the cells is evident. The vascular endothelial cells posses a high affinity and specific protoglycan receptor for xanthine oxidase (XO) [161]. Released circulating XO can bind to endothelial cells and serve as a temporary locus of enhanced tissue $O_2^{\cdot-}$ and H_2O_2 production. Similarly, it has been reported that exposure of EC to H_2O_2 causes a dose and time dependent loss of viability [162], and stimulates a rearrangement of membrane components which may alter membrane function [163]. H_2O_2 was found to stimulate endocytosis in cultured aortic endothelial cells [164]. In this study, H_2O_2

added extracellularly stimulated the uptake of macromolecules by the endothelial cells. Moreover, it has been found that intracellular XO is activated during oxidant injury of the endothelial cells, which may result in the generation of more $O_2^{\bar{\cdot}}$, and may function in the conversion of extracellular Hb to toxic intermediates [154,165].

Previous observations suggest that under the same oxygen free radical condition (i.e., H_2O_2), the presence of Hb or peroxidase will amplify the endothelial cell oxidative damage, or alternatively, the damage will occur at much lower levels of H_2O_2. In normal physiological situations, the H_2O_2 generated within the cells can decompose to H_2O by the enzymatic activities of catalase (CAT) and glutathione peroxidase (GSHPx) [166]. In the presence of transition metals (i.e., Fe^{3+}), $O_2^{\bar{\cdot}}$ reduces Fe^{3+} to Fe^{2+} by the iron-catalyzed Haber-Weiss reaction. The reduced ferrous iron reacts with H_2O_2 via a Fenton reaction to generate the highly reactive hydroxyl radicals ($^{\cdot}OH$). Iron, the breakdown product of extracellular Hb, is the most likely candidate for stimulating radical reactions in vivo [167,168]. To date however, many statements have been made claiming that the Fenton reaction is not the main source of Hb-mediated oxidative damage because its reaction rate constant is too low to have biological significance, and that ferryl and not $^{\cdot}OH$ is the reactive species formed [15,16,95,169–172]. In fact, the Hb-induced oxidative damage was not entirely prevented by $^{\cdot}OH$ scavengers, such as mannitol and thiourea [173]. Therefore, it was suggested that the reaction of Hb with peroxides may form a ferryl species, particularly a ferryl heme iron ($Fe^{+4}{=}O$) [15,95,96,168–171,174].

Ferryl Radicals

In the early 1990s, the ferryl Hb become a central focus in the investigation of Hb-mediated oxidative reactions. While the scientists at the FDA explored the reactions of Hb and its cross-linking derivatives with H_2O_2 [95,96,171,174], Texas Tech University investigators provided the evidence that ferryl-Hb is responsible for endothelial cellular injury [15,130]. In the Texas Tech study, ferryl Hb produced the most toxic effect to the human umbilical vein endothelial cells [15]. The authors suggest that Fenton and Haber-Weiss reactions can no longer be used to explain the mechanism of the endothelial oxidative stress introduced by Hb, and more scientific attention must be focused on the role of ferryl-Hb [15]. Soon after, the researchers from the FDA reported that in fact ferryl-Hb is cytotoxic to the endothelial cells, thus verifying the previous observation [175]. Moreover, they found that Hb forms a ferryl intermediate in the absence of any exogenuosly added oxidant, and contributes to the oxidative burden experienced by endothelial cells after hypoxia-reoxygenation [176]. The subsequent research conducted at the FDA resulted in establishing the differences in susceptibility of the modified Hb solutions to oxidative modification and in their ability to form toxic ferryl species [46,95,96]. This research provides the compelling evidence that alpha-alpha cross-linking induces an increased tendency to form ferryl-Hb in the presence of H_2O_2 and stabilizes the radical once formed [171,174]. According to another FDA study, the glutaraldehyde modification procedure also alters Hb autoxidation kinetics and redox properties, which may cause greater toxicity when, used as an oxygen transport fluid [47]. A similar study conducted at Texas Tech University, revealed that the glutaraldehyde modification procedure increased the Hb autoxidation rate, accelerated the reactivity with H_2O_2 and ferryl species formation, and produced severe lipid peroxidation of the human coronary artery endothelial cells [177].

It is well recognized that the reaction between Hb and H_2O_2 generates a series of steps that involve cycling between ferric- and ferryl-forms [178], and it is now believed that the conversion of the ferryl- to ferric-form is one of the most important steps in diminishing Hb pseudoperoxidase-like activity [179]. However, it was also observed that this chemical conversion could be mediated by the residual H_2O_2 present in the reaction volume. In fact, after chromatographic removal of residual H_2O_2 from the reaction mixture, the ferryl-Hb showed to be a long living species, not converting to the ferric-form [175]. In contrast, continuous access to H_2O_2 completely converted ferryl-Hb into the ferric-form [174,175]. This creates the situation in which the massive infusion of Hb-based oxygen carriers can be associated with the formation of long living toxic ferryl species. The concentration of H_2O_2 in normal human plasma is between 4 and 5 μM [180], whereas activated phagocytic cells can generate 100–600 μM [181]. Therefore, the injection of Hb-based oxygen carriers in a concentration of, for instance, 1,000 μM (6.4 g%) can be associated with the continuous presence of ferryl species in the vasculature. It was demonstrated that even low concentrations of H_2O_2 are extremely effective in the production of this toxic Hb species [182].

Ferryl-Hb can withdraw electrons from unsaturated fatty acids that, in the presence of oxygen, can catalyze a chain reaction leading to extensive lipid peroxidation of the plasma membranes [169,170]. Moreover, the alkoxyl radicals ($LO^{\bullet}$) and peroxyl radicals ($LOO^{\bullet}$) formed during the interaction between Hb and lipid hydroperoxides (LOOH), by inducing chain oxidation, may be additional contributors to endothelial damage [183].

Globin Radicals

In recent years, more evidence has been presented that besides ferryl heme ($Fe^{4+}{=}O$), other toxic products of the reaction of Hb with peroxides can be formed. This reaction, which can occur in vivo, is known to produce a globin tyrosyl radical ($gl(tyr^{\bullet})Fe^{4+}$) [184]. The ferryl heme has showed to be extremely reactive with membrane lipoproteins, unsaturated fatty acids, carbohydrates, and proteins that largely contribute to postischemic reperfusion tissue injury [169,185]. A gl(tyr$^{\cdot}$)Fe^{4+} was found to be a potent oxidizer and cross-linker of human low density lipoproteins (LDL) [182]. The clinical implication of this late discovery is that extracellular Hb may induce oxidation and structural modification of LDL's, thus activating endothelial cells and accelerating atherogenic event [186]. The current Texas Tech University study revealed that unmodified bovine Hb, when reacted with a 2.5-fold excess of H_2O_2, can easily be converted into both a ferryl-iron and globin radicals [28,187]. In this study, the formation of gl(tyr$^{\cdot}$)Fe^{4+}, was detected indirectly by monitoring the degree of apolipoprotein B (a protein part of the LDL) cross-linking. These results are in full agreement with the study done by other investigators [182,184]. The observed structural and oxidative modification of LDLs by ferryl heme and gl(tyr$^{\cdot}$)Fe^{4+} will inevitably influence their natural catabolism. It has also been suggested that modification of LDL in the presence of endothelial cells and smooth muscle cells is associated with the production of superoxide by Hb [188]. The incubation of LDL with Hb under hypoxic conditions produces the increased Relative Electrophoretic Mobility (REM) associated with LDL oxidation [188]. Oxidatively modified LDL looses its ability to be recognized by the apo B receptor and becomes recognized by a macrophage scavenger receptor leading to foam cell formation [189]. The high reactivity of Hb toward LDLs suggests its potential as an atherogenic factor [182]. A recent study has demonstrated that oxidized LDL can modulate many endothelial responses [186].

Apoptosis

Additionally, oxidized LDL increases apoptosis in vitro in a dose-dependent fashion [190]. In the cardiovascular system, apoptosis has been recently found associated with ischemic cardiomyopathies, myocardial cell death after infarction, coronary artery disease and other conduction system disorders. Apoptosis is a highly controlled mechanism of cell death in which cells undergo shrinkage, dissolution of membranes, and chromatin condensation, followed by proteolysis of cellular contents, and finally, obliteration. The pathways of apoptosis signaling converge on the activation of effector enzymes known as caspases [191]. In 1998, FDA scientists suggested that the reaction of modified Hbs (alpha-alpha cross-linked Hb and its polymerized form), but not HbA0, with H_2O_2 induced endothelial apoptosis [175]. In this study, the endothelial apoptotic death was associated with the formation of ferryl-Hb. Soon after, the investigators from the University of Mississippi provided compelling evidence that unmodified oxy-Hb, one of the most important spasmogens in the cerebral vasospasm, also induces apoptosis in cultured endothelial cells [192]. Another study showed that the ferric-ferryl redox cycling of Hb was responsible for endothelial G2/M arrest and apoptosis

[193]. Subsequent research from the University of Mississippi described, for the first time, the mechanism of Hb-induced endothelial apoptotic event [194]. The results of this study suggest that the caspase cascade, particularly caspase-8 and -9, participate in the oxy-Hb induced apoptosis that can be attenuated with a caspase inhibitor [195]. The investigators at Texas Tech University found that unmodified oxy-Hb has pro-apoptotic potential toward brain capillary endothelial cells and that this effect is controlled by intracellular GSH [112]. Other studies imply that while endothelial cells may undergo apoptosis after exposure to bilirubin [196], the carbon monoxide generated by HO-1 suppresses such events via the activation of p38 MAP kinase [197]. It is difficult to accept that the main products of the enzymatic degradation of heme, bilirubin and CO, have such an opposite effect on endothelial cells. The role of apoptosis however, in Hb-mediated toxicity in vivo, remains to be proven.

Oxidized Lipids and Free Fatty Acids

The Hb induced peroxidation of lipid membranes may also lead to the oxidation of arachidonic acid and production of 8-isoprostanes, which have been recently implicated in Hb-mediated vasoconstriction. The scientists at Texas Tech University, demonstrated that the endothelium (coronary artery and brain capillary) incubated with ferrous-Hb significantly increased the production of 8-iso $PGF_{2\alpha}$, which is formed via the non-cyclooxygenase pathway under the condition of oxidative stress [21,112,139]. Earlier studies linked cerebral vasospasm with severe lipid peroxidation [199]. In this study, prolonged arterial contraction mediated by Hb, peroxides of linoleic acid and arachidonic acid, and hydrogen peroxide, was associated with a remarkable destruction of the endothelial cells. Therefore, it is highly probable that 8-iso $PGF_{2\alpha}$ could be one of the mediators of the vasoconstrictive events mediated by Hb. The oxidized lipids, particularly the oxidation products of arachidonic acid are now considered to be the main players in the dysregulation of vascular tone and induction of endothelial dysfunction [135,150,199].

Heme Oxygenase Byproducts

Besides oxidized lipids, another dysregulator of vascular tone that can be formed during severe endothelial oxidative stress originated by the HO pathway. It is well known that HO and ferritin are important components of the defense mechanism recruited by vasculature under injurious, oxidative Hb-mediated stress [16,29,32,33,35,52–57]. In fact, HO is the only known enzymatic means for the catabolism of a heme moiety of hemoproteins, including Hb and various P-450 type cytochromes. In oxidant conditions, induced HO degrades the heme molecule, a most effective prooxidant to biliverdin and subsequently to bilirubin, which is potent antioxidant [33]. The HO protective mechanism also includes inhibition of nitric oxide synthase

(NOS) with a consequent reduction of NO production [33]. Potentially, preventing the formation of toxic ONO_2^-, which is formed from the reaction of NO and $O_2^{\cdot-}$ [157–160]. It is possible that during injurious oxidative stress, the inhibitory effect of Hb on NO, could be compensated by the release of CO, a by-product of the enzymatic decomposition of heme [32,33]. Supposedly, CO could take the control of vascular tone, by activating sGC, increasing cGMP and promoting relaxation [200]. Therefore, it is conceivable, that the never explained disappearance of Hb-mediated in vivo vasoconstriction (time depends on the product), may be connected with endothelial oxidative stress, expression of the HO system, decomposition of heme with subsequent production of the vasodilatory molecule—CO [201]. However, such a molecular protective response, can be considered as a result of a serious oxidative injury to the vasculature. The balance between vasoconstrictive and vasodilatory agents produced by the endothelial cells during Hb-mediated oxidative stress, remains to be determined.

The mentioned expression of HO isoenzymes and ferritin is a transcriptionally regulated process. The nuclear extracts from heme-treated cells exhibit induction of the HO-1 gene [202]. This is clear evidence that Hb-mediated endothelial oxidative stress modulates the cellular trancriptional response.

Glutathione and Redox Balance

Besides HO isoenzymes and ferritin, glutathione is the major cellular protector against heme-mediated endothelial injury. GSH plays the most important role in controlling the endothelial redox balance [203]. GSH is synthesized from its constituent amino acids by the action of gamma-glutamylcysteine synthetase and GSH synthetase. Glutathione exists in a reduced (GSH) and an oxidized (GSSG) form and participates in redox reactions through the reversible oxidation of its active thiol group [204]. The intracellular GSH redox homeostasis is strictly regulated to protect the cells against oxidative stress. GSH is a critical cytoplasmic scavenger of inorganic and organic peroxides serving as a substrate of many enzymes, including glutathione peroxidase (GSH-Px), controlling the intracellular production of reactive oxygen species [205]. Cellular glutathione has been demonstrated to participate in cellular division, membrane stabilization and protein folding [203]. More importantly, glutathione by participation in cell signaling and DNA transcription, is the main regulator of gene expression [206–209].

The first indication that Hb can deplete the intracellular GSH came from Texas Tech University in 1994/95 [210]. In this study, a massive (40% TBV) injection of Hb solution produced a serious depletion of GSH. The highest depletion of intracellular GSH was noted in the liver (by 39%) and heart tissues (by 25%), the organs most susceptible for lipid peroxidation. To that time, there was no published information regarding the effects of Hb administration on the intracellular GSH status. Soon after, Texas Tech University investigators described the same Hb effect in human endothelial cells [21,177]. In these studies, unmodified- and glutaraldehyde polymerized bovine Hb produced significant depletion of endothelial GSH, which they connected with the induction of transcription factors [177] and the propagation of endothelial inflammatory responses [17,21]. Other blood substitutes investigators much later showed interest in GSH research. Since 1999, however, FDA scientists become the leading forces in further exploration of the effects of Hb and its cross-linking derivatives on the endothelial GSH [211–213]. Their detailed studies on pro-oxidative effects of Hb solutions done in normal and GSH depleted endothelial cells helped to formulate the conclusion that the use of cell-free Hb as an oxygen therapeutic in patients who may lack the antioxidant protective mechanism may have serious medical consequences [211–213]. At the same time, Texas Tech University researchers have reported that Hb had a devastating effect on GSH depleted human brain capillary endothelial cells [42,112]. In this study, the depletion of endothelial GSH has accelerated the toxic effects of Hb by increasing lipid peroxidation, production of vasoconstrictive 8-isoprostanes and altering membrane permeability. These effects were associated with pro-apoptotic and pro-inflammatory event [112]. It is well established that alterations in the endothelial cells function has been linked with the increased generation of free radicals [150,203,214].

Early Antioxidant Strategies

Realizing that the pro-oxidative activity of Hb is a huge and yet unresolved problem, some investigators have implemented various strategies to overcome this unwanted effect of Hb. In 1990, Texas Tech University scientists demonstrated that while pro-oxidative and inflammatory responses of phagocytic cells can be effectively suppressed by the addition of SOD, catalase and mannitol [26], the lipid peroxidation of human erythrocytes can be eliminated by pretreatment with vitamin E and GSH [173]. Their subsequent research has shown that the addition of mannitol and vitamin E can markedly reduce the Hb pro-oxidative potential also in vivo [152]. Between 1994–1995, they discovered that the complete elimination of Hb induced lipid peroxidation in vivo can be achieved by pre-treatment of animals with selenium [210]. In this experimental study, selenite supplementation has shown to be an effective treatment of oxidative injury associated with the injection of Hb solutions. Selenium appeared to give full protection to all vital organs. The result of this study raised several issues of importance in the potential use of selenite and other selenium compounds as the perfect anti-oxidative agents used in vivo in conjunction with Hb-based oxygen carrier [210]. Eight years later, the researchers from the University of Arizona confirmed that selenium indeed could eliminate the oxidative reactions of Hb [78]. In their in vitro study, selenite reduced the oxidation rate of DBBF-Hb in the presence of oxidants and reduced DBBF-Hb-induced microvascular leakage in the rat mesentery. Other researchers investigated the effects of Trolox (an analog of vitamin E), deferoxamine (iron chelator), Hp, and other enzymatic and non-enzymatic antioxidants to attenuate the pro-oxidant effects of Hb [1,44].

While in scientific literature, nothing was published on the "antioxidant strategy" used in clinical trials of the first generation Hb-based oxygen carriers, it can be assumed that some of these products were spiked with the chemicals that posses antioxidative characteristics. The analysis of patent literature and chemical composition of the first generation Hb-based oxygen carriers revealed that Biopure's product contains a substrate for the biosynthesis of GSH, N-acetyl-L-cysteine (NAC), used as a stabilizer, but Northfield's PolyHeme contains GSH, that is added to the Hb solution during polymerization with glutaraldehyde [215,216]. At this moment, however, it is almost impossible to assess if and to what extent these agents added to the Hb solutions are able to suppress the Hb-mediated oxidative reactions. According to patent literature, other first generation products do not contain any antioxidants. Yet, the published in vivo and in vitro studies revealed that all of the first generation Hb-based oxygen carriers possesses the pro-oxidative potential which may limit their use in ischemic patients with a diminished ability to control the oxidative reactions [1–8,15,17,47,93,171,174–177,193, 211–213].

Participation of Hemoglobin in Endothelial Cell Signaling, Transcriptional and Translational Events

Gene Expression

Gene expression is a highly complex process involving cell signaling, transcriptional and translational events. In higher eukaryotes, the genome can contain up to about 70,000 genes. The regulation of gene expression involves a cascade of steps [217]. In general, to alter gene expression, an extracellular signal must trigger the cell by binding to a specific receptor expressed on the cell surface which creates an intracellular signal, including increases in second messengers, activation of kinases, activation or creation of transcription factors. The end result is the creation of a signaling molecule that accumulates within the nucleus. The transcription factors interact with very specific binding sites expressed in the structure of genes in the genomic DNA. If the transcription factors repress gene expression, transcription is prevented. If the transcription factors enhance gene expression, the transcriptional initiation complex (transcription factor plus RNA polymerase II) forms at the promoter region of the gene that allows transcription. The transcriptional initiation complex causes the coiled DNA to unwind and transcription to proceed. Upon reaching a termination code in the DNA sequence, the full-length pre-mRNA is released and the initiation complex separates. Pre-mRNA undergoes post-transcriptional processing which results in mature mRNA. The mature mRNA is then transported into the cytoplasm where it is translated to protein that in order to gain activity is subjected to the post-transcriptional process [217].

Redox Balance and Gene Expression

Endothelial cells, like all eukaryotic cells, have developed sophisticated mechanisms to regulate gene expression. One of the most powerful regulators of gene expression is based on redox balance [206–209,218–221]. Two steps in transcriptional activation can be regulated by redox balance: (1) the mechanism of activation of transcription factors, which induces/suppresses translocation into the nucleus, and (2) the binding of transcription factors to the promoter region of the gene and allowing transcription to occur [206–209,217–221].

Enzymatic and non-enzymatic antioxidants serve to balance the intracellular production of reactive oxygen species. The cellular redox state homeostasis depends upon the adaptive coordination of responses among redox-associated signaling pathways, genetic regulatory factors, and antioxidants. These processes either scavenge reactive oxygen species, or block their production. Besides reactive oxygen species detoxifying enzymes (SOD, catalase, GSH-Px), GSH plays the most important role in controlling the cellular redox balance. In endothelial cells, GSH is a critical cytoplasmic scavenger of inorganic and organic peroxides serving as a substrate (coenzyme) of many enzymes [21,177,203–213]. More importantly, GSH is the main regulator of the expression and activation of redox sensitive transcription factors [21,177,218–223]. Variations in the intracellular redox state mediated by oxidative stress can therefore transiently modify the activity of several transcription factors. Depending on the transcription factor and its own mechanism of activation, this modulation can be positive or negative and therefore can up-regulate or down-regulate gene expression [222–228].

Redox and Oxygen Regulated Transcription Factors

Research aimed at understanding the mechanisms by which oxidative stress modulates gene expression has focused on the known to date, redox and oxygen sensitive transcription factors: nuclear factor kappa B (NF-κB), hypoxia inducible factor 1α (HIF-1α) and activator protein-1 (AP-1). These are transcription factors that are activated through PKC, MAP kinase and other pathways and mediate endothelial cell gene responses to oxidant stress [150].

NF-κB is an inducible eukaryotic transcription factor which promotes the expression of over 150 target genes including: inflammatory cytokines, chemokines, immunoreceptors, cell adhesion molecules, acute phase proteins, stress response genes, cell surface receptors, regulators of apoptosis, growth factors and their regulators, early response genes, transcription factors and enzymes [229]. In endothelial cells, functional NF-κB sites are found in many genes whose expression is increased in response to inflammation, including adhesion molecules, interleukin (IL)-1, IL-6, IL-8, selectins, tissue factor, colony stimulating factors and others [23]. In resting endothelium, NF-κB exists in an inactive cytostolic form in which the Rel protein complex p50-p65 is bound to the inhibitory protein kappa B (IκB) [230]. Nuclear NF-κB activity is induced by many stimuli, including changes in intracellular redox balance [231]. This process is triggered by the phosphorylation of IκB by IκB kinase, which is activated by reactive oxygen species [232,233]. Phosphorylated IκB is subjected for ubiquitynation, and proteosome degradation, allowing the p50-p65 heterodimer to translocate into the nucleus where it binds κB sites (5′-GGGAN/NYYCC-3′) on the DNA [234]. It was also reported, that the regulation of p38-MAPK and p44/p42 MAPKs (ERK1/2)-mediated cytokine transcription and biosynthesis is redox/reactive oxygen species/NF-κB-dependent [235]. There is also an indication that reactive oxygen species mediated increases in intracellular Ca^{2+} concentration may activate calcium dependent proteases, which may be responsible for the degradation of IκB PEST sequence, and subsequent activation of NF-κB [236]. In contrast, oxidized free fatty acids and oxidized LDL can activate MAP kinase, which may promote NF-κB induction [237,238]. NF-κB can be stimulated by several stimuli relevant to endothelial stimulation, such as TNFα, IL-1, endotoxin, phorbol ester, UV, viral products, Hb, reactive oxygen and lipid species, and others [229,230]. These agents may initiate nuclear translocation with subsequent DNA binding of the active, nuclear form of NF-κB and gene induction. Next, mRNA makes its way from the nucleus to the cytoplasm to be translated into acute phase proteins.

While NF-κB is activated through IκB degradation by oxidative stress, its DNA binding is accelerated in the redox state. NF-κB is linked to the glutathione equilibrium. Shifting GSH/GSSG into the reduction equilibrium will stabilize NF-κB (prevent nuclear translocation). Shifting GSH/GSSG into an oxidative equilibrium will activate NF-κB. However, high GSSG concentrations will also promote the formation of a NF-κB disulfide complex, which inhibits DNA binding activity of this transcription factor [221,222,226]. Anti-oxidants have been shown to inhibit activation of NF-κB, however many of them, including NAC suppresses IκB degradation, but not DNA binding [207,232].

HIF-1 (hypoxia-inducible factor) transcriptionally regulates the expression of several dozens of target genes, including the genes involved in glycolysis, erythropoiesis (erythropoietin, EPO), angiogenesis (vascular endothelial growth factor, VEGF), and vascular remodeling (HO-1, NOS, ET-1) [239,240]. The HIF-1 transcription factor is a heterodimer composed of HIF-1α and HIF-1β. While the HIF-1β protein is readily found in all cells, HIF-1α is virtually undetectable in normal oxygen conditions [241]. Studies have shown that, under normoxic conditions, HIF-1α is hydroxylated (proline residue) and rapidly degraded by the ubiquitin-proteasome system. However, in normoxia HIF-1α can be stabilized by phosphorylation. A non-hypoxic, reactive oxygen species-sensitive pathway mediates cytokine-dependent (TNF-α, IL-1β) regulation of HIF-1α. Other factors known to stabilize HIF-1α under normoxic conditions include: transforming growth factor-β (TGF-β), NO, platelet derived growth factor (PDGF), and oxLDL [242,243]. The molecular pathway that governs HIF-1α-normoxic regulation is mediated by reactive oxygen species, PI_3K-, TOR and MAP kinases, particularly ERK1/2 [207,224,227,244].

Recently, in addition to NF-κB and HIF-1α, oxidant stress has been shown to modulate the activity of another transcription factor, activator protein-1 (AP-1). AP-1 is composed of a mixture of heterodimeric complexes of proteins derived from the Fos and Jun families, respectively c-Fos, FosB, Fra-1, Fra-2 and c-Jun, JunB and JunD. Jun-Jun and Jun-Fos dimers bind to the TPA-response element (TRE) with different affinities and subsequent transcriptional activities [245,246]. Changes in the composition of AP-1 complexes modulate transcriptional control of numerous genes governing cell proliferation, apoptosis and differentiation. Any changes in the ratio between GSH and GSSG activate AP-1 that lead to a transcriptional up-regulation of a number of genes [221,225,226].

Taken together, the oxidative conditions in the endothelial cytoplasm may activate NF-κB, HIF-1α and AP-1, while the reduced nuclear conditions favor the binding of these transcription factors to DNA, thus promoting gene expression. The mechanism of such toxicity is based, in large part, on reactive oxygen species which in turn could up-regulate NF-κB, HIF-1 and AP-1 target genes, involving IκB kinase, PKC, MAP kinases, and/or the SAPK/JNK1/2 signaling pathway. This oxidant stress-related signal transduction event may increase vascular cell permeability, promote leukocyte adhesion and inflammation, change vascular tone, and in extreme situations may cause cellular injury and death [150].

Hemoglobin and Nuclear Factor kappa B

In scientific literature there is limited information on signaling potency of the Hb molecule. Texas Tech University has initiated research in this area. In the late 1980s, the Texas Tech scientists established that Hb mediates the inflammatory response of human monocytes and mouse peritoneal macrophages, and that the addition of oxygen radical scavengers alleviates this inflammatory stimulus [26]. In this study, the degree of Hb autoxidation and the generation of reactive oxygen species correlated with the extent of inflammatory cellular responses. Subsequent work from the Texas Tech laboratory has shown that Hb can be classified as an active molecule, able to stimulate the human reticulo-endothelial cell system to express inflammatory cytokines [15,27,247]. These studies have linked Hb's pro-oxidative potential with the expression of inflammatory cytokines and the magnitude of cellular injury. Soon after, others confirmed this new observation. The scientists at the Letterman Army Institute of Research verified that indeed Hb is involved in the production of inflammatory cytokines [248,249]. The oxidative reactions of Hb were quickly established, yet the mechanism of Hb's pro-inflammatory action had not been provided.

It took a few years of extensive research to identify the molecular mechanism by which Hb mediates cellular inflammatory responses. In the 1990s, the Texas Tech researchers discovered that Hb is a potent inducer of the redox-regulated transcription factor NF-κB that is involved in the regulation of genes involved in inflammation [17,21,177]. They found that the activation of the endothelial NF-κB might be dependent on Hb's pro-oxidant potential and the extent of Hb mediated cellular oxidative stress that shifts GSH/GSSG into an oxidative equilibrium. In this study, however, the high GSSG did not prevent the expression of inflammatory cytokines (i.e., IL-1, TNF-α) and adhesion molecules (i.e., ICAM-1, VCAM-1). The glutaraldehyde polymerized bovine Hb, however, appeared to be a more potent inducer of NF-κB than unmodified Hb [17,177]. The authors linked this effect with the fact that glutaraldehyde polymerized Hb produced the highest endothelial lipid peroxidation and the largest depletion of intracellular GSH [177]. Based on these studies, the Texas Tech investigators suggested that the activation of NF-κB could be considered as a "bridge" between Hb-induced oxidative stress and Hb-mediated inflammatory responses [15,17,21,27,42,112,152,177,187]. Besides, this discovery established the foundation for seeing Hb as a signaling molecule [21,177,229,250]. Presently, a group of investigators from Universite Henri Poincare-Nancy, verified this finding by reporting that in fact Hb-based oxygen carriers induce expression of ICAM-1 that is consistent with the endothelial cell activation/cell signaling mechanism [251].

At this moment, the best explanation of the mechanism of Hb-mediated endothelial NF-κB induction is that this heme protein may shift the redox equilibrium into the oxidative state, allowing a build up of reactive oxygen species that are known to activate IκB kinase. The activated IκB kinase phosphorylates IκB inhibitory protein, allowing the NF-κB p50-/p65 heterodimer to translocate. It is also possible that Hb by increasing the endothelial intracellular calcium may activate calcium dependent proteases that are known to degrade IκB PEST sequence. Another possibility is that oxidized LDL and 8-isoprostanes via MAP kinases may promote NF-κB induction. It is also highly probable that Hb-generated peroxynitrite may destabilize IκB structure.

The expression of cytokines and adhesion molecules represents a key step in the propagation of inflammatory reaction [252]. Therefore, Hb in a higher concentration can be considered a potent stimulator of endothelial inflammatory responses.

Hemoglobin, Hypoxia Inducible Factor1α, and Erythropoietic Response

It has become apparent, that Hb by affecting the cellular redox-equilibrium and oxygen content may induce other redox- and oxygen-regulated transcription factors and their target genes. Soon, the scientists from the University of Alberta discovered that ferrous-Hb-mediated signaling utilizes a protein tyrosine kinase-based mechanism [113]. The investigators at the University of Virginia established that the signaling mechanism by which deoxy-Hb activates HIF-1α involves NO [253]. This research, which linked Hb with HIF-1 was of great importance, since HIF-1α is the transcription factor that regulates the genes that are in control of many basic function of the endothelium and the erythropoietic events.

Recently, the FDA investigators reported that Hb under hypoxic conditions increases the expression of HIF-1α [254]. Using a bovine aortic endothelial cell model and the Western Blot method for the detection of HIF-1α, they noted that the higher expression of HIF-1 is connected with the loss of ferrous- and accumulation of ferric-Hb, in both unmodified and chemically modified Hb solutions. This observation, perhaps, may provide more molecular details for an earlier suggestion, that prolonged exposure of endothelial cells to ferric-Hb, but not ferrous-Hb, renders these cells remarkably resistant to the secondary oxidant challenge via increased production of mRNA for HO-1 and ferritin, that are now known to be HIF-1α regulated [29,53,54].

In a novel study, using human coronary artery and brain capillary endothelial cells, the Texas Tech investigators were able to observe that under normoxia HIF-1α stability and DNA binding to the EOP gene was tightly regulated by oxidative and inflammatory events [255,256]. Hb solutions with high pro-oxidative potential accelerated NF-κB nuclear translocation and DNA binding, thus promoting inflammation. In normoxia, these Hb solutions were also found to decrease HIF-1 DNA binding to the erythropoietin (EPO) gene. These effects were more pronounced in GSH-depleted endothelium [255,256].

Because efficacious Hb-based oxygen carriers must be able to counteract the hypoxic/anoxic conditions associated with hemorrhagic shock, the FDA findings may only apply to those products that aggravate hypoxia, thus inducing HIF-1α. In fact, the first generation Hb-based oxygen carriers possessed well-documented vasoconstrictive potential [1–7]. It is not surprising that some of these products have been found to stimulate erythropoiesis [257,258]. Since HIF-1α governs the induction of the EPO gene, the erythropoietic response of these products could be mediated by hypoxic conditions. For instance, the glutaraldehyde polymerized bovine Hb solutions (Oxyglobin, Hemopure) with strong vasopressor effects [1,2,4,6,7,147,148,259], have been characterized as products that stimulate erythropoiesis [258,259]. Since the hypoxic environment induces (preserve) HIF-1α, it is possible that Hb-based oxygen carriers that promote vasoconstriction, shut down capillary flow and produce hypoxic/anoxic conditions might accelerate the expression of HIF-1α regulated genes, including EPO. It is also possible that Hb-based oxygen carriers, which in vivo alter the cellular redox state and have a strong hyperoxic effect, might trigger NF-κB and suppress HIF-1α [255,256].

The pioneering observation that Hb through redox-changes regulates the transcription factor NF-κB, and a newer finding on Hb-mediated stabilization/degradation of HIF-1α can be reflected in the current emergency statement from the scientists at University of Toronto [259]. They indicate that iron signals through the generation of reactive oxygen species activate NF-κB, whereas iron removal or disruption of its oxygen transport capability influences gene expression through HIF-1α. This statement perfectly illustrates the Hb-mediated endothelial transcriptional events.

Summary of the Endothelial Transcriptional and Translational Events

It seems that Hb is an extremely active molecule, with the ability of targeting of endothelial transcriptional and translational mechanisms. The oxidative stress mediated by Hb may injure endothelial cells and by changing the cellular redox-state, induce pathological responses on transcriptional level. Induction of NF-κB seems to be a process regulated by Hb's pro-oxidative potential, shifting the redox equilibrium into the oxidative state. Perhaps, the apoptotic reactions seen together with inflammatory events are related to the suppression of anti-apoptotic genes by oxidized lipids (oxLDL) or simultaneous induction AP-1. HIF-1α appears to be tightly linked with the availability of oxygen and endothelial redox potential. Hb solutions with a strong hyperoxic effect (high p50) will participate in the degradation of cytoplasmic HIF-1α. Increases in endothelial oxidative stress and inflammatory reactions (NF-κB activation) will significantly decrease HIF-1α binding to the promoter region of the EPO gene, therefore, decreasing Hb's erythropoietic effects. On the other hand, Hb that promotes vasoconstriction and shuts down capillary flow especially in the kidney and liver may stabilize HIF-1α, producing erythropoiesis and inducing other genes that are regulated by this transcription factor. This effect, however, can be considered pathological. The observed differences in molecular responses of the first generation Hb-based oxygen carriers could be linked to their physiological and physico-chemical characteristics, and to the presence/absence of active compounds affecting such responses (i.e., NAC, GSH).

Perhaps, the key strategy to control these transcriptional events is in the type of Hb chemical modification procedure that addresses Hb's intrinsic toxicity, particularly pro-oxidative and vasoconstrictive reactions.

New Generation of Hemoglobin-Based Oxygen Carriers: Is the "Endothelial Problem" Resolved?

The careful and detailed analysis of the scientific status of current activities in the blood substitute field, leads to the conclusion that the field is saturated with outdated ideas. For instance, the most frequently used Hb chemical modifications reagent, glutaraldehyde, was introduced more than 25 years ago. The first generation Hb-based oxygen carriers trigger a complex array of pathophysiological reactions such as; interaction with cell surface, cellular activation, cell signaling, transcriptional and catalytic activities, generation of free oxygen-, lipid-, heme- and globin-radicals, NO binding, and etc. Moreover, many observed pathophysiological events following injection of these Hb solutions can be mediated indirectly by polypeptide (i.e., cytokines) and/or lipid (i.e., 8-isoprostane) mediators.

Since currently tested free Hb-based oxygen carriers were only designed as a "vehicle", with prolonged intravascular persistence, for transporting oxygen and carbon dioxide, without any other designed pharmacological activities, vasoconstriction will remain an unacceptable result of their transfusion. Another problem with these products is the aggravation of oxidative stress and amplification of systemic inflammatory reactions, often described as elevation of liver enzymes, pancreatitis, gastrointestinal effects, flu-like symptoms, and myocardial lesions. In the course of designing these products, no theoretical connection between the Hb molecule surface and its reactivity with the reticulo-endothelial system had been made. The concept of a modified Hb molecule with specific pharmacological activities that suppress its natural (intrinsic) toxic effect has not been developed.

Currently used chemicals for intra- and intermolecular modification can only alter the physicochemical properties of Hb molecules such as: (1) decrease oxygen affinity (bovine Hb has a naturally low oxygen affinity); (2) stabilize tetramer and/or forms polymers without producing uniform pI; (3)

decrease or increase Hb's immunogenic effect; and (4) reduce or increase Hb's pro-oxidant potential. However, these chemical reagents combined with Hb molecules cannot produce the desired pharmacological effects (i.e., vasodilatory, anti-inflammatory, etc.). Besides toxicity, the currently used (in first-generation products) Hb chemical modification agents do not represent (by itself) any distinctive medicinal property [1].

Thus, there is emerging needs for an improved substitute of human blood that is safe, effective and lacks toxicity. Some research laboratories are already engaged in the development of new generations of free Hb-based oxygen carriers. The developers of these new products are hoping to eliminate the intrinsic toxic effect of Hb. Some of these new products are in preclinical or early clinical stages of development. Each of the products used different approaches to eliminate unwanted intrinsic toxic effects of Hb.

To date, the most clinically advanced new generation product is MP4, a non-vasoactive polyethylene glycol (PEG)-Hb conjugate (Sangart, San Diego, CA, USA) [2,7]. MP4 is made by reaction of human Hb with a monofunctional maleimide-activated PEG [260–262]. The theoretical basis for the design of this blood substitute product is "autregulation theory". This theory suggests that increased diffusive oxygen delivery paradoxically decrease oxygen uptake by tissue because of vasoconstriction [7,263]. The Sangart investigators, believe that control of facilitation of the oxygen transport by lowering p50 (5–10 mmHg) and increasing viscosity and oncotic pressure will result in non-vasoactive Hb-based oxygen carrier. In fact this product shows to be non-vasoactive in animals and humans. Now, MP4 is entering the Phase II clinical trial in elective surgery patients [2]. At this moment, it is unknown if this new product can interact with the endothelial cells. It will be interesting to see if MP4, with extremely low p50, will deliver enough oxygen to the ischemic tissue and have no impact on the endothelial redox equilibrium.

Another new product under pre-clinical development is human albumin-synthetic heme adduct invented by the scientists at Keio University and Waseda University [264–269]. This ingenious idea was based on the fact that human albumin is the most abundant plasma protein which maintains the colloid osmotic pressure and transports many endogenous and exogenous compounds, including under certain pathological circumstances—heme. This totally synthetic oxygen carrying solution is the recombinant human serum albumin with incorporated synthetic heme. The pre-clinical research demonstrated that this product satisfies the initial clinical requirements for an oxygen-carrying resuscitative fluid and did not induce an acute increase in blood pressure. The Keio-Waseda Joint Project investigators believe that the lack of vasoconstriction is due to the low permeability of the albumin-heme adduct through the vascular endothelium [264–269]. Therefore, the Japanese scientists successfully addressed the "endothelial issue". Other toxicological tests are under way [265]. It will be interesting to see, if the synthetic heme-recombinant albumin adduct has a lower pro-oxidative potential than that of the natural albumin-heme complex, formed during intravascular hemolysis after saturation of hemopexin. In the next couple of years, this exciting product should enter the human testing and more information of its "endothelial" performance will be available [265].

Another promising free-Hb red cell substitute product is a glutaraldehyde polymerized bovine Hb with covalently attached catalase and SOD (polyHb-SOD-CAT), developed by the scientists at McGill University [270–275]. This product attempts to reduce ischemia-reperfusion injury by removing and detoxifying reactive oxygen species, while delivering oxygen. In animal and in vitro studies, the polyHb-SOD-CAT shows promise of being an effective blood substitute, especially in ischemic patients. In fact, polyHb-SOD-CAT has a potency to reduce formation of oxygen radicals caused by glutaraldehyde polymerized bovine Hb (polyHb) [271,272]. In the recent study, using a global cerebral ischemia-reperfusion model, the polyHb-SOD-CAT markedly attenuated the severity of the blood brain barrier disruption as compared to saline, unmodified Hb and polyHb solution [274]. It seems, that this product is "endothelial friendly", because polyHb-SOD-CAT destroyed free radicals which are the worse enemies of the endothelial cells. It will be interesting to see, to which extent the conjugation of Hb with SOD and CAT affects the Hb isoelectric point and if such changes are uniform. The vasopressor potency of this product has not yet been established. Now, this novel blood substitute product is in pre-clinical stage of development and soon should enter human testing [2,275].

Another free Hb-oxygen carrier under preclinical development is the polynitroxylated human Hb, HemoZyme (SynZyme Technologies, LLC, Irvine CA, USA). This product has been constructed by the synthesis of Hb with nitroxides that have antioxidant enzyme-mimetic activities [276]. This product inhibits peroxide and superoxide-mediated neutrophil adherence to human endothelial cells and exhibits the SOD- and catalase-activity [277,278]. In the recent in vivo study, HemoZyme showed to inhibit microcirculatory dysfunction and reduce cerebral infarction following transient cerebral artery occlusion [279,280]. Now this product is being tested as a "small volume" hemorrhagic trauma protectant [281]. In the previous in vivo study, this product was used in resuscitation of severe chest trauma [282]. According to the University of Tennessee investigators, the pressor action of polynitroxylated Hb was lower than unmodified Hb, but this chemical modification had no effect on mortality. The authors suggest that the pressor action of Hb-based oxygen carriers must be attenuated by strategies other than polynitroxylation, to be safe, effective resuscitant in humans' [283]. Therefore, it will be interesting to see if HemoZyme is completely free of the pressor effect and does not extravasate.

A novel second-generation recombinant hemoglobin solution (rHb2.0) developed by Baxter Healthcare (Boulder, CO, USA) is still in preclinical testing [2,149]. The substitution of selected amino acids into the heme pocket of α and β subunits reduced the rate of reaction with NO [284,285]. The preclinical experiments conducted with this product have demonstrated that the pulmonary and systemic hemodynamic responses can be reduced and the gastrointestinal effects and myocardial lesions can be lessened [149,286]. Time will tell if this recombinant product with a lower NO scavenging potency also has anti-oxidant and anti-inflammatory properties and is friendly to the endothelium. Since it is still unclear as to which extent the heme scavenging effect on the endothelial NO contributes to the Hb-induced vasoconstriction, some experts are asking for more evidence that the observed reduction in blood pressure with this product [287] is indeed a result of reduced vasoconstriction [7].

Scientists at Texas Tech University have developed a novel Hb modification procedure to formulate a non-toxic product. The theoretical basis for this development was in contradiction to the popular theory about blood substitutes, which led others to design ineffective, even toxic products. The Texas Tech investigators have learned that in order to diminish intrinsic toxic effects of Hb; the free Hb-based oxygen carriers should possess additional pharmacological properties [288,289]. They developed a novel concept of "pharmacological cross-linking". This pharmacological cross-linking has shown to be an effective strategy for eliminating the pathological responses of vascular endothelium to Hb solutions. It addresses problems such as vasoconstriction, oxidative stress, and inflammation that have stymied the development of the first generation Hb-based oxygen carriers.

The Texas Tech product (HemoTech), recently licensed to HemoBioTech. (Dallas, TX, USA), is composed of purified bovine Hb, cross-linked intramolecularly with *o*-adenosine triphosphate (*o*-ATP) and intermolecularly with *o*-adenosine, and combined with reduced glutathione (GSH) [290–296]. The idea behind the use of *o*-adenosine was to counteract the vasoconstrictive and pro-inflammatory properties of Hb with the activation of adenosine A_2 and A_3 receptors, which would produce vasodilatation and moderation of inflammatory reactions [13,15,17,21,26–28,42,130,137,177,247,255,256, 288–297]. The additional idea of conjugation of Hb with GSH was to introduce more electronegative charges onto the surface of the Hb molecule, which would block Hb's transglomerular and transendothelial passage, and would make it less visible to phagocytes [21,27,28,31,42,177]. At the same time, GSH would shield heme from the reactive oxygen species and NO, therefore lowering the Hb pro-oxidant and vasoconstrictive potential [15,17,21,28,42,

130,152,177,187,210,288–297]. The reaction with *o*-ATP would stabilize the Hb tetramer and prevent its dimerization, and the reactions with *o*-adenosine (an affinity directed β–β cross-linker) would allow the formation of Hb-oligomers and avoid the formation of toxic high molecular weight polymers [15,21,27,84,288–296].

HemoTech was subjected to preclinical and clinical testing. Preclinical testing included research done at Texas Tech University and the IND study conducted in Italy [15,17,21,27,28,31,42,130,177,187,210,247,255,256,288,289, 297,316–318]. The research based on in vivo animal study and in vitro testing, using various human cell lines, including coronary artery and brain capillary endothelial cells, was focused on the product's: toxicity, vasoactivity, immunological, oxidative and inflammatory reactions; and therapeutic potential. The results of these studies are favorable, indicating that HemoTech has vasodilatory activity and can reduce vasoconstriction that follows hemorrhage, has erythropoietic activity, and produces no adverse nephrotoxic, neurotoxic, oxidative and inflammatory reactions [15,17,21,27,28,31,42,130,177, 187,210,247,255,256,288,289,297,316–321]. The human clinical trial indicated no toxic or allergic reactions and beneficial effects in all patients tested [316–318,322].

With this product the endothelial pathological responses have been avoided. The alteration of surface charge of Hb polymers and tetramers to the same extent is one of the essential features of this novel Hb modification procedure [288–297,317,318]. The electrophoretic mobility study demonstrated that all Hb polymers and 5% of chemically modified tetramers found in the solution have a uniform electronegative surface charge with a pI of 6.1–6.2 [289–296,317]. This new electrostatic property of Hb molecules has blocked their transglomerular and transendothelial passage, thus attenuating endothelial pathological responses and nephrotoxic reactions [21,31,42, 297,316,317,321,322]. HemoTech was found to reduce the peripheral vascular resistance, an action mediated by adenosine A_2 receptor through cyclic AMP dependent mechanism [21,177,297]. Thus, it is assumable that HemoTech may produce vasodilation by a NO/cGMP independent mechanism. It is also possible that the endothelial NO has reacted with the molecules of GSH, which are chemically attached to the Hb surface, producing S-nitroso-GSH, thus preventing the oxidation of heme and preserving NO in its active form [99–102,314–315]. In fact, the current study revealed that HemoTech produces a lower conversion of NO into nitrite/nitrate than that of unmodified Hb [21].

HemoTech did not appear to aggravate endothelial oxidative stress, or to activate the endothelial inflammatory responses [15,17,21,130,177,187,255, 256,320]. Reduction of the natural pro-oxidative potential of Hb was achieved by selective targeting amino acids residues of Hb β chains with *o*-adenosine, and incorporation of GSH [288–296,317]. HemoTech when reacted with H_2O_2 did not oxidatively modify LDLs or cross-link apo B [28]. It seems that "steering effect" and acceleration of the preferential reaction at the β–β interface makes tyrosine unavailable for the reaction with H_2O_2, thus preventing the formation of heme globin radicals. This chemical/pharmacological modification procedure also significantly decreased the formation of heme ferryl iron [15,28,177,187]. HemoTech did not change the endothelial redox equilibrium nor did it activate apoptotic responses [21,42,177,187,255,256]. This product was found to eliminate, through the cyclic AMP/IκB kinase, the endothelial NF-κB-induction and blocked the endothelial production of cytokines and adhesion molecules [21,17,177]. Even in the GSH depleted cells; HemoTech did not activate endothelial inflammatory responses [42,255,256]. Another element that contributed to HemoTech anti-inflammatory action was low endothelial Ca^{2+} flux and low formation of 8-isoprostanes, well known activators of protein kinases that destabilize NF-κB [21]. It is also possible that HemoTech stimulates the adenosine A_3 receptor, responsible for endothelial cytoprotection. It was demonstrated that stimulation of this receptor activates the endothelial anti-oxidant enzyme system, thus stabilizing the redox state [305–307]. In the recent study, using GSH depleted human brain capillary and coronary artery endothelial cells, HemoTech prevented the NF-κB induction and facilitated HIF-1α stabilization and DNA binding to the EPO gene (through cyclic AMP-mediated pathway), under normoxia [255,256]. In fact, the clinical trial showed that HemoTech not only alleviates inflammatory reactions in sickle cell anemia patients, but also produces effective erythropoietic response [322].

Together, based on preclinical and clinical testing, it can be concluded that this novel pharmacological modification method has allowed the preparation of an non-toxic and "endothelium friendly" solution, which promises to be an effective, second generation, Hb-based human red cell substitute.

Concluding Remarks

Despite tremendous progress in the research on Hb cellular and molecular responses, the current understanding of Hb's overall intrinsic toxicity is still limited. In particular, there is a lack of understanding of some of the fundamental biological events that trigger the induction of genes upon Hb treatment. Also the complete mechanism of Hb-induced vasoconstriction has not yet been established, especially non-NO-mediated pathways. It is still unknown to what extent the rise in blood pressure, observed after transfusion of the first generation Hb-based oxygen carriers, affects the perfusion rate of the vital organs. Some reports are alarming that the first generation products tend to shut down capillary flow. Besides, the pro-oxidative potential of these products is not under control, and they tend to extravasate.

What we have learned is that Hb-based oxygen carriers can no longer only be considered as 'vehicles' for transporting oxygen and carbon dioxide, but they should possess pharmacological properties which can diminish intrinsic toxic effects of Hb and help eliminate the pathological reactions associated with hemorrhagic shock.

The effective Hb-based blood substitutes, besides physiological properties of Hb, should possess additional "pharmacological" characteristic that effectively eliminate blood vessel constriction, improve the release of oxygen, and produce anti-oxidant and anti-inflammatory effects. These products should also have altered surface charge to prevent extravasation and the interaction with the reticulo-endothelium.

Therefore, the future of blood substitutes is in second generation products. Soon many of them will enter clinical trials. A pharmacological cross-linking of the Hb molecule with adenosine and GSH, pegylation of the native Hb molecule, linkage of the Hb molecule with nitroxide moiety, conjugation with SOD and catalase, creation of the synthetic heme-albumin adduct, or decreasing NO-heme binding by recombinant technology; these are the key strategies to attenuate the Hb intrinsic toxicity problems. It is reasonable to suggest that any Hb chemical modification procedure, which may attenuate natural Hb toxicity toward endothelium, should be considered as an important milestone in the development of an effective free Hb-based blood substitute. It will be interesting to see, within the next couple of years, whether these new products are viable substitutes for human red blood cells.

While some blood substitute experts are enthusiastic about the clinical future of free Hb-based oxygen carriers, others are more skeptical. Prof. Chang (McGill University) believes that all Hb-based oxygen carriers in clinical trial and new products under development will eventually prove their clinical usefulness [323]. Dr. Klein (The Johns Hopkins School of Medicine), however, is convinced that the Hb-based oxygen carriers in current clinical trials are unlikely to replace transfusions or drugs that stimulate erythropoiesis for chronic anemia [324]. Yet, Dr. Reid (Walter Reed Army Institute of Research) is hopeful that with the recent submission of one application for product licensure after more than 30 years of effort, we are close, very close [2]. However, Dr. Fratantoni reminds, that the future of blood substitutes will depend on the course taken, not on the courses that might have been chosen [325]. Nonetheless, blood substitutes are no longer science fiction; they are a reality and a necessity [326–333].

The findings discussed herein introduce a new understanding of the toxicity of Hb and suggest that the development of a non-toxic free Hb-based oxygen carrier is possible. Nonetheless, the advantages of Hb-based oxygen carriers over transfused human red blood cells will become more evident as our knowledge increases.

Conflict of Interest Statement. Dr. Simoni, is an Associate Professor of Surgery (Research) at Texas Tech University Health Sciences Center, School of Medicine (Lubbock, TX, USA) and co-inventor of the Texas Tech blood substitute (HemoTech), which is now licensed to HemoBioTech, Inc.

Acknowledgments. The author is grateful to Professor Koichi Kobayashi, Professor Eishun Tsuchida, Dr. Hirohisa Horinouchi and other Organizing Committee Members for the invitation and opportunity to address the audience of this scientifically exciting, 13th Keio University International Symposium for Life Sciences and Medicine. The author is also thankful to the Administration Officials of the Texas Tech University Health Sciences Center for their support, and the Office of Technology Transfer and Intellectual Property and HemoBioTech, Inc. for their efforts in the commercial development of the Texas Tech blood substitute product.

References

1. Riess JG (2001) Oxygen carriers ("blood substitutes")—raison d'etre, chemistry, and some physiology. Chem Rev 101(9):2797–2919
2. Reid TJ (2003) Hb-based oxygen carriers: are we there yet? Transfusion 43:280–287
3. Workshop on Criteria for Safety and Efficacy Evaluation of Oxygen Therapeutics as Red Cell Substitutes. Held under the joint auspices of the Food and Drug Administration, National Institute of Health and the Department of Defense. September 27–28, 1999, Natcher Building, National Institute of Health, Bethesda, MD. http://www.fda.gov/cber/minutes/oxygen092799.doc
4. Winslow RM (1994) Vasoconstriction and the efficacy of hemoglobin-based blood substitutes. Transf Clin Biol 1(1):9–14
5. Hess JR, Macdonald VW, Gomez CS, et al (1994) Increased vascular resistance with hemoglobin based oxygen carriers. Artif Cells Blood Substit Immobil Biotechnol 22:361–372
6. Kasper S, Walter M, Grune F, et al (1996) Effects of hemoglobin-based oxygen carrier (HBOC-201) on hemodynamics and oxygen transport in patients undergoing preoperative hemodilution for elective abdominal aortic surgery. Cardiovasc Anesth 83:921–927
7. Winslow RM (2003) Current status of blood substitute research: towards a new paradigm. J Intern Med 253(5):508–517
8. Alayash AI (1999) Hemoglobin-based blood substitutes: oxygen carriers, pressor agents, or oxidants? Nature Biotech 17:545–549

9. Twenty four of fifty two die in tests of (Baxter's) blood substitute. Chicago Tribune, April 12, 1998
10. Staples S (2003) Canada watch. Canada establishes competition for research funds. Gen Eng News 23(13):70–73
11. Viele MK, Weisopf RB, Fisher D (1997) Recombinant human hemoglobin does not affect renal function in humans: analysis of safety and pharmacokinetics. Anesthesiology 86:848–858
12. Feuerstein A. Northfield's new trial likely to be "traumatic". The Street.com, February 6, 2003, http://biz.yahoo.com/tsp/030206/10067047_1.html
13. Feola M, Simoni J, Fishman D, et al (1989) Biocompatibility of hemoglobin solutions: I. Reactions of vascular endothelial cells to pure and unpure hemoglobins. Artif Organs 13:209–215
14. Hess JR (1996) Blood substitutes. Sem Hematol 33:369–378
15. Simoni J, Simoni G, Lox CD, et al (1994) Reaction of human endothelial cells to bovine hemoglobin and tumor necrosis factor. Artif Cells Blood Substit Immobil Biotechnol 22:777–787
16. Motterlini R, Foresti R, Vandegriff K, et al (1995) Oxidative stress response in vascular endothelial cells exposed to acellular hemoglobin solutions. Am J Physiol 269:H648–654
17. Simoni J, Simoni G, Lox CD, et al (1997) Expression of adhesion molecules and von Willebrand factor in human coronary artery endothelial cells incubated with differently modified hemoglobin solutions. Artif Cells Blood Substit Immobil Biotechnol 25:211–225
18. Toda N (1990) Mechanism of contracting action of oxyhemoglobin in isolated monkey and dog cerebral arteries. Am J Physiol 258:H57–63
19. Kim HW, Greenburg AG (1997) Ferrous hemoglobin scavenging of endothelium derived nitric oxide is a principal mechanism from hemoglobin mediated vasoactivities in isolated thoracic aorta. Artif Cells Blood Substit Immobil Biotechnol 25:121–133
20. Schultz SC, Grady B, Cole F, et al (1993) A role of endothelin and nitric oxide in the pressor response to diaspirin cross-linked hemoglobin. J Lab Clin Med 122:301–308
21. Simoni J, Simoni G, Martinez-Zaguilan R, et al (1998) An improved blood substitute. Evaluation of its effects on human endothelial cells. ASAIO J 44:M356–M367
22. Vane JR, Anggard EE, Botting RM (1990) Regulatory functions of the vascular endothelium. N Engl J Med 323:27–36
23. Mantovani A, Bussolino F, Dejana E (1992) Cytokine regulation of endothelial cell function. FASEB J 6:2591–2599
24. Moncada S, Palmer RMJ, Higgs EA (1991) Nitric oxide physiology, pathophysiology, and pharmacology. Pharmacol Rev 43:109–142
25. Bunn HF, Forget BG (1986) Hemoglobin: molecular, genetic and clinical aspects. W.B. Saunders, Philadelphia, PA
26. Simoni J, Feola M, Tran R, et al (1990) Biocompatibility of hemoglobin solutions: II The inflammatory reactions of human monocytes and mouse peritoneal macrophages. Artif Organs 14:98–109
27. Simoni J, Simoni G, Lox CD, et al (1994) Cytokines and PAF release from human monocytes and macrophages: effects of hemoglobin and contaminants. Artif Cells Blood Substit Immobil Biotechnol 22:525–534
28. Simoni J, Simoni G, Wesson DE, et al (2000) A novel hemoglobin-adenosine-glutathione based blood substitute: Evaluation of its effects on human blood ex vivo. ASAIO J 46:679–692

29. Balla J, Jacob HS, Balla G, et al (1993) Endothelial-cell heme uptake from heme proteins: induction of sensitization and desensitization to oxidant damage. Proc Nat Acad Sci 90:9285–9289
30. Pimstone NR (1972) Renal degradation of hemoglobin. Semin Hematol 9:31–42
31. Simoni J, Simoni G, Hartsell A, et al (1997) An improved blood substitute. In vivo evaluation of its renal effects. ASAIO J 43:M714–M725
32. Tenhunen R, Marver HS, Schmid R (1969) Microsomal heme oxygenase. Characterization of the enzyme. J Biol Chem 244:6388–6394
33. Kutty RK, Daniel RF, Ryan DE, et al (1988) Rat liver cytochrome P-450b, P-450b, and P-420c are degraded by to biliverdin by heme oxygenase. Arch Biochem Biophys 260:638–644
34. Miller YI, Smith A, Morgan WT, et al (1996) Role of hemopexin in protection of low-density lipoproteins against hemoglobin-induced oxidation. Biochemistry 35:13112–13117
35. Balla G, Jacob HS, Eaton JW, et al (1991) Hemin: a possible physiological mediator of low-density lipoprotein oxidation and endothelial injury. Arterioscler Thromb 11(6):1700–1711
36. Regalado MM, Simoni J, Wesson DE (1999) Chronic hemodialysis patients (CHP) have increased cell-free plasma hemoglobin. Am J Kidney Dis 33:A52
37. Ross R (1995) Cell biology and atherosclerosis. Annu Rev Physiol 57:791–804
38. Reeder BJ, Sharpe MA, Kay AD, et al (2002) Toxicity of myoglobin and haemoglobin: oxidative stress in patients with rhabdomyolysis and subarachinoid haemorrhage. Biochem Soc Trans 30(4):745–748
39. Saxena R, Wijnhoud AD, Carton H, et al (1999) Controller safety study of a hemoglobin-based oxygen carrier, DCLHb, in acute ischemic stroke. Stroke 30:993–996
40. Regan RF, Panter SS (1993) Neurotoxicity of hemoglobin in cortical cell culture. Neurosci Lett. 153(2):219–222
41. Wang X, Mori T, Sumii T, et al (2002) Hemoglobin-induced cytotoxicity in rat cerebral cortical neurons: caspase activation and oxidative stress. Stroke 33(7):1882–1888
42. Simoni J, Simoni G, Wesson DE, et al (2003) Combining hemoglobin with adenosine and reduced glutathione attenuates its direct and indirect neurotoxic potential. Artif Blood 11(1):96
43. Tam SC, Wong JT (1980) Modification of hemoglobin upon covalent coupling to dextran: enhanced stability against acid denaturation and reduced affinity for haptoglobin. Can J Biochem 58(9):732–736
44. Panter SS, Vandegriff KD, Yan PO, et al (1994) Assessment of hemoglobin-dependent neurotoxicity: alpha-alpha crosslinkied hemoglobin. Artif Cells Blood Substit Immobil Biotechnol 22(3):399–413
45. Iwashita Y (1992) Relationship between chemical properties and biological properties of pyridoxylated hemoglobin-polyoxyethylene. Biomat Artif Cells Immobil Biotechnol 20(2–4):299–307
46. Alayash AI, Patel RP, Cashon RE (2001) Redox reactions of hemoglobin and myoglobin: biological and toxicological implications. Antioxid Redox Signal 3(2):313–327
47. Summers AG, Wood F, Jia Y, et al (2001) Effects of glutaraldehyde polymerization on oxygen transport and cytotoxicity of bovine hemoglobin. Artif Cells Blood Substit Immobil Biotechnol 29(2):167
48. Faivore-Fiorina B, Caron A, Fassot C, et al (1999) Presence of hemoglobin inside aortic endothelial cells after cell-free hemoglobin administration in guinea pigs. Am J Physiol 276(2 Pt 2):H766–770

49. McLeod LL, Alayash AI (1999) Detection of a ferrylhemoglobin intermediate in an endothelial cell model after hypoxia-reoxygenation. Am J Physiol 277(1 Pt 2): H92–99
50. Custer G, Balcerzak S, Reinchart J (1982) Human macrophage hemoglobin-iron metabolism in vivo. Am J Hematol 13:23–36
51. Deiss A (1983) Iron metabolism in reticuloendothelial cells. Sem Hematol 20:81–90
52. Balla J, Jacob HS, Balla G, et al (1992) Endothelial cell heme oxygenase and ferritin induction by heme proteins: a possible mechanism limiting shock damage. Trans Assoc Am Physicians 105:1–6
53. Balla G, Jacob HS, Balla J, et al (1992) Ferritin: a cytoprotective antioxidant stratagem of endothelium. J Biol Chem 267(25):18148–18153
54. Balla J, Vercellotti GM, Nath K, et al (2003) Haem, haem oxygenase and ferritin in vascular endothelial injury. Nephrol Dial Transplant 18(Suppl. 5):V8–V12
55. Jeny V, Balla J, Yachie A, et al (2002) Pro-oxidant and cytotoxic effects of circulating heme. Hemost Thromb Vasc Biol 100(3):879–887
56. Eguchi D, Weiler D, Alam J, et al (2001) Protective effect of heme oxygenase-1 transfer against oxyhemoglobin-induced endothelial dysfunction. J Cereb Blood Flow Metab 21(10):1215–1222
57. Abraham NG, Lavrowsky Y, Schwartzman ML, et al (1995) Transfection of the human heme oxygenase gene into rabbit coronary microvessel endothelial cells: protective effect against heme and hemoglobin toxicity. Proc Natl Acad Sci USA 92(15): 6798–6802
58. Simionescu M, Simionescu N (1986) Function of the endothelial cell surface. Ann Rev Physiol 48:279–293
59. Hardebo JE, Kahrstrom J (1985) Endothelial negative surface charge areas and blood-brain barrier function. Acta Physiol Scand 125:495–499
60. Vehasakari VM, Chang CTC, Stevens JK, et al (1984) The effect of polycations on vascular permeability in the rat. J Clin Invest 73:1053–1061
61. Nagy Z, Petres H, Huttner I (1983) Charge-related alternations of the cerebral endothelium. Lab Invest 49:662–671
62. Bass PS, Drake AF, Wang Y, et al (1990) Cationization of bovine serum albumin alters its confirmation as well as its charge. Lab Investig 62:185–188
63. Pietra GG, Sampson P, Lanken PN, et al (1983) Transcapillary movement of cationized ferritin in the isolated perfused rat lung. Lab Invest 49:54–61
64. Rippe B, Haraldsson B (1994) Transport of macromolecules across microvascular walls: the two-pore theory. Physiol Rev 74:163–219
65. Karmakar N, Dhar P (1996) Effect of steady shear stress on fluid filtration through the rabbit arterial wall in the presence of macromolecules. Clin Exp Pharmacol Physiol 23(4):299–304
66. Wilson J, Winter M, Shasby DM (1990) Oxidants, ATP depletion, and endothelial permeability to macromolecules. Blood 76(12):2578–2582
67. Yamashita T, Mimura K, Umeda F, et al (1995) Increased transendothelial permeation of albumin by high glucose concentration. Metabolism 44(6):739–744
68. Watanabe K (1985) Vascular permeability to macromolecules changes qualitatively in inflammation? Jpn J Pharmacol 39(30):398–401
69. Anda T, Yamashita H, Khalid H, et al (1997) Effect of tumor necrosis factor-alpha on the permeability of bovine brain microvessel endothelial cell monolayers. Neurol Res 19(4):369–376
70. Haselton FR, Alexander JS, Mueller SN (1993) Adenosine decreases permeability of in vitro endothelial monolayer. J Appl Physiol 74(4):1581–1590

71. Green K, Kearse EC, Yokogaki S, et al (2001) Human and rabbit corneal endothelial permeability after different chemical forms of glutathione. Ophthalmic Res 33(3): 151–155
72. Liu SM, Sundqvist T (1997) Nitric oxide and cGMP regulate endothelial permeability and F-actin distribution in hydrogen peroxide-treated endothelial cells. Exp Cell Res 235(1):238–244
73. Kampp M (1971) Transcapillary exchange of large molecules: mammals. In: Altman PL, Dittmer DS (eds) Respiration and circulation, FASEB, Bethesda, MD, Chapter 131, pp 504–509
74. Skopp G, Potsch L, Lutz R, et al (1998) Hemoglobin diffusion across a venous wall: an experimental study. Am J Forensic Med Pathol 19(4):372–376
75. Milici AJ, Bankston PW (1982) Fetal and neonatal rat intestinal capillaries: permeability to carbon, ferritin, hemoglobin, and myoglobin. Am J Anat 165(2):165–186
76. Nakai K, Sakuma I, Ohta T, et al (1998) Permeability characteristics of hemoglobin derivatives across cultured endothelial cell monolayers. J Lab Clin Med 132(4): 313–319
77. Baldwin AL (1999) Modified hemoglobin produce venular interendothelial gaps and albumin leakage in the rat mesentery. Am J Physiol 277(2 Pt 2):H650–659
78. Baldwin AL, Wiley EB, Summers AG, et al (2003) Sodium selenite reduces hemoglobin-induced venular leakage in the rat mesentery. Am J Physiol Heart Circ Physiol 284(1):H81–91
79. Bunn HF, Esham WT, Bull RW (1969) The renal handling of hemoglobin. I. Glomerular filtration. J Exp Med 129:909–924
80. Bunn HF, Jandl JH (1969) The renal handling of hemoglobin. II. Catabolism. J Exp Med 129:925–934
81. Bucci E, Razynska A, Urbaitis B, et al (1989) Pseudo cross-link of human hemoglobin with mono-93,5,-dibromosalicyl) fumarate. J Biol Chem 264:6191–6195
82. Thomas M, Matheson-Urbanitis B, Kwansa H, et al (1997) Introduction of negative charges to a crosslinked hemoglobin: lack of effect on plasma half time. Artif Cells Blood Substit Immobil Biotechnol 25(3):309–314
83. Hess JR (1996) Blood substitutes. Semin Hematol 33:369–378
84. Simoni J, Simoni G, Feola M (1993) Chromatographic analysis of biopolymers distribution in "poly-hemoglobin", an intermolecularly crosslinked hemoglobin solution. Anal Chim Acta 279:73–88
85. Levick JR (2000) An introduction to cardiovascular physiology, 3rd edn. Oxford University Press
86. Mohrman DE, Heller LJ, Heller LJ (2002) Cardiovascular physiology, 5th edn. McGraw-Hill/Appleton & Lange
87. Aitd WC (2003) Endothelial cell heterogeneity. Crit Care Med 31(4 Suppl.):S221–230
88. Zuberbuhlr RC, Bohr DF (1965) Responses of coronary smooth muscle to catecholamines. Circulat Res 16:431–440
89. Harder DR, Belardinelli L, Sperelakis N, et al (1979) Differential effects of adenosine and nitroglycerin on the action potentials of large and small coronary arteries Circulat Res 44:176–182
90. Schnaar RL, Sparks HV (1972) Response of large and small coronary arteries to nitroglycerin, $NaNO_3$, and adenosine. Am J Physiol 223:223–228
91. Tsukada T, Rubio R, Berne RM (1984) Pharmacological differentiation between large and small coronary vessels. Arch Int Pharmacodyn 270:255–267
92. Vanhoutte PM, Scott-Burden T (1994) The endothelium in health and disease. Texas Heart Inst J 21:62–67

93. Hess JR (1995) Review of modified hemoglobin research at Letterman: attempts to delineate the toxicity of cell free tetrameric hemoglobin. Artif Cells Blood Substit Immobil Biotechnol 23(3):277–289
94. Alayash AI, Fratantoni JC, Bonaventura C, et al (1993) Nitric oxide binding to human ferrihemoglobins cross-linked between either alpha or beta subunits. Arch Biochem Biophys 303(2):332–338
95. Alayash AI, Cashon RE (1994) Reactions of nitric oxide and hydrogen peroxide with hemoglobin-based blood substitutes. Ann NY Acad Sci 17:378–381
96. Alayash AI, Ryan BA, Fratantoni JC, et al (1994) Redox reactivity of modified hemoglobins with hydrogen peroxide and nitric oxide: toxicological implications. Artif Cells Blood Substit Immobil Biotechnol 22(3):373–378
97. Radomski M, Moncada S (1993) Regulation of vascular homeostasis by nitric oxide. Thromb Haemost 70:36–41
98. Toothill C (1967) The chemistry of the in vivo reactions between haemoglobin and various oxides and nitrogen. Br J Anaesth 39:405–412
99. Jia L, Bonaventura C, Bonaventura J, et al (1996) Protein S-nitrosohemoglobin: a dynamic activity of blood involved in vascular control. Nature 380:221–226
100. Huang Z, Ucer KB, Murphy T, et al (2002) Kinetics of nitric oxide binding to R-state hemoglobin. Biochem Biophys Res Commun 292(4):812–818
101. Huang Z, Louderback JG, Goyal M, et al (2001) Nitric oxide binding to oxygenated hemoglobin under physiological conditions. Biochim Biophys Acta 1568(3):252–260
102. Hobbs AJ, Gladwin MT, Patel RP, et al (2002) Hemoglobin: NO transporter, NO inactivator or none of the above? Trends Pharmacol Sci 23(9):406–411
103. Joshi MS, Ferguson TB Jr, Han TH, et al (2002) Nitric oxide is consumed, rather than conserved, by reaction with oxyhemoglobin under physiological condition. Proc Natl Acad Sci USA 99(16):10341–10346
104. Rohlfs RJ, Bruner E, Chiu A, et al (1998) Arterial blood pressure responses to cell-free hemoglobin solutions and the reaction with nitric oxide. J Biol Chem 273(20): 12128–12134
105. Kavdia M, Tsoukias NM, Popel AS (2002) Model of nitric oxide diffusion in an arteriole: impact of hemoglobin-based blood substitutes. Am J Physiol Heart Circ Physiol 282(6):H2245–2253
106. Zang H, Weir BKA, Macdonald L (1996) Mechanism of $[Ca^{++}]_i$ elevation induced by erythrocyte components in endothelial cells. J Pharmacol Exp Ther 277:1501–1509
107. Shasby DM, Yorek M, Shasby SS (1988) Exogenous oxidants initiate hydrolysis of endothelial cell inositol phospholipids. Blood 72:481–499
108. Berridge MJ, Irvine RF (1984) Inositol triphosphate, a novel second messenger in cellular signal transduction. Nature 312:315–319
109. Somers M, Gawryl M, Siegel NJ, et al (1994) Interaction of ultrapure hemoglobin (Hb) with renal epithelial cells. Artif Cells Blood Substit Immobil Biotechnol 22:A163
110. Suttorp N, Weber U, Welsch T, et al (1993) Role of phosphodiesterases in the regulation of endothelial permeability in vivo. J Clin Invest 91:1421–1428
111. Horovitz A, Menice CB, Laporte R, et al (1996) Mechanism of smooth muscle contraction. Physiol Rev 76:963–1003
112. Simoni J, Simoni G, Wesson DE, et al (2002) A novel hemoglobin-adenosine-glutathione based red cell substitute: its effects on human brain capillary endothelial cells. ASAIO J 48(2):193
113. Vollrath B, Cook D, Megyesi J, et al (1998) Novel mechanism by which Hb induces constriction of cerebral arteries. Eur J Pharmacol 361(2–3):311–319

114. Wickman G, Lan C, Vollarth B (2003) Functional roles of the rho/rho kinase pathway and protein kinase C in the regulation of cerebrovascular constriction mediated by hemoglobin: relevance to subarachinoid hemorrhage and vasospasm. Circ Res 92(7):809–816
115. Wickman G, Vollrath B (2000) Effects of tamoxifen on oxyhemoglobin-induced cerebral vasoconstriction. Eur J Pharmacol 390(1–2):181–184
116. Laher I, Zhang JH (2001) Protein kinase C and cerebral vasospasm. J Cereb Blood Flow Metab 21(8):887–906
117. Defouw LW, Defouw DO (2001) Protein kinase C activity contributes to endothelial hyperpermeability during early angiogenesis in the chick chorioallantoic membrane. Tissue Cell 33(2):135–140
118. Kim HW, Greenburg AG (2003) Hemoglobin mediated contraction of isolated blood vessels: why is precontraction necessary? Artif Blood 11(1):80
119. Cocks TM, Malta E, King SJ, et al (1991) Oxyhemoglobin increases the production of endothelin-1 by endothelial cell in culture. Eur J Pharmacol 196(2):177–182
120. Ohlstein EH, Storer BL (1992) Oxyhemoglobin stimulation of endothelin production in cultured endothelial cells. J Neurosurg 77(2):274–278
121. Yanagishawa M, Kurihara H, Kimura S, et al (1988) A novel potent vasoconstrictor peptide produced by vascular endothelial cells. Nature (Lond.) 332:411–415
122. Masaki T, Yanahishawa M, Goto K (1992) Physiology and pharmacology of endothelins. Med Res Rev 12:391–421
123. Gandhi CR, Berkowitz DE, Watkins D (1994) Endothelins: biochemistry and pathophysiologic actions. Anesthesiology 80:892–905
124. Kohno M, Yasunari K, Murakawa K, et al (1990) Plasma immunoreactive endothelin in essential hypertension. Am J Med 88:614–618
125. Boulanger C, Luscher TF (1990) Release of endothelin from porcine aorta. J Clin Invest 85:587–590
126. Gulati A, Singh G, Rebello S, et al (1995) Effect of diaspirin crosslinked and stroma-reduced hemoglobin on mean arterial pressure and endothelin-1 concentration in rats. Life Sci 56(17):1433–1442
127. Gulati A, Sen AP, Shrama AC, et al (1997) Role of ET and NO in resuscitative effect of diaspirin cross-linked hemoglobin after hemorrhage in rat. Am J Physiol 273(2 Pt 2):H827–836
128. Saxena R, Wijnhoud AD, Man in't Veld AJ, et al (1998) Effect of diaspirin cross-linked hemoglobin on endothelin-1 and blood pressure in acute ischemic stroke in man. J Hypertens 16(10):1459–1465
129. Hemsen A, Lundberg JM (1992) Free hemoglobin interferes with detection of endothelin peptides. Biochem Biophys Res Commun 189:777–781
130. Simoni J, Simoni G, Lox CD, et al (1995) Evidence for the direct inhibition of endothelin-1 secretion by hemoglobin in human endothelial cells. ASAIO J 41(3): M641–M651
131. Tai J, Kim HW, Greenburg AG (1997) Endothelin-1 is not involved in hemoglobin associated vasoactivities. Artif Cells Blood Substit Immobil Biotechnol 25(1–2): 135–140
132. Lin G, Macdonald RL, Marton LS, et al (2001) Hemoglobin increases endothelin-1 in endothelial cells by decreasing nitric oxide. Biochem Biophys Res Commun 280(3):824–830
133. Libertal W, Wolf EF, Merril EW, et al (1987) Hemodynamic effects of stroma free hemolysates in the isolated perfused rat kidney. Life Sci 41:2525–2533

134. Zilletti L, Ciufi M, Franchi-Micheli S, et al (1994) Cyclo-oxygenase activity of hemoglobin. In: Everse J, Winslow RM, Vandegriff KD (eds) Methods in Enzymology, Part B, Vol. 231. Academic Press, San Diego, CA, pp. 562–573
135. Takenaka K, Kassell NF, Foley PL, et al (1993) Oxyhemoglobin-induced cytotoxicity and arachidonic acid release in cultured bovine endothelial cells. Stroke 24(6): 839–845
136. Burhop KE, Farrel L, Nigro C, et al (1992) Effects of intravenous infusion of diaspirin cross-linked hemoglobin (DCLHb) on sheep. Biomat Artif Cells Immobil Biotechnol 20:581–585
137. Feola M, Simoni J, Canizaro PC, et al (1988) Toxicity of polymerized hemoglobin solutions. Surg Gynecol Obstet 166:211–222
138. Feola M, Simoni J, Tran R, et al (1989) Toxic factors in the red blood cell membrane. J Trauma 29(8):1065–1075
139. Simoni J, Simoni G, Wesson DE, et al (2001) Free hemoglobin (Hb) mediates the synthesis of 8-iso prostaglandin $F_{2\alpha}$, a vasoconstrictive isoprostane. Artif Cells Blood Substit Immobil Biotechnol 29(2):162
140. Morrow JD, Hill KE, Burk RF, et al (1990) A series of prostaglandin F2 like compounds are produced in vivo in humans by a non-cyclooxygenase free radical-catalyzed mechanism. Proc Natl Acad Sci USA 87:9383–9387
141. Morrow JD, Roberts LJ 2nd (1996) The isoprostanes: current knowledge and directions for future research. Biochem Pharmacol 51:1–9
142. John GW, Valentin P (1997) Analysis of the pulmonary hypertensive effects of the isoprostane derivative, 8-iso $PGF_{2\alpha}$ in the rat. Br J Pharmacol 122:899–905
143. Mohler ER, Franklin MT, Adam LP (1996) Intracellular signaling by 8-epi-prostaglandin F2 alpha is mediated by thromboxane A2/prostaglandin endoperoxidase receptors in porcine carotid arteries. Biochem Biophys Res Commun 225: 915–923
144. Sametz W, Prasthofer S, Wintersteiger R, et al (1999) Vascular effects of isoprostanes after endothelial damage. Prostaglandins Leukot Essent Fatty Acids 61:369–372
145. Jourdan KB, Evans TW, Curzen N, et al (1997) Evidence of dilator function of 8-iso prostaglandin $F_{2\alpha}$ in rat pulmonary artery. Br J Pharmacol 120:1280–1285
146. Mian KB, Martin E (1995) Differential sensitivity of basal and acetylocholine-stimulated activity of nitric oxide to destruction by superoxide anion in rat aorta. Br J Pharmacol 115:993–1000
147. Cheung ATW, Jahr JS, Driessen B, et al (2001) The effect of hemoglobin glutamer-200 (bovine) on the microcirculation in a canine hypovolemia model: an intravital microscopy study. Artif Cells Blood Substit Immobil Biotechnol 29(2):118
148. Cheung ATW, Jahr JS, Driessen B, et al (2003) Blood substitute resuscitation as a treatment modality for moderate hypovolemia. Artif Blood 11(1):73
149. Burhop KE (2003) The development of a second generation, designer, recombinant hemoglobin. Keio J Med 52(Suppl. 1):12
150. Lum H, Roebuck KA (2001) Oxidant stress and endothelial dysfunction. Am J Physiol Cell Physiol 280:C719–C741
151. Faassen AE, Sunby SR, Panter SS, et al (1988) Hemoglobin: a lifesaver and oxidant; how to tip the balance. Biomat Artif Cells Artif Organs 16:93–104
152. Simoni J, Feola M, Canizaro PC (1990) Generation of free oxygen radicals and the toxicity of hemoglobin solutions. Biomat Artif Cells Artif Organs 18:189–202
153. Mishra HP, Fridowich I (1972) The generation of superoxide radicals during autoxidation of hemoglobin. J Biol Chem 247:6960–6964

154. Sutton HC, Roberts PB, Witerbourn CC (1976) The rate of reaction of superoxide radical ion with oxyhaemoglobin and methaemoglobin. Biochem J 155:503–510
155. Halliwell B, Gutteridge JMC (1984) Oxygen toxicity, oxygen radicals, transition metals and diseases. Biochem J 219:1–14
156. Zhu L, Gunn C, Beckman JS (1992) Bactericidal activity of peroxynitrite. Arch Biochem Biophys 298:452–457
157. Radi R, Beckman JS, Bush KM, et al (1991) Peroxynitrite-induced membrane lipid peroxidation: The cytostolic potential of superoxide and nitric oxide. Arch Biochem Biophys 288:481–487
158. Marshall JJ, Knots HA (1990) Endothelial-derived relaxing factor. A prospective from in vivo data. Hypertension 16:371–386
159. Beckman JS, Beckman TW, Chen J, et al (1990) Apparent hydroxyl radical production by peroxynitrite; implications for endothelial injury from nitric oxide and superoxide. Proc Natl Acad Sci USA 87:1620–1624
160. Alayash AI, Ryan BA, Cashon RE (1998) Peroxynitrite-mediated heme oxidation and protein modification of native and chemically modified hemoglobins. Arch Biochem Biophys 349(1):65–73
161. McAdams M, Freeman B (1993) Receptor mediated binding of xanthine oxidase to vascular endothelium. Free Radic Biol Med 15(5):521
162. Ciolino HP, Levine RL (1993) Protein oxidation is an early event in oxidant injury to endothelial cells in vitro. Free Radic Biol Med 15(5):519
163. Partridge CA, Philips PG (1993) Exposure of pulmonary microvascular endothelial cells to hydrogen peroxide alters distribution of surface glycoproteins. Free Radic Biol Med 15(5):526
164. Sundquist T, Liu SM (1993) Hydrogen peroxide stimulates endocytosis in cultured bovine aortic endothelial cells. Acta Physiol Scand 149(2):127–131
165. Minetti M, Mallozzi C, Scorza G, et al (1993) Role oxygen and carbon radicals in hemoglobin oxidation. Arch Biochem Biophys 302:233–244
166. Pryor WA (1976) The role of free radical reactions in biological systems. In: Pryor WA (ed.), Free Radicals in Biology, Academic Press, New York, NY, pp 1–49
167. Gutteridge JMC (1986) Iron promoters of the Fenton reaction and lipid peroxidation can be released from hemoglobin by peroxides. FEBS Lett 201:291–295
168. Gutteridge JMC (1987) The antioxidant activity of haptoglobin towards haemoglobin-stimulated lipid peroxidation. Biochim Biophys Acta 917:219–223
169. Kanner J, Harel S (1985) Initiation of membranal lipid peroxidation by activated metmyoglobin and methemoglobin. Arch Biochem Biophys 237:314–321
170. Harel S, Kanner J (1988) The generation of ferryl or hydroxyl radicals during interaction of haemoproteins with hydrogen peroxide. Free Radic Res Comms 5:21–33
171. Alayash AI, Fratantoni JC, Bonaventura C, et al (1992) Consequences of chemical modification on the free radical reactions of human hemoglobin. Arch Biochem Biophys 298:114–120
172. Yamada T, Volkmer C, Grisham MB (1991) The effect of sulfasalazine metabolites on hemoglobin-catalyzed lipid peroxidation. Free Rad Biol Med 10:41–49
173. Simoni G, Simoni J, Feola M (1991) Oxidative hemolysis of erythrocytes incubated with purified modified bovine hemoglobin. Protective effect of plasma and radical scavengers. Biomat Artif Cells Immobil Biotechnol 19(2):486
174. Cashon RE, Alayash AI (1995) Reaction of human hemoglobin HbA0 and two cross-linked derivatives with hydrogen peroxide: Differential behavior of the ferryl intermediate. Arch Biochem Biophys 316(1):461–469

175. Goldman DW, Breyer RJ 3rd, Yeh D, et al (1998) Acellular hemoglobin-mediated oxidative stress toward endothelium: a role for ferryl iron. Am J Physiol 275(3 Pt 2): H1046–1053
176. McLeod LL, Alayash AI (1999) Detection of a ferrylhemoglobin intermediate in an endothelial cell model after hypoxia-reoxygenation. Am J Physiol 277(1 Pt 2):H92–99
177. Simoni J, Simoni G, Lox CD, et al (1997) Modified hemoglobin solution, with desired pharmacological properties, does not activate nuclear transcription factor NF-kappa B in human vascular endothelial cells. Artif Cells Blood Substit Immobil Biotechnol 25(1–2):193–210
178. Giulivi C, Davies KJA (1990) A novel antioxidant role for hemoglobin. The comproportionation of ferrylhemoglobin with oxyhemoglobin. J Biol Chem 265:19453–19460
179. Alayash AI, Brockner-Rayan BA, Eich RF (1999) Reaction of sperm whale myoglobin with hydrogen peroxide. J Biol Chem 274:2029–2037
180. Yamamato Y, Brodsky MH, Baker JC, et al (1987) Detection and characterization of lipid hydroperoxides at picomole level by high performance liquid chromatography. Anal Biochem 160:7–13
181. Grisham MB, Gaginella TS, Ritter von C, et al (1990) Effects of neutrophil-derived oxidants on intestinal permeability, electrolyte transport and epithelial viability. Inflammation 14:531–542
182. Miller YI, Felikman Y, Shaklai N (1996) Hemoglobin induced apolipoprotein B crosslinking in low-density lipoprotein peroxidation. Arch Biochem Biophys 326: 252–260
183. Yoshida Y, Kashiba K, Nikki E (1994) Free radical mediated oxidation of lipids induced by hemoglobin in aqueous dispersion. Biochim Biophys Acta 120:165–172
184. Svistunenko DA, Patel RP, Voloshchenko SV, et al (1997) The globin based free radical of ferryl hemoglobin is detected in normal human blood. J Biol Chem 272(11): 7114–7121
185. Halliwell B, Gutteridge JM (1990) Role of free radicals and catalytic metal ions in human disease: an overview. Methods Enzymol 186:1–85
186. Weis JR, Pitas RE, Wilson BD, et al (1991) Oxidized low-density lipoprotein increases cultured human endothelial cell tissue factor activity and reduces protein C activation. FASEB J 5(10):2459–2465
187. Simoni J, Simoni G, Wesson DE, et al (2001) Oxidative reactions of hemoglobin crosslinked with adenosine and conjugated with reduced glutathione. Artif Cells Blood Substit Immobil Biotechnol 29(2):164
188. Balagopalakrishna C, Nirmala R, Rifkind JM, et al (1997) Modification of low density lipoprotein by erythrocytes and hemoglobin under hypoxic conditions. Adv Exp Med Biol 411:337–345
189. Ross R (1995) Cell biology of atherosclerosis. Annu Rev Physiol 57:791–804
190. Dimmeler S, Haendler J, Galle J, et al (1997) Oxidized low density lipoprotein induced apoptosis of human endothelial cells by activation of CPP32-like protease. A mechanistic clue to the "response to injury" hypothesis. Circulation 95:1760–1763
191. Best PJM, Hasdai D, Sangiorgi G, et al (1999) Apoptosis. Basic concepts and implication in coronary artery disease. Arterioscler Thromb Vasc Biol 19:14–22
192. Ogihara K, Zubkow AY, Bernake DH, et al (1999) Oxyhemoglobin-induced apoptosis in cultured endothelial cells. J Neurosurg 91(3):495–465
193. D'Agnillo F, Alayash AI (2001) Redox cycling of diaspirin cross-linked hemoglobin induces G2/M arrest and apoptosis in cultured endothelial cells. Blood 98(12): 3315–3323

194. Megero T, Chen B, Lancon J, et al (2001) Oxyhemoglobin induces caspase-mediated death in cerebral endothelial cells. J Neurochem 77(4):1128–1135
195. Meguro T, Chen B, Parent AD, et al (2001) Caspase inhibitors attenuate oxyhemoglobin-induced apoptosis in endothelial cells. Stroke 32(2):561–566
196. Akin E, Clower B, Tibbs R, et al (2002) Bilirubin produces apoptosis in cultured bovine brain endothelial cells. Brain Res 93(2):168–175
197. Brouard S, Otterbein LE, Anrather J, et al (2000) Carbon monoxide generated by heme oxygenase 1 suppresses endothelial cell apoptosis. J Exp Med 192(7):1015–1026
198. Sano K, Asano T, Tanishima T, et al (1980) Lipid peroxidation as a cause of cerebral vasospasm. Neurol Res 2(3–4):253–272
199. Patrignani P (2001) Oxidized lipids. Ital Heart J 2(12):873–877
200. Morita T, Kourembanas S (1995) Endothelial cell expression of vasoconstrictors and growth factors is regulated by smooth muscle cell-derived carbon monoxide. J Clin Invest 96(6):2676–2682
201. Motterlini R, Gonzalez A, Foresti R, et al (1998) Heme oxygenase-1-derived carbon monoxide contributes to the suppression of acute hypertensive responses in vivo. Circ Res 83(5):568–577. Erratum in: Circ Res 83(12):1289
202. Lavrovsky Y, Schwartzman ML, Levere RD, et al (1994) Identification of binding sites for transcriptional factors NF-kappa B and AP-2 in the promoter region of the human oxygenase 1 gene. Proc Natl Acad Sci USA 91:5987–5991
203. Gilmont RR, Dardano DO, Young M, et al (1998) Effects of glutathione depletion on oxidant-induced endothelial cell injury. J Surg Res 80:62–68
204. Meister A (1988) Glutathione metabolism and its selective modification. J Biol Chem 263:17205–17208
205. Olson CE (1988) Glutathione modulates toxic oxygen metabolite injury of canine chief cell monolayer in primary culture. Am J Physiol 254(1 Pt 1):G49–56
206. Krenz-Remy C, Arrigo A-P (2002) Gene expression and thiol redox state. Methods Enzymol 348:200–215
207. Haddad JJE, Olver RE, Land SC (2000) Antioxidant/Pro-oxidant equilibrium regulates HIF-1α and NF-κB redox sensitivity. J Biol Chem 275(28):21130–21139
208. Haddad JJ (2002) Oxygen-sensitive pro-inflammatory cytokines, apoptosis signaling and redox-responsive transcription factors in development and pathophysiology. Cytokine Cell Mol Ther 7(1):1–14
209. Haddad JJ (2002) Antioxidant and prooxidant mechanism in the regulation of redox(y)-sensitive transcription factors. Cell Signal 14(11):879–897
210. Simoni J, Simoni G, Garcia EL, et al (1995) Protective effect of selenium on hemoglobin mediated lipid peroxidation in vivo. Artif Cells Blood Substit Immobil Biotechnol 23(4):469–486
211. D'Agnillo F, Wood F, Porras C, et al (2000) Effects of hypoxia and glutathione depletion on hemoglobin- and myoglobin-mediated oxidative stress toward endothelium. Biochim Biophys Acta 1495(2):150–159
212. D'Agnillo F, Alayash AI (2000) Interactions of hemoglobin with hydrogen peroxide alters thiol levels and course of endothelial cell death. Am J Physiol Heart Circ Physiol 279(4):H1880–1889
213. Alayash AI (2001) Oxidative mechanisms of hemoglobin-based blood substitutes. Artif Cells Blood Substit Immobil Biotechnol 29(6):415–425
214. Kozar RA, McKenoe BJ, Pownall HJ (1994) Free radical-induced alterations in endothelial cell function. J Surg Res 56:32–36

215. Gawryl MS, Houtchens RA, Light WR (2001) Method for preserving a hemoglobin blood substitute. USA Patent 6,271,351
216. Sehgal LR, De Woskin RE, Moss GS, et al (2003) Acellular red blood cell substitute. USA Patent 6,552,173
217. Watkins LR, Hansen MK, Nguyen KT, et al (1999) Dynamic regulation of the proinflammatory cytokine, interleukin-1beta: Molecular biology for non-molecular biologists. Minireview. Life Sci 65(5):449–481
218. Filomeni G, Rotilio G, Ciriolo MR (2002) Cell signaling and the glutathione redox system. Biochem Pharmacol 64(5–6):1057–1064
219. Gabbita SP, Robinson KA, Steward CA, et al (2000) Redox regulatory mechanism of cellular signal transduction. Arch Biochem Biophys 376(1):1–13
220. Michelis C, Minet E, Mottet D, et al (2002) Regulation of gene expression by oxygen: NF-kappa B and HIF-1, two extremes. Free Radic Biol Med 33(9)1231–1242
221. Galter D, Mihm S, Droge W (1994) Distinct effects of glutathione disulfide on nuclear transcription factor kappa B and the activator protein-1. Eur J Biochem 221(2): 639–648
222. Pineda-Molina E, Klatt P, Vazquez J, et al (2001) Glutathionylation of the p50 subunit of NF-kappa B: a mechanism for redox-induced inhibition of DNA binding. Biochemistry 40(47):14134–14142
223. Renard P, Delaive E, Van Steenbrugge M, et al (2001) Is the effect of interleukin-1 on glutathione oxidation in cultured human fibroblasts involved in nuclear factor kappa B activation? Antioxid Redox Signal 3(2):329–340
224. Haddad JJE, Land SC (2000) O_2-evoked regulation of HIF-1alpha and NF-kappa B in perinatal lung epithelium requires glutathione biosynthesis. Am J Physiol Lung Cell Mol Physiol 278:L492–503
225. Yang G, Shegog ML, Dennery PA (2002) Effect of glutathione on lung activator protein-1 activation and heme oxigenase-1 induction in the immature rat. Pediatr Res 52(1):34039
226. Henderson WR, Chi EY, Teo JL, et al (2002) A small molecule inhibitor of redox-regulated NF-kappa B and activator protein-1 transcription blocks allergic airway inflammation in mouse asthma model. J Immunol 169(9):5294–5299
227. Lando D, Pongratz I, Poellinger L, et al (2000) A redox mechanism controls differential DNA binding activities of hypoxia-inducible factor (HIF) 1 alpha and the HIF-like factor. J Biol Chem 275(7):4618–4627
228. Huang EL, Arany Z, Livingston DM, et al (1996) Activation of hypoxia-inducible transcription factor depends primarily upon redox-sensitive stabilization of its alpha subunit. J Biol Chem 271(50):32253–32259
229. Pahl HL (1999) Activators and target genes of Rel/NF-kappa B transcriptional factors. Oncogene 18:6853–6866
230. Barkett M, Gilmore TG (1999) Control of apoptosis by Rel/NF-kappa B transcription factors. Oncogene 18(49):6910–6924
231. Flohe L, Brigelius-Flohe R, Saliou C, et al (1997) Redox regulation of NF-kappa B activation. Free Radic Biol Med 22(6):1115–1126
232. Schreck R, Albermann K, Baeuerle PA (1992) Nuclear factor kappa-B: an oxidative stress responsive transcription factor of eukaryotic cells. Free Radic Res Commun 17: 221–237
233. Li N, Karin M (1999) Is NF-kappa B the sensor of oxidative stress? FASEB J 13(10): 1137–1143

234. Chen FE, Gosh G (1999) Regulators of DNA binding by Rel/NF-kappa B transcription factors: structural views. Oncogene 18(49):6845–6852
235. Haddad JJ, Land SC (2002) Redox/ROS regulation of lipopolysaccharide-induced mitogen-activated protein kinase (MAPK) activation and MAPK-mediated TNF-alpha biosynthesis. Br J Pharmacol 135(2):520–536
236. Sen CK, Roy S, Packer L (1996) Involvement of intracellular Ca^{2+} in oxidant-induced NF-kappa B activation. FEBS Lett 385:58–62
237. Andalibi A, Liao F, Imes S, et al (1993) Oxidized lipoproteins influence gene expression by causing oxidative stress and activating the transcription factor NF-kappa B. Biochem Soc Trans 21(Pt 3)(3):651–655
238. Hennig B, Toborek M, Joshi-Barve S, et al (1996) Linoleic acid activates nuclear transcription factor-kappa B (NF-kappa B) and induced NF-kappa B-dependent transcription of cultured endothelial cells. Am J Clin Nutr 63(3):322–328
239. Wenger RH (2002) Cellular adaptation to hypoxia: O_2-sensing protein hydroxylases, hypoxia-inducible transcription factors, and O_2-regulated gene expression. FASEB J 16:1151–1162
240. Gleadle JM, Ratcliffe PJ (1997) Induction of hypoxia-inducible factor-1, erythropoietin, vascular endothelial growth factor, and glucose transporter-1 by hypoxia: evidence against regulatory role for Src kinase. Blood 89:503–509
241. Schroedl C, McClintock DS, Budinger GR, et al (2002) Hypoxic but not anoxic stabilization of HIF-1 alpha requires mitochondrial reactive oxygen species. Am J Physiol Lung Cell Mol Physiol 283:L922–931
242. Chandel NS, McClintock DS, Feliciano CE, et al (2000) Reactive oxygen species generated at mitochondrial complex III stabilize hypoxia-inducible factor 1 alpha during hypoxia. J Biol Chem 275(33):25130–25138
243. Kallio PJ, Wilson W, O'Brien S, et al (1999) Regulation of the hypoxia-inducible transcription factor 1 alpha by the ubiquitin-proteasome pathway. J Biol Chem 274(10): 6519–6525
244. Richard DE, Berra E, Gothie E, et al (1999) p/42/p44 mitogen-activated protein kinase phosphorylate hypoxia-inducible factor 1 alpha and enhance the transcriptional activity of HIF-1. J Biol Chem 274(46):32631–32637
245. Shaulian E, Karin M (2002) AP-1 as a regulator of cell life and death. Nat Cell Biol 4(5):E131–136
246. Shaulian E, Karin M (2001) AP-1 in cell proliferation and survival. Oncogene 20(19): 2390–2400
247. Simoni J, Simoni G, Lox CD, et al (1991) Reaction of human monocytes and macrophage-leukocytes to bovine hemoglobin. Biomat Artif Cells Immobil Biotechnol 19(2):487
248. McFaul SJ, Bowman PD, Villa VM, et al (1994) Hemoglobin stimulates mononuclear leukocytes to release interleukin-8 and tumor necrosis factor alpha. Blood 84: 3175–3181
249. McFaul SJ, Bowman PD, Villa VM (2000) Hemoglobin stimulates the release of proinflammatory cytokines from leukocytes in whole blood. J Lab Clin Med 135:263–269
250. Gilmore TD: Inducers of NF-κB activity. http://people.bu.edu/gilmore/nf-kb/inducers
251. Toussaint-Hacquard M, Devaux Y, Longrios D, et al (2003) Biological response of human aortic endothelial cells exposed to acellular hemoglobin solutions developed as potential blood substitutes. Life Sci 72(10):1143–1157
252. Benton LD, Khan M, Greco RS, et al (1993) Integrins, adhesion molecules and surgical research. Surg Gynecol Obstet 177:311–327

253. Palmer LA, Gaston B, Johns RA (2000) Normoxic stabilization of hypoxia-inducible factor-1 expression and activity: redox dependent effect of nitrogen oxides. Mol Pharmacol 58:1197–1203
254. Yeh LH, Alayash AI (2003) Redox reactions of haemoglobin and cell signaling mechanism. J Intern Med 253:518–526
255. Simoni J, Simoni G, Griswold JA, et al (2003) Hemoglobin, transcriptional activator and suppressor. How to tip the balance? Artif Blood 11(1):69
256. Simoni J, Simoni G, Griswold JA, et al (2003) Activatory and suppressive roles of hemoglobin-based blood substitutes at the transcriptional level. ASAIO J 49(2):181
257. Raush CW, Feola M (1992) Extra pure semi-synthetic blood substitute. US Patent 5, 084, 558
258. Gawryl MS (2003) Hemopure™: clinical development and experience. Artif Blood 11(1):46
259. Templeton DM, Liu Y (2003) Genetic regulation of cell function in response to iron overload or chelation. Biochim Biophys Acta 1619(2):113–124
260. Vandegriff KD, Malavalli A, Wooldridge J, et al (2003) MP4, a new nonvasoactive PEG-Hb conjugate. Transfusion 43(4):509–516
261. Vandegriff K, Bellelli A, Malavalli A, et al (2003) Kinetics of ligand binding to MP4, a polyethylene glycol conjugated hemoglobin. Artif Blood 11(1):60
262. Winslow RM (2003) MP4, a new non-vasoactive polyethylene glycol-hemoglobin conjugate. ASAIO J 49(2):224
263. Winslow RM, Tsai AG, Vandegriff KD, et al (2003) Target oxygen delivery by low p50 hemoglobin: a new basis for hemoglobin-based oxygen carriers. Artif Blood 11(1):45
264. Tsuhida E, Komatsu T, Masukawa Y, et al (2003) Human serum albumin incorporation synthetic heme: red blood cell substitute without hypertension by nitric oxide scavenging. J Biomed Mater Res 64A(2):257–261
265. Kobayashi K, Tsuchida E (2003) Safety and efficacy of hemoglobin-vesicles and albumin-hemes. Keio J Med 52(1):32
266. Komatsu T, Yamamoto H, Huang Y, et al (2003) Exchange transfusion of albumin-heme as an artificial oxygen carrier into anesthetized rats physiological responses and oxygen delivery. Keio J Med 52(1):45
267. Komatsu T, Tsuchida E (2003) Serum albumin including synthetic hemes as an oxygen-carrying hemoprotein. Keio J Med 52(1):46
268. Tsuchida E (2003) Serum albumin including hemes as novel oxygen carrying hemoprotein and its medical applications. ASAIO J 49(2):222
269. Kobayashi K (2003) Evaluation of artificial oxygen carriers in vivo—History and perspective of Keio-Waseda joint project of oxygen infusions. Artif Blood 11(1):27
270. D'Agnillo F, Chang TMS (1997) Modified hemoglobin blood substitute from cross-linked hemoglobin-superoxide dismutase-catalase. US Patent 5,606,025
271. Chang TMS, D'Agnillo F, Razack S (1998) A second-generation hemoglobin based blood substitute with antioxidant activities. In: Chang TMS (ed) Blood substitutes: principles, methods, products and clinical trials. vol. 2. Karger, Basel, pp 178–186
272. D'Agnillo F, Chang TMS (1998) Polyhemoglobin-superoxide dismutase—catalase as a blood substitute with antioxidant properties. Nature Biotechnol 16:667–671
273. Chang TMS (2002) Oxygen carriers. Curr Opinion Invest Drugs 3:1187–1190
274. Powanda D, Chang TMS (2002) Cross-linked polyhemoglobin-superoxide dismutase-catalase supplies oxygen without causing blood brain barrier disruption or brain edema in a rat model of transient global brain ischemia-reperfusion. Artif Cells Blood Substit Immobil Biotechnol 30:25–42

275. Chang TMS (2003) Future generations of red cell substitutes. J Int Med 253:527–535
276. Hsia JC (1997) Composition and methods using nitroxides to avoid oxygen toxicity, particularly in stabilized, polymerized, conjugated or encapsulated hemoglobin used as red cell substitute. USA Patent 5,591,710
277. Okayama N, Park JH, Coe L, et al (1999) Polynitroxyl αα-hemoglobin (PNH) inhibits peroxide and superoxide-mediated neutrophil adherence to human endothelial cells. Free Radic Res 31(1):53–58
278. Krishna MC, Ma L, Samuni A, et al (1996) Superoxide dismutase- and catalase-mimetic activity of a polynitroxyl hemoglobin (PNH). Artif Cells Blood Substit Immobil Biotechnol 24:369
279. Saezler RK, Arfors KE, Tuma RF, et al (1999) Polynitroxylated hemoglobin-based oxygen carrier: inhibition of free radical-induced microcirculatory dysfunction. Free Radic Biol Med 27(1–2):1–6
280. Patel PM, Harada H, Ma L, et al (1998) Polynitroxyl hemoglobin (PNH) reduces cerebral infarction following transient cerebral artery occlusion in the HRS rat. Shock 9:61
281. Hsia C, Li M (2003) HemoZyme as battlefield hemorrhagic trauma protectant. Artif Blood 11(1):49
282. Maxwell RA, Gibson JB, Fabian TC, et al (2000) Resuscitation of severe chest trauma with four different hemoglobin-based oxygen-carrying solutions. J Trauma 49(2): 200–211
283. Hartl M, Bader AG, Bister K (2003) Molecular targets of the oncogenic transcription factor jun. Curr Cancer Drug Targets 3(1):41–55
284. Looker D, Abbott-Brown D, Cozart T, et al (1992) A human recombinant hemoglobin designed for use as a blood substitute. Nature 356:258–260
285. Doherty DH, Doyle MP, Curry SR, et al (1998) Rate of reaction with nitric oxide determines the hypertensive effect of cell-free hemoglobin. Nat Biotechnol 16: 672–676
286. Burhop KE, Doyle M, Schick M, et al (2003) The development and preclinical testing of a novel second generation recombinant hemoglobin solution. Artif Blood 11(1):50
287. Malhotra AK, Kelly ME, Miller PR, et al (2003) Resuscitation with a novel hemoglobin-based oxygen carrier in a swine model of uncontrolled perioperative hemorrhage. J Trauma 54(5):915–924
288. Simoni J, Simoni G, Weinstock S, et al (1998) An improved blood substitute. Emerg Ther Targets 2(1):85–92
289. Feola M, Simoni J (2001) Hemoglobin-adenosine-glutathione complex as a red cell substitute. Is this a perfect match? Artif Cells Blood Substit Immobil Biotechnol 29(2):143
290. Feola M, Simoni J (2003) Improved blood substitute. Japanese Patent 3,437,572
291. Feola M, Simoni J, Canizaro PC (1999) Polyhemoglobin stabilized by purine derivatives and glutathione. Korean Patent 702,403
292. Feola M, Simoni J (1998) Improved blood substitute. European Patent EP 0,586,381 B1
293. Feola M, Simoni J, Canizaro PC (1997) Polyhemoglobin stabilized by purine derivatives and glutathione. Irish Patent 459,071
294. Feola M, Simoni J, Canizaro PC (1996) Polyhemoglobine Stabilisee a l'adie de derives de Purine et de Glutathion. European Patent EP 0,507,870 B1
295. Feola M, Simoni J, Canizaro PC (1995) Blood substitute. USA Patent 5,439,882
296. Feola M, Simoni J, Canizaro PC (1994) Polyhemoglobin stabilized by purine derivatives and glutathione. Australian Patent 650,439

297. Simoni J, Simoni G, Newman G, et al (1996) An improved blood substitute: in vivo evaluation of its hemodynamic effects. ASAIO J 42(5):M773–782
298. Hori M, Kitakaze M (1991) Adenosine, the heart, and coronary circulation. Hypertension 18(5):565–574
299. Tabrizchi R, Bedi S (2001) Pharmacology of adenosine receptors in the vasculature. Pharmacol Ther 91(2):133–147
300. Linden J (2002) Autregulation of cyclic AMP in vascular smooth muscle: a role for adenosine receptors. Mol Pharm 62(5):969–970
301. Polte T, Schroder H (1998) Cyclic AMP mediates endothelial protection by nitric oxide. Biochem Biophys Res Commun 251(2):460–465
302. Bouma MG, van den Wildenberd FA, Buurman WA (1997) The anti-inflammatory potential of adenosine in ischemia-reperfusion injury: established and putative beneficial actions of a retaliatory metabolite. Shock 8(5):313–320
303. McWhinney CD, Dudley MW, Bowlin TL, et al (1996) Activation of adenosine A3 receptors on macrophages inhibits tumor necrosis factor-alpha. Eu J Pharmacol 310:209–216
304. Li C, Ha T, Liu L, et al (2000) Adenosine prevents activation of transcription factor NF-kappa B and enhances activator protein-1 binding activity in ischemic rat hart. Surgery 127(2):161–169
305. Liang BT, Jacobson KA (1998) A physiological role of the adenosine A3 receptor: sustained cardioprotection. Proc Natl Acad Sci USA 95(12):6995–6999
306. Maggirwar SB, Dhanraj DN, Somani SM, et al (1994) Adenosine acts as an endogenous activator of the cellular antioxidant defense system. Biochem Biophys Res Commun 210(2):508–515
307. Ramkumar V, Nie Z, Rybak LP, et al (1995) Adenosine, antioxidant enzymes and cytoprotection. Trends Pharmacol Sci 16(9):283–285
308. Zalewska-Kaszubska J (2002) Neuroprotective mechanism of adenosine action on CNS neurons. Neurol Neurochir Pol 36(2):329–336
309. Baxter GF (2002) Role of adenosine in delayed preconditioning of myocardium. Cardiovasc Res 55:483–494
310. Green K, Kearase EC, Yokogaki S, et al (2001) Human and rabbit corneal endothelial permeability after different forms of glutathione. Ophthalmic Res 33(3):151–155
311. Zhou D, Mayberg MR, London S, et al (1996) Reduction of intracellular glutathione levels produces sustained arterial narrowing. Neurosurgery 39(5):991–997
312. Tejedor C, Lorente JA, Delagado MA, et al (2002) Interaction between hemoglobin and glutathione in the regulation of blood flow in normal and septic pigs. Crit Care Med 30(11):2493–2500
313. Deem S, Kim JU, Manjula BN, et al (2002) Effects of S-nitrosation and cross-linking of hemoglobin on hypoxic pulmonary vasoconstriction in isolated rat lungs. Circ Res 91(7):626–632
314. Prasad A, Andrews NP, Padder FA, et al (1999) Glutathione reverses endothelial dysfunction and improves nitric oxide bio-availability. J Am Coll Cardiol 34(2):507–514
315. van der Vliet A, Hoen PA, Wong PS, et al (1998) Formation of S-nitrosothiols via direct nucleophilic nitrosation of thiols by peroxynitrite with elimination of hydrogen peroxide. J Biol Chem 273(46):30255–30262
316. Feola M, Simoni J, Angelillo R (2001) Preclinical and clinical experience with a novel hemoglobin adenosine-glutathione based red cell substitute. Artif Cells Blood Substit Immobil Biotechnol 29(2):107
317. Simoni J (1997) Texas tech blood substitute research and development; 1984–1997. A monograph, TTUHSC, Lubbock, TX, USA, pp 1–68

318. Feola M, Simoni J (2002) Hemoglobin combined with ATP, adenosine, GSH. Combat Casualty Care Research Program. Advanced Technology Applications for Combat Casualty Care (ATACCC) Conference, St. Pete Beach, FL, September 9–13
319. Simoni J, Simoni G, Wesson DE, et al (2001) Attenuation of hemoglobin neurotoxic potential by cross-linking with adenosine and conjugation with reduced glutathione. Artif Cells Blood Substit Immobil Biotechnol 29(2):128
320. Simoni J, Simoni G, Wesson DE, et al (1997) A novel free Hb-based blood substitute: in vitro evaluation of its effects on human vascular and smooth muscle cells. The VII International Symposium on Blood Substitutes, Waseda University, Tokyo, Japan, September 7–10, 1997. Program & Abstracts 2A-03:45
321. Simoni J, Simoni G, Newman G, et al (1996) A novel free Hb-based blood substitute: In vivo evaluation of its cardiovascular and renal effects. Artif Cells Blood Substit Immobil Biotechnol 24(4):427
322. Feola M, Simoni J, Angelillo R, et al (1992) Clinical trial of a hemoglobin based blood substitute in patients with sickle cell anemia. Surg Gynecol & Obstet 174(5):379–386
323. Chang TMS (2003) Future generation of red blood cell substitutes. J Int Med 253: 527–535
324. Klein HG (2002) Blood Substitutes: how close to a solution? Oncology (Huntingt) 16(9 Suppl. 10):147–151
325. Fratantoni JC (1999) Red blood cell substitutes; evolution of approaches to demonstrating efficacy. Artif Cells Blood Substit Immobil Biotechnol 27(1):1–9
326. Chang TMS (2000) Editorial: Is there a need for blood substitutes in the new millennium and what can we expect in way of safety and efficacy? Artif Cells Blood Substit Immobil Biotechnol 28(1):i–vii
327. Greenburg AG (2000) Editorial Comment: Is there a need for blood substitutes in the new millennium and what can we expect in way of safety and efficacy? Artif Cells Blood Substit Immobil Biotechnol 28(2):v–vi
328. Chen HS (2000) Editorial Comment: Is there a need for blood substitutes in the new millennium and what can we expect in way of safety and efficacy? Artif Cells Blood Substit Immobil Biotechnol 28(2):vii
329. Feola M, Simoni J (2000) Editorial Comment: Is there a need for blood substitutes in the new millennium and what can we expect in way of safety and efficacy? Artif Cells Blood Substit Immobil Biotechnol 28(2):vii–ix
330. Tsuchida E (2000) Editorial Comment: Is there a need for blood substitutes in the new millennium and what can we expect in way of safety and efficacy? Artif Cells Blood Substit Immobil Biotechnol 28(3):v–vii
331. Biro GP (2000) Editorial Comment: Is there a need for blood substitutes in the new millennium and what can we expect in way of safety and efficacy? Artif Cells Blood Substit Immobil Biotechnol 28(3):viii–xii
332. Alayash AI (2001) Editorial Comment: Is there a need for blood substitutes in the new millennium and what can we expect in way of safety and efficacy? A research perspective. Artif Cells Blood Substit Immobil Biotechnol 29(1):1–3
333. Hsia CJC (2001) Editorial Comment: Is there a need for blood substitutes in the new millennium and what can we expect in way of safety and efficacy? A development perspective. Artif Cells Blood Substit Immobil Biotechnol 29(3):vii–x

The Development of a Second-Generation, Designer, Recombinant Hemoglobin

Kenneth E. Burhop

Summary. The first-generation hemoglobin therapeutics, most of which were created more than 10 years ago, were designed to make a solution that looked identical to hemoglobin contained within a red blood cell. Numerous issues have been raised with their experimental use such as pulmonary and systemic vasoactivity, extravasation of hemoglobin, serum enzyme increases, adverse effects on gastrointestinal motility, generation of myocardial lesions, and potential interactions between hemoglobin and endotoxin. In retrospect, these physiologic effects are not unexpected, since it is now known that an inherent property of all natural (wild-type) hemoglobins is their ability to interact with nitric oxide (NO), secondary to extravasation of the hemoglobin into parenchymal tissue.

Key words. HBOC, Recombinant hemoglobin, Nitric oxide, Blood substitute, Hemoglobin

To address these issues, Baxter has modified the basic hemoglobin functionality using recombinant technology and site-directed mutagenesis of the distal heme pockets of recombinant human hemoglobin produced in *Escherichia coli*, in combination with some of the technology learned from the first-generation products (e.g., cross-linking polymerization and derivatization to enlarge the size of the molecule). A series of hemoglobin variants with reduced NO reaction rates have been constructed. Substitution of certain amino acids into the heme pockets of α and β-subunits reduced the rate constants for reaction with NO by up to 30-fold relative to wild-type hemoglobin. The systemic hemodynamic responses to these hemoglobins were

Medication Delivery, Baxter Healthcare Corporation, DF3-2W, One Baxter Parkway, Deerfield, IL 60015, USA

reduced and the magnitudes of the responses were correlated with the rates of NO scavenging. Therefore, it appears that there are now available viable approaches to modify the intrinsic biologic properties of hemoglobin and produce improved, second-generation hemoglobin products.

Historical Development of Hemoglobin Therapeutics

It is believed that physicians performed the first successful blood transfusion into a human recipient in the seventeenth century, but the practice quickly fell into disfavor when many of the subsequent patients died. While sporadic attempts to transfuse humans were made thereafter, significant progress in the field was made only after scientists gained a better understanding of the critical issues limiting the success of this procedure, such as how to prevent blood from coagulating once it is removed from the body and the fact that humans have different blood types that require all blood units to be tested for compatibility with the intended recipient. In the early part of the twentieth century most of these issues had been resolved so that by the 1920s health-care professionals widely practiced transfusion therapy. Interest in research on blood and blood storage was further stimulated by the need for the treatment of military and civilian casualties in World War II, culminating in the establishment of American Red Cross blood banks in 1947. Without question, the implementation of the modern blood banking system has been a major achievement of twentieth century medicine and provided a life saving therapy to millions of patients. On the other hand, like any medical procedure, blood transfusion has several limitations and is not without risk.

In the mid-1980s recognition that serious viral diseases, such as AIDS and hepatitis, could be transmitted by blood led scientists to intensify their work to improve the safety of the human blood supply. Subsequent industry-wide measures have made blood transfusion safer than ever. However, while the risk of direct transmission of viral diseases by most blood products has been substantially reduced as a result of increased vigilance in donor screening, blood testing, and blood processing, the specter of new potential blood borne pathogens has contributed to ongoing concern about the consequences of transfusion. In addition, there is mounting evidence that blood transfusion results in immune suppression that may make patients more susceptible to common infections such as pneumonia. Other limitations to blood collected for transfusion include the fact that it can only be stored for six weeks before it must be discarded and the fact that red cells become impaired during storage such that the ability to deliver oxygen to tissues immediately after infusion is reduced. There are also a significant number of red cells (up to 25%) that become permanently damaged during blood storage such that they survive in the circulation for only a short period of time.

These issues have spurred government, academic and industry research efforts to find a safe and effective alternative to blood transfusion. The primary focus of this research has been the identification and development of solutions that can perform the oxygen transport function of red blood cells. While such solutions have often been referred to as "blood substitutes", this nomenclature is erroneous since these solutions are incapable of performing the other functions of blood such as coagulation. Therefore, these solutions are now more appropriately denoted as oxygen carrying solutions or oxygen therapeutics. The development of such solutions has historically been based on two different technologies that can effectively transport oxygen to tissues, perfluorocarbons and hemoglobins. Perfluorocarbons are synthetic chemicals that readily dissolve gases, while hemoglobins are the pigmented proteins in red blood cells that bind oxygen and enable blood to transport oxygen from the lungs to the tissues. The primary Baxter development effort has been directed to the use of hemoglobin based formulations that are often referred to as hemoglobin based oxygen carriers (HBOCs). Since these formulations may potentially be used to treat conditions for which blood is not used, this class of agents is often referred to as hemoglobin therapeutics.

Researchers have infused solutions containing hemoglobin with varying degrees of success since 1868. However, due to a number of technical limitations, and the corresponding lack of success, research in this field languished until the 1970s when it was realized that many of the adverse side effects that plagued early efforts were due to inadequate purification. This in turn led to recognition of the fact that even highly purified hemoglobin does not function well outside of the red cell, unless it is appropriately modified. Fortunately, in the late 1970s and early 1980s, a number of modifications were identified that resulted in hemoglobins capable of functioning well when infused into the bloodstream. For the most part, all of these first-generation hemoglobin therapeutics, most of which were created more than 10 years ago, were designed to make a solution that looked identical to hemoglobin contained within a red blood cell.

Baxter Hemoglobin Therapeutics

Two first-generation hemoglobin-based oxygen carriers were under development by Baxter Hemoglobin Therapeutics and Somatogen during the 1990s (Diaspirin Cross-Linked Hemoglobin; DCLHb, trade name HemAssist) and a modified recombinant human hemoglobin (rHb1.1, trade name Optro), respectively. Each of these products had circumvented the safety concerns from dimerization of the hemoglobin tetramer by crosslinking the alpha chains (either chemically in the case of DCLHb or through recombinant engineering with rHb1.1). During the course of their respective development programs, both the Baxter product and the Somatogen product were entered into clinical trials.

Preclinical and initial clinical studies confirmed their potential utility and safety leading to further clinical development. Specifically, preclinical studies demonstrated that DCLHb and rHb1.1 were well tolerated, non-immunogenic, exhibited excellent oxygen transport properties, were retained in the circulation for clinically useful time intervals, and perfused tissues efficiently. Phase I and II studies in a variety of clinical indications found that DCLHb and rHb1.1 were safe and enhanced tissue oxygen consumption and extraction, but had significant vasopressor effects, probably due to nitric oxide (NO) binding. Furthermore, initial evidence of a potential benefit of blood transfusion avoidance and reduction was found in two Phase III surgery trials of DCLHb.

The clinical programs of these two first-generation hemoglobin products merged in 1998 with the acquisition of Somatogen by Baxter. However, the development of both first-generation hemoglobin-based oxygen carriers was discontinued by Baxter in September, 1998 after these products failed to meet the desired clinical safety endpoints. Global concerns about the clinical safety of DCLHb followed the premature termination of the Phase III US Trauma Trial due to an unfavorable imbalance of mortality results. Interestingly, these results were in contrast to the coincident European DCLHb trauma trial (HOST) involving immediate treatment at the scene of the trauma in which there was no significant increase in mortality seen among the patients receiving DCLHb. However, there were infrequently occurring but clinically significant fatal, life-threatening and serious adverse experiences observed across all trials for both DCLHb and rHb1.1 that appeared unusual or seemed to occur more often than expected for their clinical setting. These included Adult Respiratory Distress Syndrome (ARDS), Systemic Inflammatory Response Syndrome (SIRS), Multiple Organ Failures (MOF), acute pancreatitis, and myocardial ischemia.

Initially, it was believed that the vasoconstrictive effects, with the resulting increase in blood pressure seen following infusion of DCLHb or rHb1.1, would not pose a significant problem. In fact, there was considerable evidence suggesting that this pressor effect could be used to a clinical advantage, and that the first-generation products could be used as pharmacologic agents. Now it appears that the interaction of hemoglobin with nitric oxide and the physiologic and pathophysiologic consequences of this interaction may be responsible for many of the adverse effects observed with the first-generation of purified and modified hemoglobin solutions that were investigated in the clinic in the 1990s. It was hypothesized that in some vulnerable patients, the NO binding effects of the hemoglobin may have resulted in vasoconstriction in certain regional vascular beds, including the mesenteric vasculature, leading to the development of a cascade of inflammatory effects producing the eventual outcomes noted above.

Therefore, Baxter made a strategic decision to stop development of its first-generation hemoglobin products that possess significant (native) nitric oxide reactivity and to focus efforts on the development of a second-generation recombinant hemoglobin product with reduced nitric oxide scavenging.

Other HBOC Companies

Several hemoglobin-based oxygen carriers are currently undergoing product development. Biopure (Cambridge, MA, USA) is developing Hemopure (bovine hemoglobin that is glutaraldehyde cross-linked to produce a polyhemoglobin); Northfield (Northfield, IL, USA) is developing Polyheme (hemoglobin from donated human blood that is pyridoxylated to decrease the oxygen binding affinity and glutaraldehyde cross-linked to produce a polyhemoglobin); and Hemosol (Mississauga, Ontario, Canada) is developing Hemolink (hemoglobin obtained from donated human blood and O-raffinose crosslinked to produce a polyhemoglobin). All of these agents are in advanced clinical trials (Phase III) and Biopure has recently announced that they have applied for product approval with the FDA. There is limited information about the preclinical and clinical profiles of these products; however, based upon publicly available information, presentations and some publications, these products have generally been reported as effective in a variety of surgical settings for avoiding and/or reducing the requirement for allogeneic blood transfusions. The safety evaluations reported for some of these products, however, have indicated similar findings to those observed with DCLHb and rHb1.1, including hemodynamic effects (hypertension, vasoconstriction, increased systemic and pulmonary vascular resistance, bradycardia, reduced cardiac output), abdominal discomfort and adverse effects on gastrointestinal motility, skin discoloration, enzyme increases (AST, CK, LDH, lipase), pancreatitis, production of myocardial lesions, and potential interactions with endotoxin.

Baxter's Second-Generation Recombinant Human Hemoglobin Program

The Baxter Hemoglobin Therapeutics second-generation recombinant hemoglobin development program is exclusively focused on utilizing recombinant technology in the bacterium *Escherichia coli* to produce "designer" hemoglobin solutions. "Recombinant" means that the genetic information for making a therapeutic protein is inserted into the DNA of a cell such as *E. coli*. The DNA then instructs the cell to produce the desired protein, in this case, a new form of hemoglobin. This technology can be used to induce a variety of cell types to synthesize functional hemoglobin. In addition, modifications of the hemoglobin molecular structure can alter the properties of the molecule, allowing researchers to create hemoglobins with improved functionality or enhanced safety when used as hemoglobin therapeutics.

The second-generation product development effort at Baxter has been driven by the working hypothesis that many of the side effects observed after HBOC infusion are a consequence of the interaction of hemoglobin with NO. Native hemoglobin interacts very strongly with NO, a ubiquitous and potent chemical messenger found throughout the body and it appears that this scavenging of NO was associated with some of the adverse outcomes observed with the first-generation hemoglobins. Therefore, Baxter Hemoglobin Therapeutics developed a hemoglobin-based oxygen carrier with diminished NO scavenging characteristics.

Recombinant technology is the only approach known that can significantly alter the inherent interactions of hemoglobin and NO. Through recombinant technology utilizing site-directed mutagenesis, genes were constructed for several hundred hemoglobin variants. The individual hemoglobin tetramers were internally cross-linked (alpha-alpha fusions) by recombinant engineering. These variants also incorporated amino acid substitutions in the distal heme pockets of both the alpha and beta subunits of hemoglobin leading to steric hindrance for NO entry. The result of this extensive research program was the production of hemoglobin variants with markedly reduced NO reactivity that still maintained effective oxygen binding and release. Substitution of certain amino acids into the heme pockets of alpha- and beta-subunits reduced the rate constants for reaction with NO by up to 30-fold relative to wild-type hemoglobin. The systemic hemodynamic responses to these hemoglobins in rats were reduced compared to responses to hemoglobins with wild type NO scavenging rates and the magnitudes of the responses were correlated with the rates of NO scavenging. Studies in rats verified that the vasoconstrictive response (increase in mean arterial pressure) corresponded directly to the rate of NO scavenging; i.e., as NO scavenging is decreased the pressor response decreased as did most of the other adverse affects seen with the first-generation hemoglobin solutions (Fig. 1).

Baxter Hemoglobin Therapeutics determined that molecular size and its impact on extravasation were also important predictors of some of the adverse pharmacologic effects seen with the hemoglobin molecules; i.e., as the size of the molecule increased (within certain limits), some of these adverse effects diminished and circulatory half-life was increased. Therefore, Baxter Hemoglobin Therapeutics increased the molecular size of the hemoglobin through polymerization and derivatization of the individual

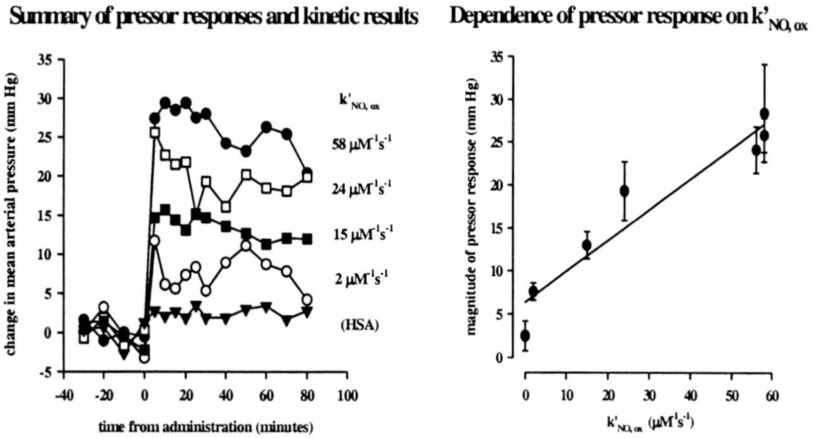

FIG. 1. Relationship between the blood pressure response in rats and NO scavenging rate of hemoglobin. 350 mg/kg topload doses ($n \geq 6$ rats/gp)

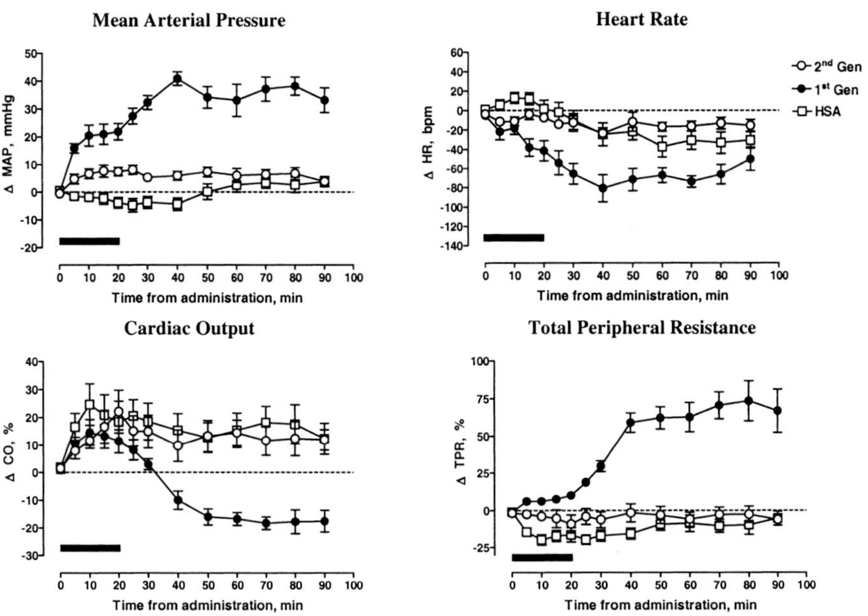

FIG. 2. Responses to 2 g/kg topload dose. *Bar* in each figure indicates duration of infusion

hemoglobin tetramers to produce larger molecular weight derivatives and polymers of the hemoglobin.

As a result of all of these specifically directed modifications to the hemoglobin molecule itself, a dramatically improved second-generation recombinant hemoglobin product has been developed. As an example, shown above (Fig. 2) are the cardiovascular responses seen following infusion of a large dose (2 g/kg) of a human serum albumin solution (HSA) oncotically matched to the second-generation hemoglobin product, or a first-generation recombinant hemoglobin product (rHb1.1), or a new and improved second-generation recombinant hemoglobin product. As seen in Fig. 2, following infusion of the second-generation Hb product, there is a dramatic decrease in the observed vasoactivity as compared to the first-generation product, there is an increase in cardiac output versus a decrease as seen with a number of the first-generation hemoglobin products, and there is no change in calculated total peripheral vascular resistance. In particular, the cardiac output and total peripheral resistance responses to the second-generation products are the same as those to HSA.

Conclusion

There is still a significant unmet medical need for HBOCs in a variety of medical situations. There are now available viable approaches to modify the intrinsic biologic properties of hemoglobin and produce improved, second-generation hemoglobin products. Testing in animals suggests that these "designer" hemoglobin products have an enhanced safety and efficacy profile as compared to first-generation products. The ultimate answer as to the value of these products will obviously lie in the results of extensive clinical testing.

Hemoglobin-Vesicles (HbV) as Artificial Oxygen Carriers

Hiromi Sakai[1], Keitaro Sou[1], Shinji Takeoka[1], Koichi Kobayashi[2], and Eishun Tsuchida[1]

Summary. Considering the physiological significance of the cellular structure of a red blood cell (RBC), it may be reasonable to mimic its structure for designing a hemoglobin (Hb)-based oxygen carrier. In this chapter, we have summarized the characteristics and performances of Hb-vesicles (HbV) that have been developed on the basis of molecular assembly. Collaborative in vitro and in vivo studies have revealed sufficient safety and efficacy of HbV.

Key words. Blood substitutes, Hemoglobin-vesicles, Red blood cells, Oxygen transport, Liposome

Introduction: Importance of Cellular Structure

When we design an artificial oxygen carrier based on hemoglobin (Hb) molecules, we may have to reconsider why Hb is encapsulated in RBCs in our body. Barcroft et al. (1923) insisted that the reasons for Hb encapsulation in RBCs were: (1) a decrease in the high viscosity of Hb and a high colloidal osmotic pressure; (2) prevention of the removal of Hb from blood circulation; and (3) preservation of the chemical environment in the cells such as the concentration of phosphates (2,3-DPG, ATP, NADPH, etc.) and other electrolytes [1]. Moreover, during the long history of development of Hb-based oxygen carriers, many side effects of molecular Hb have become apparent such as renal toxicity due to the dissociation of tetrameric Hb subunits to two dimers ($\alpha_2\beta_2 \rightarrow 2\alpha\beta$), which may induce renal toxicity and entrapment of gaseous messenger molecules (NO and CO) inducing vasoconstriction,

[1] Advanced Research Institute for Science and Engineering, Waseda University, 3-4-1 Okubo, Shinjuku-ku, Tokyo 169-8555, Japan
[2] Department of Surgery, School of Medicine, Keio University, 35 Shinanomachi, Shinjuku-ku, Tokyo 160-8582, Japan

hypertension, reduced blood flow and tissue oxygenation in the microcirculatory levels, neurological disturbances, and malfunctioning of esophageal motor function. These side effects of molecular Hb would imply the importance of cellular structure.

The pioneering work was performed by Chang (1957) [2], who started encapsulation of Hb like a RBC and prepared microcapsules (5 μm) made of nylon, collodion, etc. Toyoda (1965) [3] and Kitajima of the Kambara-Kimoto group (1971) [4] also covered Hb solution with gelatin, gum Arabic, or silicone; however, it was very difficult to regulate the particle size appropriate for blood flow in the capillaries and to obtain sufficient biocompatibility. After Bangham and Horne reported in 1964 that phospholipids assembled to form vesicles in aqueous media [5], and that they encapsulate water-soluble materials in their inner aqueous interior, it was quite reasonable to use such vesicles for Hb encapsulation. Djordjevici and Miller (1977) prepared liposome-encapsulated Hb (LEH) composed of phospholipids, cholesterol, fatty acid, etc [6]. Hunt, Kondo, Chapman, Gaber, Farmer, Beissinger, Chang, Schmidt, Farmer, Rudolph and others attempted LEH [7–16]. In the United States, Naval Research Laboratories showed the remarkable progress of LEH. Hemoglobin-vesicles (HbV), with a high efficiency production process and improved properties, have been established by Tsuchida's group, based on the technologies of molecular assembly and precise analysis of pharmacological and physiological aspects [1,17] (Fig. 1).

In this chapter we summarize the characteristics of HbV based on the science of molecular assembly and its excellent results.

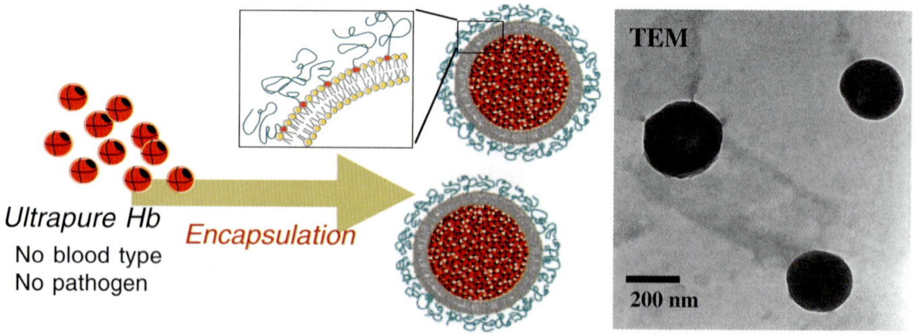

FIG. 1. Hb-vesicles (diameter, ca. 250 nm) are prepared from ultrapure Hb obtained from outdated RBC. The surface of the vesicles is modified with polyethyleneglycol that ensures the dispersion stability during storage and during circulation in the blood stream. Transmission electron micrograph (TEM) clearly demonstrates the well-regulated particle size and high Hb content within the vesicles

Preparation and Characteristics of HbV as a Molecular Assembly

Purification of Hb for the Utmost Safety

The primary advantage of using an artificial oxygen carrier should the absence of risk of infectious diseases derived from human blood. Even though strictly inspected RBCs after expiration of limitation period are used as a source of Hb, it is necessary to introduce additional procedures to inactivate and remove viruses in the process of Hb purification in order to guarantee the utmost safety from infection. In our purification process, virus inactivation was performed by pasteurization at 60°C for 12 h, which are the same conditions used for the pasteurization of human serum albumin [18,19]. This process can be introduced by utilizing the stability of carbonylhemoglobin (HbCO). The thermograms of HbCO indicated the denaturation temperature at 78°C, which is much higher than that for oxyhemoglobin (64°C) [20] (Fig. 2).

The virus inactivation efficiency was evaluated by the Hokkaido Red Cross Blood Center [21,22]. The Hb solution spiked with vesicular stomatitis virus (VSV) was treated at 60°C for 1 h under either an air or CO atmosphere. VSV was inactivated at less than 5.8 $\log_{10}$ and less than 6.0 $\log_{10}$ under the air and

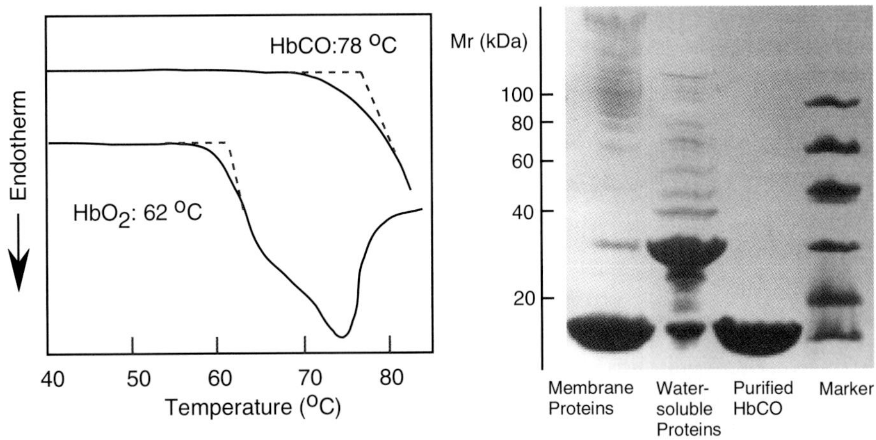

FIG. 2. **Left**, the calorimetric thermograms of HbCO solution showed the decomposition temperature at 78°C, indicating the thermal stability for pasteurization at 60°C. The amount of sample was 60 µl (6.0 g/dl). The heating speed was 1.0°C/min. **Right**, SDS-PAGE of HbCO after the heat treatment (60°C, 12 h), indicates the purity and no contamination of other proteins derived from RBC. The concentration of Hb applied to the gel was 10 mg/ml, which was 10 times higher than the maximum concentration described in the instruction manual of PhastSystem, in order to show the absence of other bands in the purified HbCO

CO atmosphere, respectively. Although the methemoglobin (metHb) rate increased after the heat treatment under the air atmosphere, no metHb formation was observed by the treatment under the CO atmosphere. Isoelectric focusing analysis revealed the denaturation of Hb after the heat treatment under the air, while the Hb band was not altered in the carbonylated condition. Some protein bands other than Hb had disappeared on sodiumdodecylsulfate-polyacrylamide gel electrophoresis (SDS-PAGE) and isoelectric focusing (IEF) after the heat treatment. During the pasteurization, all the other concomitant proteins are denatured and precipitated. As a result, we obtain ultrapure Hb solution. This high purity is essential to prevent membrane plugging during the next ultrafiltration process.

We tested ultrafiltration of HbCO solution to remove viruses with PLANOVA-35N and -15N (Bemberg Microporous Membrane: BMM; Asahi Kasei, Tokyo, Japan) [23]. The virus removal mechanism is by size exclusion through the capillary pores, and the filtration method is a depth filtration. The unit membrane which has a network structure of capillaries and voids is accumulated to form 150 layers. PLANOVA -35N and -15N have mean pore sizes of 35 nm and 15 nm, respectively. PLANOVA-35N is suitable for removing envelope-type viruses such as HIV, and HCV of which the size ranges from 40 nm to 100 nm, PLANOVA -15N can be used to remove the nonenvelope-type viruses, such as parvoviruses, of which the size is less than 40 nm. However, when the pores of the membrane filter are plugged by impurities, the PLANOVA-35N is sometimes used as a prefilter for PLANOVA-15N. The permeation flux (LMH) and the permeated ratio of HbCO solution ([Hb] = 5.6 g/dl) through PLANOVA-35N at 13°C were 36 ($L/m^2/h$) and almost 100 (%), respectively. Those through PLANOVA-15N at 13°C were 15 ($L/m^2/h$) and 95 (%), respectively. The LMH increased to 18 ($L/m^2/h$) at 25°C. Under the same conditions, a high removal efficiency of a bacteriophage, $\phi \times 174$, (>7.7 log) was confirmed. These results indicate that PLANOVA-15N is effective for the process of virus removal from Hb solutions. We also confirmed the effectiveness of other virus removal ultrafiltration systems such as Viresolve.

Thus, purified HbCO solution can be concentrated to above 40 g/dl very effectively using an ultrafiltration process. After regulation of the electrolyte concentrations, this is supplied for encapsulation procedure. The ligand of the resulting HbV, CO, is converted to O_2 by illuminating the liquid membrane of HbV suspension to a visible light under O_2 flow [24].

Other groups have selected methods to preserve the well-organized enzymatic systems originally present in the RBCs aiming at the prolonged stability of ferrous state of Hb [25,26]. However, this may cause insufficient virus removal or inactivation and cannot guarantee the utmost safety of the resulting artificial oxygen carrier. One advantage of HbV is that any reagent can be coencapsulated in the vesicles. It has been confirmed that coencapsulation of an appropriate amount of a reductant, such as glutathione or homocysteine, and active oxygen scavengers, such as catalase, effectively retards the metHb formation [27–31].

Effective Hb Encapsulation

The performance of HbV depends on the weight ratio of Hb to lipid ([Hb]/[Lipid]). This value is improved by lowering the number of bilayer membrane (lamellarity) of the vesicle and raising the concentration of Hb in the interior of the vesicle. We studied the optimal conditions for Hb encapsulation using an extrusion method and considering the behaviors of Hb and lipid assemblies as a kind of polymer electrolyte [32–35].

The maximum [Hb]/[Lipid] ratio that would relate to the isoelectric point (pI) of Hb can be obtained at ca. pH 7. The Hb molecule is negatively charged when pH is above 7.0, and the electrostatic repulsion between Hb and the negatively charged bilayer membrane results in lower encapsulation efficiency. However, the lower pH should enhance Hb denaturation by interaction with the lipid bilayer membrane and metHb formation at a lower pH. Therefore, the physiological pH, 7.0–7.4, would be optimal. It was also revealed that the higher ionic strength shields the repulsion between the negatively charged lipid bilayer membranes and increases the lamellarity.

The number of bilayer membranes decreases with increased microviscosity (decreased lipid mobility). Multilamellar vesicles are converted to smaller vesicles with smaller lamellarity during the extrusion procedure. When membrane fluidity is high, deformation of vesicles during extrusion occurs more easily, even for multilamellar vesicles, resulting in larger lamellarity in the final vesicles. Therefore, the use of lipids with higher phase transition temperature is preferred. However, these lipids would make extrusion more difficult, because a higher shear stress (high extrusion pressure) is required. Based on this reasoning, mixed lipids contain 1,2-dipalmitoyl-*sn*-glycero-3-phosphatidylcholine (DPPC) as the main component.

Based on the precise analysis of the characterization of the physicochemical properties of the components, the encapsulation efficiency of Hb solution in a size-regulated phospholipid vesicle has been improved using an extrusion method [36,37]. Mixed lipids (DPPC, cholesterol, 1,5-*O*-dioctadecyl-*N*-succinyl-L-glutamate (DPEA), and 1,2-distearoyl-*sn*-glycero-3-phosphoethanolamine-*N*-[monomethoxy poly(ethylene glycol) (5,000)] (PEG-DSPE)] at a molar ratio of 5, 5, 1, and 0.033 were hydrated with a NaOH solution (7.6 mM) to obtain a polydispersed multilamellar vesicle dispersion (50 nm–30 μm in diameter). The polydispersed vesicles were converted to smaller vesicles having an average diameter of ca. 500 nm with a relatively narrow size distribution by freeze-thawing at a lipid concentration of 2 g/dl and cooling rate of −140°C /min. The lyophilized powder of the freeze-thawed vesicles was rehydrated into a concentrated Hb solution (40 g/dl) and retained the average size and distribution of the original vesicles. The resulting vesicle dispersion smoothly permeated through the membrane filters during extrusion. The average permeation rate of the freeze-thawed vesicles was ca. 30 times faster than that of simple hydrated vesicles. During the extrusion process, Hb solution was encapsulated into the reconstructed vesicles effectively with a diameter of 250 ± 20 nm, and the [Hb]/[lipid] ratio reached 1.7–1.8.

Regulation of Oxygen Affinity

Oxygen affinity of purified Hb (expressed as P_{50}, O_2 tension at which Hb is half-saturated with O_2) is about 5 Torr, and Hb strongly binds O_2 and does not release O_2 at 40 Torr (partial pressure of mixed venous blood). Historically, it has been regarded that the O_2 affinity of an Hb-based O_2 carrier (HBOC) should be regulated similarly to that of RBC, namely about 25–30 Torr, using an allosteric effector, or by a direct chemical modification of the Hb molecules. Theoretically, this allows sufficient O_2 unloading during blood microcirculation, as could be evaluated by the arterio-venous difference in O_2 saturation in accordance with an O_2 equilibrium curve. It has been expected that decreasing the O_2 affinity (increasing P_{50}) results in an increase in the O_2 unloading. This expectation is supported by the result that the RBC with a high P_{50} shows an enhanced O_2 release for improved exercise capacity in a mouse model [38].

If this theory is correct, P_{50} of Hb in HbV should be equivalent to that of human RBCs, i.e., 28 Torr, or higher. Pyridoxal 5′-phosphate (PLP) is coencapsulated in HbV as an allosteric effector to regulate P_{50} [39]. The main binding site of PLP is the *N*-terminal of the α- and β-chains and β-82 lysine within the β-cleft, which is part of the binding site of natural allosteric effector, 2,3-diphosphoglyceric acid (2,3-DPG) [40]. The bound PLP retards the dissociation of the ionic linkage between β-chains of Hb during conversion of deoxy to oxyHb in the same manner as does 2,3-DPG. Thus, oxygen affinity of Hb decreases in the presence of PLP. The P_{50} of HbV can be regulated to 5–150 Torr by coencapsulating the appropriate amount of PLP or inositol hexaphosphate as an allosteric effector [41]. Equimolar PLP to Hb (PLP/Hb = 1/1 by mol) was coencapsulated, and P_{50} was regulated to 18 Torr. When the molar ratio PLP/Hb was 3/1, P_{50} was regulated to 32 Torr. The O_2 affinities of HbV can be regulated quite easily without changing other physical parameters, whereas in the case of the other modified Hb solutions their chemical structures determine their O_2 affinities, thus regulation is difficult. The appropriate O_2 affinities for O_2 carriers have not yet been completely decided;

however, the easy regulation of O_2 affinity may be useful to meet the requirement of the clinical indications such as oxygenation of ischemic tissues (see section "Improved Oxygenation in Ischemic Hamster Flap Tissue by Hemodilution with HbV").

Surface Modification of HbV and Its Stability During Long-Term Storage

Since Hb autoxidizes to form metHb and loses its oxygen-binding ability during storage as well as in blood circulation, the prevention of metHb formation is required. The conventional long-term preservation methods are to store modified Hbs in a frozen state or to store them as a freeze-dried powder with some cryoprotective or lyoprotective agents such as saccharides or polyols [42,43]. Some groups have recently reported a method to preserve deoxygenated Hbs in a liquid state [44], using the well-known intrinsic characteristic of Hb that the Hb oxidation rate in a solution is dependent on the oxygen partial pressure and deoxyHb essentially is not autoxidized at ambient temperature [45,46].

In the case of HbV, not only the inside Hb, but also the cellular structure has to be physically stabilized in order to prevent intervesicular aggregation, fusion, and leakage of encapsulated Hb and other reagents. Phospholipid vesicles are molecular assemblies and generally regarded as unstable capsules which require some reinforcement. We studied the γ-ray polymerization in the bilayer membranes of phospholipids bearing dienoyl groups, and the resulting polymerized phospholipid membrane significantly stabilized HbV [47–49]. The polymerized vesicles preserved the particle diameter and function of the inside Hb even after 10 repeated freeze-thawings and freeze-dryings and rehydrations [50,51]. However, the relatively slow rate of metabolism of the polyphospholipid in the reticuloendothelial systems is considered to be a problem. Cryoprotection and lyoprotection of the HbV were performed by the addition of saccharides such as trehalose [52] or glycolipid [53]. However, preservation of the oxygen carriers in a liquid state may be more useful for infusion in emergency situations than the time-consuming procedures such as redissolving the Hb powder or thawing several hundred milliliters of the frozen Hb solution stored in a freezer.

Surface modification of phospholipid vesicles with the poly(ethylene glycol) (PEG)-conjugated lipid is a well-known method to prolong the circulation time of the vesicles in vivo for drug delivery systems [54,55]. For HbV, the surface of HbV was also modified with PEG chains to improve its dispersion state of the vesicles when mixed with blood components [56]. The PEG-modified HbV has shown an improved blood circulation and tissue oxygenation due to the absence of HbV aggregate formation and viscosity ele-

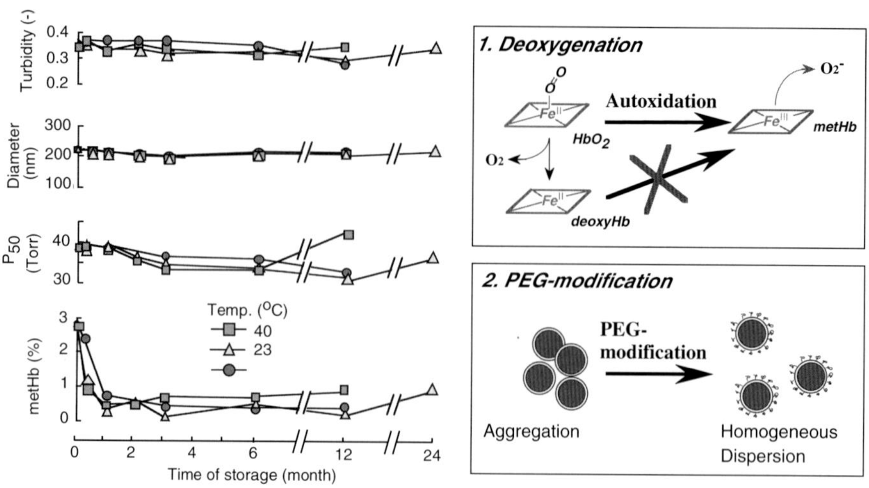

FIG. 3. Stability of HbV during storage for up to 24 months. Deoxygenation is important to prevent autoxidation to metHb, and PEG-modification suppresses aggregation and fusion of HbV to stabilize the dispersion condition. Both techniques are essential for the long-term storage of HbV. A reductant coencapsulated in HbV not only consumed a *trace amount of oxygen* but also gradually reduced metHb

vation [57,58] and prolonged circulation persistence in vivo [59]. However, little attention has been paid to the ability of PEG modification for the long-term preservation of vesicles or liposomes in the liquid state [60,61].

We studied the possibility of the long-term preservation of HbV by the combination of two technologies, i.e., surface modification of HbV with PEG chains and deoxygenation during storage for 2 years [62] (Fig. 3). The samples stored at 4° and 23°C showed a stable dispersion state for 2 years, although the sample stored at 40°C showed the precipitation and decomposition of vesicular components, a decrease in pH, and 4% leakage of total Hb after 1 year. The PEG chains on the vesicular surface stabilize the dispersion state and prevent the aggregation and fusion due to their steric hindrance. The original metHb content (ca. 3%) before the preservation gradually decreased to less than 1% in all the samples after 1 month due to the presence of homocysteine inside the vesicles which consumed the residual oxygen and gradually reduced the trace amount of metHb. The rate of metHb formation was strongly dependent on the partial pressure of oxygen, and no increase in metHb formation was observed due to the intrinsic stability of the deoxygenated Hb. These results indicate the possibility that HbV suspension can be stored at room temperature for at least 2 years.

Generally, phospholipid vesicles are regarded as unstable capsules; however, the establishment of this pivotal technology will enhance the application of PEG-modified vesicles in other fields. The long-term preservation of oxygen carriers overcomes the limitation of the blood transfusion system and will be of benefit to clinical medicine.

Interaction of Lipopolysaccharide (LPS) with HbV and Quantitative Measurement of LPS

The production process of HbV has to be guaranteed with a good manufacturing practice (GMP) standard as a biological product regarding the strict regulation of impurity and viral and bacterial contamination. It is required to strictly monitor the content of the lipopolysaccharide (LPS), known as an endotoxin, a component of the outer membrane of gram-negative bacteria possessing a large variety of biological influences on numerous mammalian cells and tissues. Endotoxin is an extremely potent toxin with a lethal dose (LD_{50}) of 3 mg/kg and 1 mg/kg in rats and dogs, respectively [63,64]. The U.S. Food and Drug Administration (FDA) has established a guideline on human maximum endotoxin dose permissible for parenteral products (5 EU/kg) [65] that may include Hb-based oxygen carriers. This limit is based on the endotoxin activity (Endotoxin Unit: EU; 1 EU = 100 pg), and can be measured via the *Limulus* amebocyte lysate (LAL) assay, in which LAL clots and forms a gel in the presence of LPS [66]. In general, the LAL method has advantages over rabbit pyrogen testing, because the LAL method requires a smaller sample, and the assays can easily be repeated [67]. Since the volume of oxygen carriers to be infused for shock resuscitation or acute hemodilution is estimated to be less than 20 ml/kg, the specific endotoxin limits per millimeter should be 0.25 EU/ml (= 5/20), similar to that for water for injection (0.25 EU/ml).

Bacterial LPS is an amphiphilic macromolecule; therefore, it hydrophobically interacts with protein and biomembranes [68]. Hb strongly interacts with LPS showing synergistic toxicity [69,70]. The constituent of endotoxin that causes LAL gelation is a glycophospholipid-designated lipid-A [71]. Lipid-A possesses several fatty acid constituents that are readily inserted into the bilayer membrane of the phospholipid vesicles. The inclusion of lipid-A in the phospholipid vesicles markedly reduces several functions of lipid-A such as its LAL gelation activity [72]. Using isothermal titration calorimetry (ITC), we quantitatively clarified for the first time that LPS from the *Salmonella minnesota* wild type (smooth form) was inserted into the phospholipid vesicles with an enthalpy change (ΔH) of −80 kcal/mol and the maximum incorporation of 7.6 mol% on the outer surface of the vesicles [73]. To our knowledge, the ΔH value of PEG_{5000}-DSPE (MW of PEG = 5 kDa) for the same phospholipid vesicles is only −13 kcal/mol. This comparison indicates that LPS inserted into the bilayer membrane is thermodynamically more stabi-

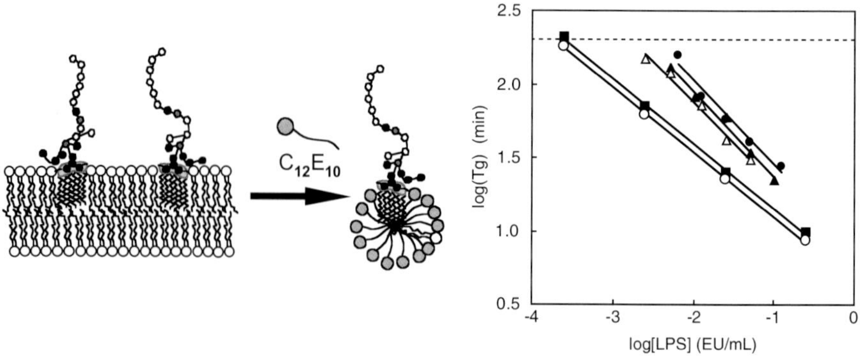

FIG. 4. (*Left*) Solubilization of LPS-contaminated vesicles with a detergent to form mixed micelles. (*Right*) Calibration curves for the quantitative measurement of LPS in the presence of $C_{12}E_{10}$ at various concentrations (vol%); 2.0 (●), 0.8 (▲), 0.4 (△), 0.1 (■), 0 (○). [LPS] is the final concentration in the test tube for turbidimetry. Dilution factors should be multiplied to obtain [LPS] in the HbV suspension at [Hb] = 10 g/dl. For example, [LPS] should be multiplied with 400 at [$C_{12}E_{10}$] = 0.1 wt%. The *broken line* indicates the gelation time limit for Toxinometer (200 min)

lized than PEG_{5000}-DSPE. The large difference in ΔH is probably due not only to the hydrophobic interactions by the eight alkyl chains of LPS but also to the hydrogen bonding of the amide bonds into the interface of the hydrophobic and hydrophilic regions that contribute to the interaction of LPS with the phospholipid bilayer membrane. As for the interaction between Hb and LPS, the ITC analysis was recently reported by Jurgens et al. [74], who clarified that 3–5 LPS molecules bind to one Hb molecule. As a consequence, the researchers who study HbV or other phospholipid vesicles for delivering other functional molecules encountered a problem in measuring the LPS content for the quality control of these materials [75–77].

Considering this background information, we tested the solubilization of HbV with deca(oxyethylene) dodecyl ether ($C_{12}E_{10}$) to release the LPS entrapped in the vesicles as a pretreatment for the succeeding LAL assay of the kinetic-turbidimetric gel clotting analysis using Toxinometer (Wako Pure Chem. Ind. Ltd., Tokyo, Japan) (detecting wavelength, 660 nm) [73] (Fig. 4). The $C_{12}E_{10}$ surfactant interferes with the gel clotting in a concentration-dependent manner, and the optimal condition was determined in terms of minimizing the dilution factor and $C_{12}E_{10}$ concentration. We clarified the condition that allowed the measurement of LPS higher than 0.1 EU/ml in the HbV suspension. This modified LAL assay using $C_{12}E_{10}$ and the Toxinometer is routinely used in our production system of HbV. Significant attention is paid to the quality control of HbV for preclinical studies, and all the HbV prepared under sterile conditions showed an LPS content less than 0.1 EU/ml at [Hb] = 10 g/dl.

Moreover, the utilization of the histidine-immobilized agarose gel (Pyrosep; Wako Pure Chem. Ind. Ltd., Tokyo, Japan) effectively concentrated the trace amount of LPS from the $C_{12}E_{10}$-solubilized HbV solution and washed out $C_{12}E_{10}$ as an inhibitory element [78]. The LAL assay with the LPS-adsorbed gel resulted in the detection limit of 0.0025 EU/ml. The pretreatment with $C_{12}E_{10}$ would be applicable not only to HbV but also to other drug delivery systems using phospholipid vesicles encapsulating or incorporating functional molecules.

Interaction with Active Oxygen Species

It has been pointed out that that heme-mediated reactions of chemically modified Hbs such as ligand coordinations and redox reactions could cause organ dysfunction and/or tissue damage. Especially, redox reactions may affect the physiological protection against reactive oxygen species [79]. The oxidation of oxyHb by H_2O_2 is known to generate ferrylHb and metHb accompanied by heme degradation and the release of free iron. Furthermore, during the autoxidation of oxyHb to metHb, reactive oxygen species such as superoxide, hydrogen peroxide, and the hydroxyl radical are generated to damage not only the remaining oxyHb but also living cells and organs. Especially, ferrylHb is known to be a potent oxidant which catalyzes the peroxidation of lipids comprising the biomembrane and other biomaterials [80,81]. In normal human plasma, the concentration of H_2O_2 is 4–5 μM [82] and elevates to 100–600 μM under inflammatory [83] or ischemia/reperfusion conditions [84]. In fact, ferrylHb can be found both in the RBCs [85] and in the endothelial cells model after hypoxia reoxygenation [86,87]. Several *in vitro* studies suggest that free radicals or degradation products catalyzed by ferrylHb could damage the endothelial cells in the presence of acellular-type Hb modifications. Hb-mediated cytotoxicity via ferrylHb is one of the important safety issues of HBOCs [88].

On the other hand, in the cellular-type HbV, reactive oxygen species generated within the HbV during metHb formation were completely consumed by Hb. Although such a reaction leads to Hb oxidation, no reactive oxygen species have been detected outside the vesicles. However, reaction of Hb inside the vesicle with exogenous H_2O_2 is one of the important safety issues to be clarified and compared with a free Hb solution. We confirmed that during the reaction of the Hb solution with H_2O_2, metHb and ferrylHb are produced, and H_2O_2 is decomposed by the catalase-like reaction of Hb [89]. The aggregation of discolored Hb products due to heme degradation is accompanied by the release of iron (ferric ion). On the other hand, the concentrated Hb within the vesicles reacts with H_2O_2 that permeated across the bilayer membrane, and the same products as the Hb solution were formed inside the vesicles. However, there is no turbidity change, no particle diameter change of the HbV, and no peroxidation of lipids comprising the vesicles after the reaction with H_2O_2. Furthermore, no free iron is detected outside the vesicle, though ferric ion is released from the denatured Hb inside the vesicle, indicating the barrier effect of the bilayer membrane against the permeation of ferric ion. When vesicles composed of egg yoke lecithin (EYL) as unsaturated lipids are added to the mixture of Hb and H_2O_2, the lipid peroxidation is caused by ferrylHb and hydroxyl radical generated from reaction of the ferric iron with H_2O_2. However, no lipid peroxidation is observed in the case of the HbV dispersion because the saturated lipid membrane of the HbV should prevent the interaction of the ferrylHb or ferric iron with the EYL. These results indicate the high safety of the Hb vesicles which enclose the reactive Hb products in the reaction with H_2O_2.

Influence of HbV on Clinical Laboratory Tests and Countermeasures

One of the remaining issues of the chemically modified acellular Hbs is the interference during clinical laboratory tests by the presence of Hbs in the serum. This topic has been extensively discussed in the field of clinical chemistry and laboratory medicine [90–94]. Even though clinical laboratory assays of blood serum components play an important role in the diagnosis and the care of many peri- or postoperative and traumatic patients, both hemolysis and lipemia are well known to cause interference in many colorimetric and spectrophotometric methods in routine automated assays. Accordingly, the presence of HBOCs interferes with the measurements due to the strong optical absorbances attributed to the Hb species (400–600 nm in wavelength). An appropriate pretreatment or calculation to subtract the deviation should be required to obtain accurate concentrations of the analytes. HbV particles (diameter, 250 nm), which possess both the Hb absorption and light scattering, show strong interference in various measurements [95]. It is important to clarify the interference of the HbV suspension in clinical laboratory tests performed on serum and to establish a pretreatment method to avoid such interference (Fig. 5).

The HbV suspension, acellular Hb solution ([Hb] = 10 g/dl) or saline, was mixed with a pooled human serum at various ratios up to 50 vol% ([Hb] = 5 g/dl), and the magnitude of the interference effect of HbV and Hb on 30 analytes was studied. The mixture of the HbV suspension and serum was ultracentrifuged (50,000 g, 20 min) to remove the HbV particles as precipitate, and the supernatant was analyzed and compared with the saline control group. The HbV particles were also removed by centrifugation (2,700 g, 30 min) in the presence of dextran (Mw 200 kDa). The HbV suspension showed considerable interference effects in most analytes. The majority of these

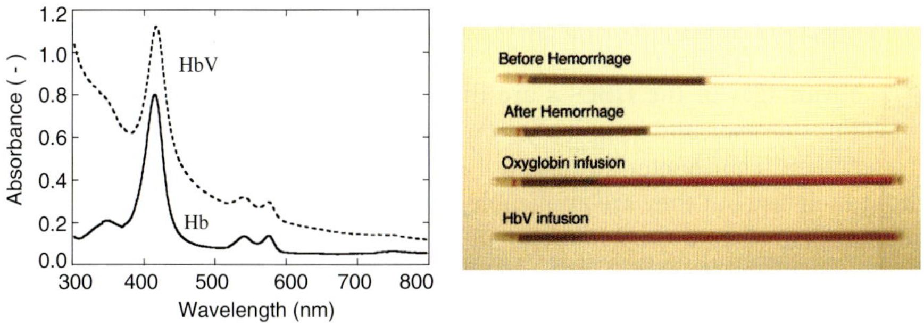

FIG. 5. **Left**, absorption spectrum of Hb and HbV at [Hb] = 0.01 g/dl in a 10 mm cuvette measured using a UV/vis spectrophotometer. The significant turbidity is confirmed especially at shorter wavelength for an HbV suspension. **Right**, glass capillaries for the hematocrit measurements during the resuscitation of hemorrhagic shocked hamsters. The centrifuged glass capillary containing blood after the infusion of glutaraldehyde-polymerized bovine Hb showed a red colored supernatant due to the presence of Hb components. In the case of HbV infusion, HbV does not precipitate at the normal centrifugation condition (10,000 g, 5 min), therefore, the supernatant is red and turbid

effects were more serious than those of the acellular Hb solution. These findings are thought to be due to the light absorption of Hb in HbV and/or the light scattering generated in the suspension that interferes with the colorimetric and turbidimetric measurements. The components of HbV may also interfere with the chemical reactions of the studied assays. However, removal of the HbV from the supernatant diminished the interference in most of the assays. This pretreatment of plasma allows accurate measurements of total protein, albumin, globulin, AST, ALT, LDH, ALP, γ-GTP, bilirubin, creatinine, urea nitrogen, uric acid, amylase, lipase, creatinine phosphokinase, total cholesterol, free cholesterol, β-lipoprotein, HDL-cholesterol, total lipid, free fatty acid, phospholipid, and electrolytes (Na, K, Cl, Ca, inorganic phosphate, Mg, Fe, and Cu). Neutral fat was not measured accurately due to the sedimentation by ultracentrifugation.

This pretreatment may be applicable to the removal of perfluorocarbon particles as another type of O_2 carrier, because it is reported that the particles form aggregation in the presence of dextran [96]. We currently utilize the pretreatment of ultracentrifugation for the safety study of HbV in animal tests. Addition of Dex may be an alternative way to facilitate the precipitation of HbV at a lower centrifugal force that is more convenient for a clinical situation, because not all clinical laboratories are equipped with an ultracentrifuge. In this research, we studied the major analytes only. Further research is necessary to clarify the interference for the other measurements of analytes including hydrophobic or amphiphilic drugs or biological components that may interact with the hydrophobic bilayer membrane of HbV.

Efficacy of HbV as Oxygen Carriers in Vivo

The advantages of the HBOCs are the absence of blood-type antigens and infectious viruses, and stability for long-term storage that overwhelm the RBC transfusion. The shorter half lives of HBOCs in the blood stream (2–3 days) limit their use but they are applicable for a shorter period of use such as: (1) a resuscitative fluid for hemorrhagic shock in an emergency situation for a temporary time or bridging until the packed RBCs are available, (2) a fluid for preoperative hemodilution or perioperative O_2 supply fluid for a hemorrhage in an elective surgery to avoid or delay allogeneic transfusion, (3) a priming solution for the circuit of an extracorporeal membrane oxygenator (ECMO), and (4) other potential indications, e.g., so-called O_2 therapeutics to oxygenate ischemic tissues.

One particle of HbV (diameter, ca. 250 nm) contains about 30,000 Hb molecules. Since HbV acts as a particle in the blood, not as a solute, the colloid osmotic pressure of the HbV suspension is nearly zero. It requires the addition of a plasma expander for a large substitution of blood to maintain blood volume. The candidates of plasma expanders are human serum albumin (HSA), hydroxyethyl starch, dextran, or gelatin depending on the clinical setting, cost, countries and clinicians. The absence of any infectious disease from humans is the greatest advantage of recombinant human serum albumin (rHSA) and it will soon be approved as an alternative for clinical use in Japan. Moreover, there should be no immunological and hematological abnormalities that are often seen in the use of dextran and hydroxyethyl starch. Aiming at application of HbV suspended in a plasma expander to the above indications, HbV was tested for resuscitation from hemorrhagic shock [97–100] and extreme hemodilution [57,58,101–105] in the Waseda-Keio group and with Prof. Intaglietta at the University of California, San Diego. Moreover, HbV was tested for oxygenation of an ischemic skin flap by Dr. Erni et al. at Inselspital University Hospital, Bern [106,107], and this implies the further application of HbV for other ischemic diseases such as myocardial and brain infarction and stroke. Some of the published results are summarized in this section.

Resuscitation from Hemorrhagic Shock with HbV Suspended in Recombinant Human Serum Albumin [100]

Objective. The ability of the suspension of HbV to restore the systemic condition after hemorrhagic shock was evaluated in anesthetized Wistar rats for 6 h after resuscitation.

Methods. The HbV was suspended in a 5 g/dl recombinant human serum albumin solution (HbV/rHSA) at an Hb concentration of 8.6 g/dl. Forty male

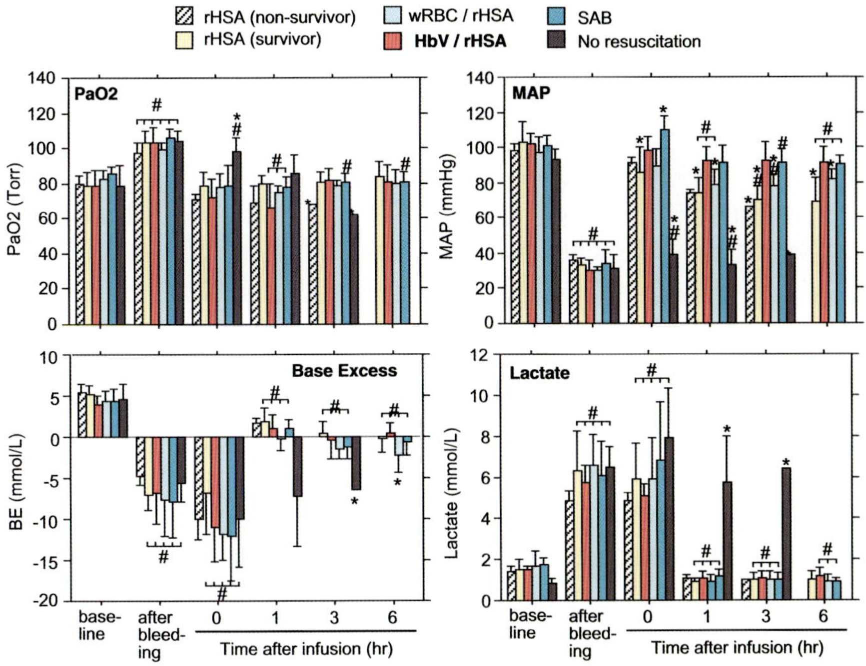

FIG. 6. Changes in mean arterial pressure (MAP) and blood gas parameters during hemorrhagic shock and resuscitation with infusion of HbV suspended in recombinant human serum albumin (HbV/rHSA), shed autologous blood (SAB), washed red blood cells suspended in recombinant human serum albumin (wRBC/rHSA), and recombinant human serum albumin (rHSA) alone. The sham group did not receive a resuscitative fluid after the hemorrhage, and died within 3 h. The number of surviving rats was 3 at 1 h. In the rHSA group, 2 of the 8 rats died between 1 and 6 h. Accordingly, the rHSA group was divided into the rHSA(survivor) group and the rHSA(non-survivor) groups until they died. Therefore, the number of rats (n) for the rHSA(survivor) and rHSA(non-survivor) groups were 6 and 2, respectively. # significantly different from baseline ($p < 0.05$), * significantly different versus the HbV/rHSA group ($p < 0.05$)

Wistar rats were anesthetized with 1.5% sevoflurane inhalation throughout the experiment. Polyethylene catheters were introduced through the right jugular vein into the right atrium for infusion and into the right common carotid artery for blood withdrawal and mean arterial pressure (MAP) monitoring.

Measurements and Main Results. Shock was induced by 50% blood withdrawal. The rats showed hypotension (MAP = 32 ± 10 mmHg) and significant metabolic acidosis and hyperventilation (Fig. 6). After 15 min, they received HbV/rHSA, shed autologous blood (SAB), washed homologous red blood cells (wRBC) suspended in rHSA (wRBC/rHSA, [Hb] = 8.6 g/dl), or rHSA alone.

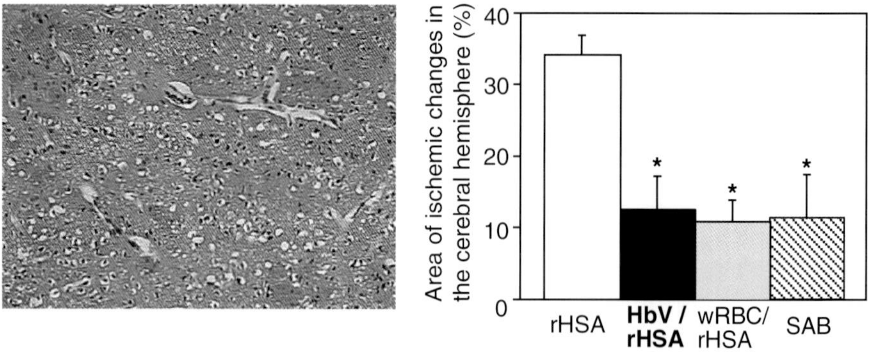

FIG. 7. Resuscitation from hemorrhagic shock with HbV suspended in rHSA in comparison with rHSA, wRBC/rHSA. The cerebral hemisphere on the right side of the rHSA group showed significant ischemic changes, a pyknotic change of the nuclei and an edematous change (34 ± 3% of the total section area) as shown in the left picture, relating to the ligation of the right carotid artery. However, the other groups that were resuscitated with O_2-carrying fluids showed minimal changes (* $p < 0.001$ vs. rHSA; HbV/rHSA, 13 ± 5%; SAB, 11 ± 6%; wRBC/rHSA, 11 ± 3%). The non-resuscitated rats did not show such ischemic changes

The HbV/rHSA group restored MAP to 93 ± 8 mmHg at 1 h, similar to the SAB group (92 ± 9 mmHg), which was significantly higher compared with the rHSA (74 ± 9 mmHg) and wRBC/rHSA (79 ± 8 mmHg) groups. There was no remarkable difference in the blood gas variables between the resuscitated groups; however, two of eight rats in the rHSA group died before 6 h. After 6 h, the rHSA group showed significant ischemic changes in the right cerebral hemisphere relating to the ligation of the right carotid artery followed by cannulation, whereas the HbV/rHSA, SAB, and wRBC/rHSA groups showed less changes (Fig. 7). These results indicate that HbV suspended in recombinant human serum albumin provides restoration from hemorrhagic shock that is comparable with that obtained using shed autologous blood.

90% Exchange Transfusion with HbV Suspended in Human Serum Albumin [58,103,104]

Objective. The effect of surface modification of HbV with poly(ethylene glycol) (Mw. 5 kDa) on hemodynamics and O_2 transport was studied by 90% exchange transfusion with the PEG-modified HbV and unmodified HbV suspended in 5% HSA in anesthetized Wistar rats.

Methods. Male Wistar rats were anesthetized with an intraperitoneal injection of sodium pentobarbital (50 mg/kg). Catheters (PE-20) were introduced into the right jugular vein for infusion (1 ml/min) and the right common carotid artery for blood withdrawal (1 ml/min) and MAP measurements. MAP and heart rate were monitored through the arterial catheter. Arterial blood samples for gas analyses were also obtained from the arterial catheter. Abdominal aortic blood flow was measured by an ultrasonic pulsed Doppler flow meter as an indicator of cardiac output. The O_2 tension of blood withdrawn from the right atrium was measured as an indicator of mixed venous O_2 tension. These values were employed to calculate O_2 delivery and consumption. Renal cortical and skeletal muscle tissue O_2 tensions were monitored as indicators of tissue perfusion. Unmodified HbV/HSA, HSA alone, and washed rat RBC suspended in 5% HSA containing 10 g/dl of Hb (ratRBC/HSA) were employed as controls.

Measurements and Main Results. Both the PEG-modified HbV/HSA and unmodified HbV/HSA groups showed sustained MAP and blood gas parameters which were comparable with ratRBC/HSA group. Only the HSA group showed the significant decline in these parameters and resulting death within 30 min after completion of exchange. The blood flow in the abdominal aorta increased 1.5 times, and the total peripheral resistance decreased in the PEG-modified HbV/HSA-administered group in comparison with the unmodified HbV/HSA group. As for the blood gas parameters, the base excess and pH remained at higher levels in the PEG-modified HbV/HSA group, and the O_2 tension in mixed venous blood for the PEG-modified HbV/HSA group tended to be maintained at a higher level than that for the unmodified HbV/HSA group. Owing to the physicochemical properties, the PEG modification of HbV reduced the viscosity by the suppression of aggregation and resulted in prompt blood circulation in vivo.

Subcutaneous Microvascular Responses to 80% Exchange Transfusion with PEG-modified and Unmodified HbV [57]

Objective. The function of PEG-modified and unmodified HbV as a blood replacement was tested in the subcutaneous microvasculature of conscious hamsters during severe hemodilution in which 80% of the RBC mass (70 ml/kg) was substituted with suspensions of the vesicles in 5% HSA solution (Fig. 8).

Methods. Conscious male Syrian golden hamsters (60–70 g) with dorsal skinfold preparation were used. Blood withdrawal and sample infusions were simultaneously performed at a rate of 0.3 ml/min. At 30%, 60%, and 80% blood exchange levels, MAP, heart rate, blood gases, and microvascular parameters were measured.

Measurements and Main Results. Both materials yielded normal MAP, heart rate, and blood gas parameters at all levels of exchange, which could not be

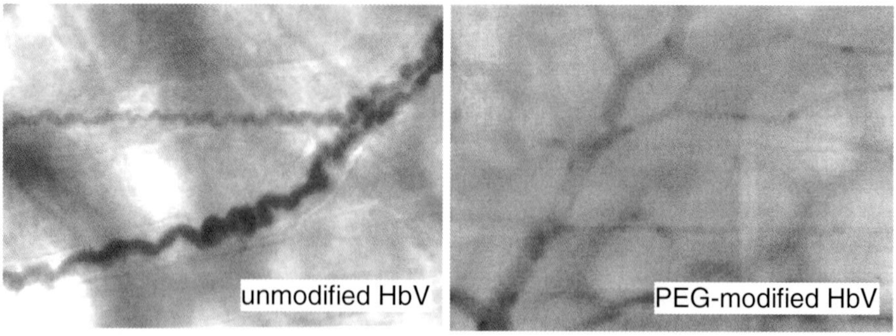

FIG. 8. Micrographs of microvasculature after 80% exchange transfusion with unmodified HbV or PEG-modified HbV suspended in 5% HSA. A high contrast was obtained by illumination with a wavelength range of around 420 nm, being absorbed at the Soret band of Hb molecules in HbV and RBC. **Left**, the aggregated vesicles block and chains in collecting venules were observed. **Right**, the microvasculature of postcapillaries is blackened owing to the homogeneous dispersion of PEG-modified HbV particles in the plasma phase. This is effective for better blood flow in the microcirculation

achieved with HSA alone. Subcutaneous microvascular studies showed that PEG-modified HbV/HSA significantly improved microhemodynamic conditions (flow rate, functional capillary density, vessel diameter, and oxygen tension) relative to unmodified HbV/HSA. PEG-modified HbV was homogeneously dispersed in the plasma phase while the unmodified HbV showed aggregation in venules and capillaries. PEG reduced vesicular aggregation and viscosity, improving microvascular perfusion relative to the unmodified type. However, the microvascular perfusion with PEG-modified HbV/HSA was lower than the blood perfused one.

Improved Oxygenation in Ischemic Hamster Flap Tissue by Hemodilution with HbV [107]

Objective. The aim of this study was to test the influence of oxygen affinity of HbVs and level of blood exchange on the oxygenation in collateralized, ischemic, and hypoxic hamster flap tissue during normovolemic hemodilution.

Methods. Microhemodynamics were investigated with intravital microscopy. Tissue oxygen tension was measured with Clark-type microprobes. HbVs with a P_{50} of 15 Torr (HbV_{15}) and 30 Torr (HbV_{30}) were suspended in 6% Dextran 70 (Dx70). The Hb concentration of the solutions was 7.5 g/dl. A stepwise replacement of 15%, 30%, and 50% of total blood volume was performed, which resulted in a gradual decrease in total Hb concentration.

Measurements and Main Results. In the ischemic tissue, hemodilution led to an increase in microvascular blood flow to maximally 141%–166% of baseline in all groups (median; $P < 0.01$ vs. baseline, not significant between groups). Tissue oxygen tension was transiently raised to 121 ± 17% after the 30% blood exchange with Dx70 ($P < 0.05$), whereas it was increased after each step of hemodilution with HbV15-Dx70 and HbV30-Dx70, reaching 217 ± 67% ($P < 0.01$) and 164 ± 33% ($P < 0.01$ vs. baseline and other groups), respectively, after the 50% blood exchange. From these results it can be concluded that despite a decrease in total Hb concentration, the oxygenation in the ischemic, hypoxic tissue could be improved with increasing blood exchange with HbV solutions. Furthermore, better oxygenation was obtained with the left-shifted HbVs.

Safety of HbV (In Vitro and In Vivo Tests)

Rheological Property and Oxygen Releasing Behavior

The rheological property of an artificial oxygen carrier is important because the infusion amount should be significantly large and that may affect the blood viscosity and hemodynamics. It has been suggested that the higher viscosity and the resulting higher perfusion pressure would be beneficial to increase the shear stress on the vascular wall for vasorelaxation and to homogeneously transmit the pressure to microvascular networks and thus to supply blood to whole capillaries [108]. PEG-modified HbV suspended in 5% HSA solution was mixed with human blood and the viscosity was measured. The viscosity was similar to that of blood, and the mixtures at various mixing ratios showed a viscosity of 3–4 cP. RBC is the main component to determine blood viscosity and the results indicate no significant interaction between HbV and RBC [39]. To observe the flow pattern of the mixture of HbV and RBC, they were mixed in various volume ratios at [Hb] = 10 g/dl in isotonic saline containing 5% HSA, and the suspension was perfused at the centerline flow velocity of 1 mm/s through an O_2 permeable fluorinated ethylenepropylene copolymer tube (inner diameter, 28 μm) exposed to a deoxygenated environment [109]. The mixtures of acellular Hb solution and RBC were also tested. Since HbV was homogeneously dispersed in the HSA solution, increasing the volume of the HbV suspension resulted in a thicker marginal RBC-free layer (Fig. 9).

In the same experimental model, measurement of the O_2 release from the narrow tube was performed using a scanning-grating spectrophotometer with a photon count detector, and the rate of O_2 release was determined based on the visible absorption spectrum in the *Q* band of Hb [109]. Irrespective of the mixing ratio, the rate of O_2 release from the HbV-RBC mixtures was

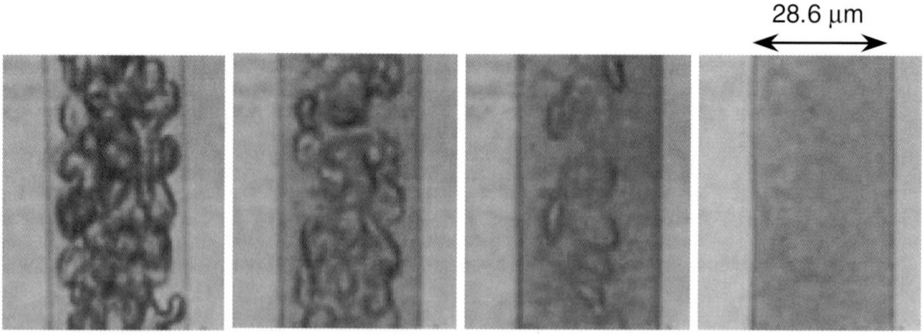

Fig. 9. Flow patterns of the mixture of HbV and RBC suspended in HSA in a narrow tube. HbV particles were homogeneously dispersed in a suspension medium. They tended to distribute in the marginal zone of the flow. The thickness of the RBC-free layer increased with the increasing amount of HbV. The RBC-free phase becomes darker and more semi-transparent, indicating the presence of HbV. Diameter of the tube = 28 μm; [Hb] = 10 g/dl; centerline flow velocity = 1 mm/s

similar with that from RBC alone. On the other hand, the addition of 50 vol% acellular Hb solution to RBC significantly enhanced the rate of deoxygenation. This outstanding difference in the rate of the O_2 release between the HbV suspension and the acellular Hb solution should mainly be due to the difference in the particle size (250 vs. 8 nm) that affects their diffusion for the facilitated O_2 transport. It has been suggested that the faster O_2 unloading from the HBOCs is advantageous for tissue oxygenation [110]. However, this concept is controversial regarding the recent finding that an excess O_2 supply would cause autoregulatory vasoconstriction and microcirculatory disorders [111–113]. We confirmed that HbV does not induce vasoconstriction and hypertension, due to not only the reduced inactivation of nitric oxide as an endothelium-derived vasorelaxation factor, but also possibly the moderate O_2 releasing rate similar to RBC as confirmed in this study.

Effects on Hematological Functions

The biocompatibility of HbV is important to clinical use. Transient thrombocytopenia was one of the most significant hematological effects observed after infusion of liposome-encapsulated Hbs in rodents [114]. Exchange transfusion with unmodified HbV (containing DPPG as a lipid component) in anesthetized rats also resulted in a slightly decreased platelet count, although the change was insignificant [104]. These effects were also observed for administration of negatively charged liposomes [115,116]. The transient reduction in platelet counts caused by liposomes was also associated with sequestration of platelets in the lung and liver. Platelet activation is necessary to prevent bleeding in vivo; however, nonphysiological activation leads to initiation and modulation of inflammatory responses because platelets contain an array of potent proinflammatory substance. RANTES (Regulated upon activation, normal T-cell expressed and presumably secreted), one of the C-C chemokines, is a useful marker for platelet activation as it is stored in α-granules of platelets and was shown to be released after stimulation. Accordingly, the biocompatibility of HbV was examined by estimating their effects on agonist-induced platelet aggregation response and RANTES release from platelets in vitro [117]. This study on biocompatibility was performed in collaboration with Dr. H. Ikeda at the Hokkaido Red Cross Blood Center (Sapporo), and his colleagues.

The effect of low concentration of HbV (Hb: 5.8 mg/dl) on platelet function was assessed by examining an agonist-induced aggregation response, and that of relatively high concentrations of HbV (Hb: 0.29, 1 and 2 g/dl) by measuring the release of RANTES from platelets, which is regarded as a marker of platelet activation. The pre-incubation of platelets with HbV at 5.8 mg/dl of Hb did not affect platelet aggregation induced by collagen, thrombin, and ristocetin. The pretreatment of platelet-rich plasma (PRP) with HbV at concentration up to 2 g/dl of Hb had no aberrant effects on the collagen-induced RANTES release. Furthermore, the collagen-induced release of RANTES from PRP was not affected by longer incubation with HbV at 2 g/dl of Hb. The basal levels of RANTES from PRP were unchanged in the presence of HbV. These results suggest that HbV, at the concentrations studied, have no aberrant effects on platelet functions in the presence of plasma.

The effect of HbV on the coagulation time (PT, APTT) was tested with human plasma. HbV was mixed with human plasma at the ratios of 20%, 40% and 60% v/v. The prothrombin time (PT) and activated partial thromboplastin time (APTT) were measured automatically. The results were compared with saline and phosphate buffered saline. The PT value increased from 10 s to 15 s with increasing the mixing ratio; however, there was no significant difference between the groups. The APTT value increased from about 40 s to about 50 s with an increase of the mixing ratio; however, there were no significant differences between the groups. The delayed coagulation is due to the dilution of the blood components, and there is no significant effect on the blood coagulation system.

Polymorphonuclear neutrophils (PMNs) are essential cells in the host defense against a variety of infectious agents. Circulating PMNs require activation to migrate to inflammatory sites and then effectively kill pathogens. Previously in the field of drug delivery systems, sterically stabilized liposomes with PEG have been reported to reduce the chemotactic activity of human PMNs in response to zymosan and the bacterially derived peptide, *N*-formyl-methionyl-leucyl-phenylalanine (fMLP) [118]. Therefore, the effects of the PEG-modified HbV on human PMNs in vitro were studied, focusing on the functional responses to fMLP as an agonist [119]. The pretreatment of PMNs with HbV up to a concentration of 56 mg/dl Hb did not affect the fMLP-triggered chemotactic activity. In parallel to these results, the fMLP-induced upregulation of CD11b (Mac-1) levels on HbV-pretreated PMNs was comparable to that of untreated cells. Furthermore, the pretreatment of PMNs with HbV even at 580 mg/dl Hb did not affect the gelatinase B [Matrix methalloproteinase-9 (MMP-9)] release, suggesting that the fMLP-induced release of secondary and tertiary granules was normal. In addition, the fMLP-triggered superoxide production of PMNs was unchanged by the pretreatment of HbV at 580 mg/dl Hb. Thus, these results suggest that HbV, at the concentrations studied, have no aberrant effects on the fMLP-triggered functions of human PMNs.

Hypertension and Vasoconstriction in Relation with NO and CO

As clinical trials of the chemically modified Hbs are extended to include larger numbers of individuals, it becomes apparent that the principal side effect consistently reported in the administration of acellular Hb solutions is hypertension presumably because of vasoconstriction. Hypertension, a well-defined reaction of the acellular intramolecularly cross-linked Hb (XLHb), was proposed to be beneficial in the treatment of hypotension concomitant to hemorrhagic shock [120]. However, vasoconstriction reduces blood flow, lowering functional capillary density, and therefore affecting tissue perfusion and oxygenation [113,121]. Nitric oxide (NO) scavenging by Hb due to intrinsic high affinity of NO to Hb is the mechanism presumed to cause vasoconstriction and hypertension [122,123]. This theory was validated indirectly using exteriorized rabbit aortic rings in organ baths, where constriction was observed following the addition of acellular Hb solutions as well as an NO synthase inhibitor [124,125]. Different modifications of the Hb molecule cause hypertension that is qualitatively and quantitatively different, and red blood cells (RBCs) and cellular HbV (liposome-encapsulated Hb) do not cause either vasoconstriction or hypertension [99,100,105]. Most evidence for the pressor response is obtained from measurements of systemic pressure, and direct evidence about the mechanism involved is scarce. In previous studies in conscious hamsters fitted with a dorsal skinfold, we found that small arteries of 130–160 μm diameter, termed resistance vessels, exhibit the greatest reactivity in hemorrhagic shock [126], playing a significant role in the regulation of blood flow. Constriction of these resistance vessels in this model was also directly correlated to the pressure response following administration of NO synthase inhibitor [127].

In collaboration with Prof. Intaglietta, we analyzed the relationship between the constriction of resistance vessel and hypertension after administration of acellular Hb and the extent to which the effect is dependent on the size of acellular Hb molecules modified by polymerization, polymer conjugation, and cellular liposome encapsulation [128]. Conscious Syrian golden hamsters with dorsal skinfold preparation were used. After the top load infusion of Hb products (7 ml/kg) into arterial catheters inserted into the jugular vein, mean arterial pressure and heart rate were monitored through the jugular arterial catheter, and microvascular responses were monitored by an intravital microscopy. The Hb products included intra-molecularly crosslinked Hb (XLHb), PEG-conjugated pyridoxalated Hb (PEG-PLP-Hb), hydroxyethyl-starch-conjugated XLHb (HES-XLHb), glutaraldehyde-polymerized XLHb (Poly-XLHb), and HbV. Their molecular diameters were 7, 22, 68, and 224 nm, respectively. The top load infusion of 7 ml/kg of XLHb (5 g/dl) caused the immediate increase of MAP, which was 34 ± 13 mmHg higher 3 h after infusion. There was a simultaneous decrease in the diameter of the resistance vessels ($79 \pm 8\%$ of basal value) which caused blood flow to decrease throughout the microvascular network. The diameter of smaller arterioles did not change significantly. Infusion of O_2 carriers of greater molecular size resulted in lesser vasoconstriction and hypertension with HbV showing the smallest changes. Infusion of HSA was used as a control and produced no microvascular or systemic effects. Constriction of resistance arteries was found to be correlated to the level of hypertension, and the responses proportional to the molecular dimensions of Hb-based O_2 carriers. Since the results correlate with molecular size it is likely that the effects are related to the diffusion properties of the different Hb molecules.

The liver is a major organ that detoxifies excess amounts of heme by the action of heme oxygenase (HO). HO decomposes protoheme IX to generate biliberdin-IXα and CO. Under normal conditions, the liver contains at least two OH isozymes for physiologic degradation of the heme: HO-1 and HO-2. One of the important roles of the HO reaction is to generate CO that serves as an endogenous regulator that is necessary for maintaining microvascular blood flow [129]. Since Hb strongly binds with CO (about 200 times stronger than O_2), it is necessary to confirm the effects of HbV in hepatic microcirculation in comparison with stroma free Hb solution. Dr. Suematsu et al. studied the perfusion of a rat liver with an acellular Hb solution and HbV, and found out that the Hb solution increased vascular resistance by 30% [130]. The smaller acellular Hb molecules (7 nm) extravasate across the fenestrated endothelium with a pore size of about 100 nm, and reach to the space of Disse. Heme is excessively metabolized by HO-2 to produce CO and bilirubin. Even though CO acts as a vasorelaxation factor in the liver, the excess amount of Hb in the space of Disse rapidly binds CO, resulting in vasoconstriction and an increase in vascular resistance. On the other hand, HbV (250 nm) is large enough to maintain in the sinusoid, and the vascular resistance is maintained.

These results indicate the importance of the size of the oxygen carriers, and that the size of HbV is appropriate for the maintenance of microvascular blood flow.

Biodistribution and Metabolism of HbV, and Influence on Organ Function

In the physiological condition, free Hb released from RBC is rapidly bound to haptoglobin, and removed from the circulation by hepatocytes. However, when the Hb concentration exceeds the haptoglobin binding capacity, unbound Hb is filtered through the kidney where it is actively absorbed. When the reabsorption capacity of the kidney is exceeded, hemoglobinuria and eventually renal failure occur. The encapsulation of Hb completely suppresses renal excretion, although HbV particles as well as phospholipid vesicles (liposomes) in the blood stream are finally captured by phagocytes in the reticuloendothelial system (RES, or mononuclear phagocytic system, MPS) [131].

To examine the precise circulation persistence and biodistribution of HbV, we used radiolabelling technique, ^{99m}Tc-labelled HbV, in collaboration with Prof. Phillips at the University of Texas. The HbV co-encapsulated homocysteine (5 mM) was successfully labeled with ^{99m}Tc by using the hexamethylpropylene amine oxime. The circulation half-life of ^{99m}Tc-HbV was determined to be 35 h. In the gamma camera image, the radioactivity in the blood pool of the heart was gradually decreased and those of the liver and spleen were increased with time. The biodistribution data showed the major organs to eliminate the ^{99m}Tc-HbV from the blood circulation were the liver, bone marrow, and spleen, independent of the injection dose. [132].

The influence of HbV on RES, mainly liver and spleen, was studied with carbon clearance measurements and histopathological examination [133]. The HbV suspension was intravenously infused in male Wistar rats (200 g) at dose rates of 10 and 20 ml/kg, and the phagocytic activity was measured by monitoring the rate of carbon clearance at 8 hs, and at 1, 3, 7 and 14 days after infusion. The phagocytic activity transiently decreased one day after infusion by about 40%, but it recovered and was enhanced at 3 days, showing a maximum of about twice the original level at 7 days, and then returned to the original level at 14 days. The initial transient decreased activity indicates a partly, but not completely, suppressed defensive function of the body. The succeeding increased phagocytic activity corresponds to the increased metabolism of HbV. The histopathological examination with hematoxylin/eosin, and anti-human Hb antibody staining showed that HbV was metabolized within 7 days. Hemosiderin was slightly confirmed with Berlin blue staining at 3 and 7 days in the liver and spleen, although they disappeared at 14 days, indicating that the heme metabolism, excretion, or recycling of the iron ion proceeded smoothly and siderosis was minimal. Electron microscopic examination of the spleen and liver tissues clearly demonstrated the vesicular structure of HbV with a diameter of about 1/40 of RBCs in capillaries, and in phagosomes as entrapped in the spleen macrophages and Kupffer cells one day after infusion. The vesicular structure could not be observed at 7 days. Even though infusion of HbV modified the phagocytic activity for two weeks, it does not seem to cause any irreversible damage to the phagocytic organs from the histological point of view.

We analyzed the influence of HbV on the organ functions by laboratory tests of plasma on a total of 29 analytes [134]. The HbV suspension was intravenously infused into male Wistar rats (20 ml/kg). The blood was withdrawn at 8 hs, and 1, 2, 3, and 7 days after infusion, and the plasma was ultracentrifuged to remove HbV in order to avoid its interference effect on the analytes. Enzyme concentrations, AST, ALT, ALP, and LAP showed significant, but minor changes, and did not show a sign of a deteriorative damage to the liver as one of the main organs for the HbV entrapment and the succeeding metabolism. The amylase and lipase activities showed reversible changes; however, there were no morphological changes in the pancreas. Plasma bilirubin and iron did not increase in spite of the fact that a large amount of Hb was metabolized in the macrophages. Cholesterols, phospholipids, and β-lipoprotein transiently increased showing the maximum at 1 or 2 days, and returned to the control level at 7 days. They should be derived from the membrane components of HbV that are liberated from macrophages entrapping HbV. In conjunction with the previous report of the prompt metabolism of HbV in the reticuloendothelial system by histopathological examination, it can be concluded that HbV infusion transiently modified the values of the analytes without any irreversible damage to the corresponding organs at the bolus infusion rate of 20 ml/kg.

In the series of safety evaluations, the repeated infusion of HbV in Wistar rats was performed at the dose rate of 10 ml/kg/day for 14 days [135]. All the rats tolerated the infusion and body weight increased continuously. The hematological test, serum blood biochemistry, and histopathological examination did not raise any serious concern about the safety of HbV. One day after the final infusion spleen and liver weights increased significantly. Histopathological observation indicated significant HbV accumulation in liver and spleen; however, there was no sign of organ damage. Serum clinical laboratory tests indicated significant increases in lipid components derived provably from HbV particles. After a 2 week interval, spleen and liver weight returned to the original levels; however, a significant amount of hemosiderin was confirmed without serum iron increase. All the concentrations of the lipid components returned to the original levels. Judging from these results, there was no sign of significant toxicity of HbV at the level of dosage employed.

Summary

The efficacy of HbV as oxygen carriers and their safety have been demonstrated. The advantages of cellular HbV can be summarized as follows:

1. The encapsulated Hb is extremely purified and free from virus, endotoxin, and blood type antigen.
2. There is no chemical modification of Hb. Dissociation of Hb tetramers to dimers is restrained and there is no release of Hb from HbV, preventing renal dysfunction.
3. The oxygen affinity is adequately adjusted and the metHb formation is restrained because both the allosteric effectors and metHb reduction systems can be coencapsulated in the vesicles.
4. HbV can be stored for over 2 years at room temperature, owing to both surface modification with PEG chains and deoxygenation.
5. The surface modification of HbV with PEG chains increases high dispersion stability and is effective to prevent aggregation in blood circulation.
6. The colloid osmotic pressure of the HbV suspension is close to zero. But it is adjustable with the addition of adequate colloids such as HSA, which is important to maintain blood volume. The solution viscosity can be adjusted equivalent to that of blood. This would be important for the shear stress on the vascular wall to regulate vascular tone.
7. HbV suspended in a plasma expander such as HSA and rHSA showed sufficient oxygen transporting capacity comparable with RBC for resuscitation from hemorrhagic shock and extreme hemodilution. It is also applicable for oxygenation of ischemic tissues.
8. The physiological activity of Hb such as binding with NO and CO, production of active oxygen species, heme release, and hemeoxygenase activation, can be minimized by encapsulation. Thus there is less vasoconstriction, hypertension, and oxygen injury.

According to the above achievements, significant efforts have been made to produce HbV with a facility of GMP standard, and to start preclinical and finally clinical trials. The combination of recombinant Hb-vesicles suspended in recombinant albumin would be the most ideal "artificial red blood cells" in the future.

Acknowledgments. This work has been supported by The Ministry of Education, Culture, Sports, Science and Technology, and The Ministry of Health, Labor and Welfare, Japan. The authors gratefully acknowledge, Dr. H.

Horinouchi, Dr. M. Watanabe, Dr. Y. Izumi (Keio Univ.), Dr. H. Ikeda (Hokkaido Red Cross Blood Center), Prof. M. Suematsu (Keio Univ.), Dr. M. Takaori (Higashitakarazuka Satoh Hospital), Prof. S. Hoka (Kitasato Univ.), Prof. R. Ogawa (Nippon Med. College), Prof. M. Intaglietta (UCSD), Prof. W.T. Phillips (Univ. Texas San Antonio), and Prof. N. Maeda (Ehime Univ.), and their active colleagues for the meaningful discussions and contributions to the research.

References

1. Tsuchida E, Takeoka S (1995) Stabilized hemoglobin vesicles. In: Tsuchida E (ed) Artificial red cells. John Wiley & Sons, Chichester, pp 35–64
2. Chang TMS (1991) Blood substitutes based on modified hemoglobin prepared by encapsulation or crosslinking: An overview. Biomater Artif Cells Immobilization Biotechnol 20:159–182
3. Toyoda T (1965) Artificial blood. Kagaku 35:7–13
4. Kitajima M, Sekiguchi W, Kondo A (1971) A modification of red blood cells by isocyanates. Bull Chem Soc Jpn 44:139–143
5. Bangham AD, Horne RW (1964) Negative staining of phospholipids and their structure modification by surface-active agents as observed in the electron microscope. J Mol Biol 8:660–668
6. Djordjevich L, Miller IF (1977) Lipid encapsulated hemoglobin as a synthetic erythrocyte. Fed Proc 36:567
7. Hunt CA, Burnette RR, MacGregor RD, et al (1985) Synthesis and evaluation of a protypal artificial red cell. Science 230:1165–1168
8. Kato A, Arakawa M, Kondo T (1984) Liposome-type artificial red blood cells stabilized with carboxymethylchitin. Nippon Kagaku Kaishi 6:987–991
9. Gaber BP, Farmer MC (1984) Encapsulation of hemoglobin in phospholipid vesicles: preparation and properties of a red cell surrogate. Prog Clin Biol Res 165:179–190
10. Hayward JA, Levine DM, Neufeld L, et al (1985) Polymerized liposomes as stable oxygen-carriers. FEBS Lett 187:261–266
11. Suzuki K, Miyauchi Y, Okamoto T, et al (1988) The characteristics and ability of NRC. Jpn J Artif Organs 17:708–711
12. Rudolph AS (1988) Freeze-dried preservation of liposome encapsulated hemoglobin: A potential blood substitute. Cryobiology 25:277–284
13. Jopski B, Pirkl V, Jaroni HW, et al (1989) Preparation of hemoglobin-containing liposomes using octyl glucoside and octyltetraoxyethylene. Biochim Biophys Acta 978:79–84
14. Mobed M, Chang TMS (1991) Preparation and surface characterization of carboxymethylchitin-incorporated submicron bilayer-lipid membrane artificial cells (liposomes) encapsulating hemoglobin. Biomater Artif Cells Immobil Biotechnol 19:731–744
15. Zheng S, Zheng Y, Beissinger R (1994) Efficacy, physical properties and pharmacokinetics of sterically-stabilized liposome-encapsulated hemoglobin. Artif Cells Blood Substitutes Immobil Biotechnol 22:487–501
16. Liu L, Yonetani T (1994) Preparation and characterization of liposome-encapsulated haemoglobin by a freeze-thaw method. J Microencapsulation 11:409–421
17. Tsuchida E (1998) Blood substitutes: present and future perspectives. Elsevier, Chichester

18. Sakai H, Takeoka S, Yokohama H, et al (1993) Purification of concentrated Hb using organic solvent and heat treatment. Protein Expression Purif 4:563–569
19. Fukutomi I, Sakai H, Takeoka S, Nishide H, Tsuchida E, Sakai K (2002) Carbonylation of oxyhemoglobin solution using a membrane oxygenator. J Artif Organs 5:102–107
20. Sakai H, Masada Y, Takeoka S, et al (2002) Characteristics of bovine hemoglobin as a potential source of hemoglobin-vesicles for an artificial oxygen carrier. J Biochem 131:611–617
21. Abe H, Ikebuchi K, Hirayama J, et al (2001) Virus inactivation in hemoglobin solution by heat treatment. Artif Cells Blood Substit Immobil Biotechnol 29:381–388
22. Huang Y, Takeoka S, Sakai H, et al (2002) Complete deoxygenation from a hemoglobin solution by an electro-chemical method and heat treatment for virus inactivation. Biotechnol Prog 18:101–107
23. Naito Y, Fukutomi I, Masada Y, et al (2002) Virus removal from hemoglobin solution using Planova membrane. J Artif Organs 5:141–145
24. Chung JE, Hamada K, Sakai H, et al (1995) Ligand exchange reaction of carbonylhemoglobin to oxyhemoglobin in a hemoglobin liquid membrane. Nippon Kagaku Kaishi 1995: 123–127
25. Takahashi A (1995) Characterization of neo red cells (NRCs), their function and safety in vivo tests. Artif Cells Blood Substitutes Immobil Biotechnol 23:347–354
26. Ogata Y, Goto H, Kimura T, et al (1997) Development of neo red cells (NRC) with the enzymatic reduction system of methemoglobin. Artif Cells Blood Substitutes Immobil Biotechnol 25:417–427
27. Teramura Y, Kanazawa H, Sakai H, et al (2003) The prolonged oxygen—carrying ability of Hb vesicles by coencapsulation of catalase in vivo. Bioconjugate Chem 14:1171–1176
28. Sakai H, Onuma H, Umeyama M, et al (2000) Photoreduction of methemoglobin by irradiation in near-ultraviolet region. Biochemistry 39:14595–14602
29. Takeoka S, Sakai H, Kose T, et al (1997) Methemoglobin formation in hemoglobin vesicles and reduction by encapsulated thiols. Bioconjugate Chem 8:539–544 (1997)
30. Takeoka S, Ohgushi T, Sakai H, et al (1997) Construction of artificial metHb reduction system in Hb-vesicles. Artif Cells Blood Substitues Immobil Biotechnol 25:31–41
31. Sakai H, Takeoka S, Seino Y, et al (1994) Suppression of methemoglobin formation by glutathione in a concentrated hemoglobin solution and in a Hb-vesicles. Bull Chem Soc Jpn 67:1120–1125
32. Takeoka S, Sakai H, Nishide H, et al (1993) Preparation conditions of human hemoglobin-vesicles covered with lipid membranes. Jpn J Artif Organs 22:566–569
33. Takeoka S, Terase K, Sakai H, et al (1994) Interaction between phosphoslipid assemblies and hemoglobin (Hb). J Macromol Sci Pure Appl Chem A31:97–108
34. Takeoka S, Sakai H, Terease K, et al (1994) Characteristics of Hb-vesicles and encapsulation procedure. Artif Cells Blood Substitutes Immobilization Biotechnol 22:861–866
35. Takeoka S, Ohgushi T, Terase K, et al (1996) Layer-controlled hemoglobin vesicles by interaction of hemoglobin with a phospholipid assembly. Langmuir 12:1755–1759
36. Sakai H, Hamada K, Takeoka S, et al (1996) Physical properties of hemoglobin vesicles as red cell substitutes. Biotechnol Prog 12:119–125
37. Sou K, Naito Y, Endo T, et al (2003) Effective encapsulation of proteins into size-controlled phospholipid vesicles using freeze-thawing and extrusion. Biotechnol Prog 19:1547–1552

38. Shirasawa T, Izumizaki M, Suzuki Y, et al (2003) Oxygen affinity of hemoglobin regulates O_2 consumption, metabolism, and physical activity. J Biol Chem 278:5035–5043
39. Sakai H, Yuasa M, Onuma H, et al (2000) Synthesis and physicochemical characterization of a series of hemoglobin-based oxygen carriers: objective comparison between cellular and acellular types. Bioconjug Chem 11:56–64
40. Benesch R, Behesch RE (1967) The effect of organic phosphates from the human erythrocyte on the allosteric properties of hemoglobin. Biochem Biophys Res Commun 26:162–167
41. Wang L, Morizawa K, Tokuyama S, et al (1992) Modulation of oxygen-carrying capacity of artificial red cells (ARC). Polymer Adv Technol 4:8–11
42. Matsumura S, Yamaji K, Ohki H, et al (1992) Large scale production and characterization of lyophylized pyridoxalated hemoglobin polyoxyethylene (PHP). Biomater Artif Cells Immobil Biotechnol 20:435–438
43. Kerwin BA, Heller MC, Levin SH, et al (1998) Effects of Tween 80 and scrose on acute short-term stability and long-term storage at –20 °C of a recombinant hemoglobin. J Pharm Sci 87:1062–1068
44. Kerwin BA, Akers MJ, Apostol I, et al (1999) Acute and long-term stability studies of deoxy hemoglobin and characterization of ascorbate-induced modifications. J Pharm Sci 88:79–88
45. Levy A, Zhang L, Rifkind JM (1988) Hemoglobin: a source of superoxide radical under hypoxic conditions. Oxy-radicals Mol Pathol Proc Upjohn-UCLA Symp 11–25
46. Balagopalakrishna C, Manoharan PT, Abugo OO, et al (1996) Production of superoxide from hemoglobin-bound oxygen under hypoxic conditions. Biochemistry 35:6393–6398
47. Tsuchida E, Hasegawa E, Kimura N, et al (1992) Polymerization of unsaturated phospholipids as large unilamellar liposomes at low temperature. Macromolecules 25:207–212
48. Hosoi F, Omichi H, Akama K, et al (1997) Radiation-induced polymerization of phospholipid mixtures for the synthesis of artificial red blood cells. Nucl Instr Methods Phys Res B 131:329–334
49. Satoh T, Kobayashi K, Sekiguchi S, et al (1992) Characteristics of artificial red cells: hemoglobin encapsulated in poly-lipid vesicles. ASAIO J 38:M580–M584
50. Wang L, Takeoka S, Tsuchida E, et al (1992) Preparation of dehydrated powder of hemoglobin vesicles. Polymer Adv Technol 3:17–21
51. Sakai H, Takeoka S, Yokohama H, et al (1992) Encapsulation of Hb into unsaturated lipid vesicles and γ-ray polymerization. Polymer Adv Technol 3:389–394
52. Rudolph AS, Cliff RO (1990) Dry storage of liposome-encapsulated hemoglobin: a blood substitute. Cryobiology 27:585–590
53. Sakai H, Takisada M, Chung JE, et al (1995) Modification of hemoglobin-vesicles with oligosaccharide chains. Artif Organs Today 4:309–316
54. Woodle MC, Lasic DD (1992) Sterically stabilized liposomes. Biochim Biophys Acta 1113:171–199
55. Klibanov AL, Maruyama K, Torchilin VP, et al (1990) Amphipathic polyethylene glycols effectively prolongs the circulation time of liposomes. FEBS Lett 268:235–237
56. Yoshioka H (1991) Surface modification of haemoglobin-containing liposomes with poly(ethylene glycol) prevents liposome aggregation in blood plasma. Biomaterials 12:861–864
57. Sakai H, Tsai AG, Kerger H, et al (1998) Subcutaneous microvascular responses to hemodilution with red cell substitutes consisting of polyethylene glycol-modified vesicles encapsulating hemoglobin. J Biomed Mater Res 40:66–78

58. Sakai H, Takeoka S, Park SI, et al (1997) Surface-modification of hemoglobin vesicles with poly(ethylene glycol) and effects on aggregation, viscosity, and blood flow during 90%-exchange transfusion in anesthetized rats. Bioconjugate Chem 8:23–30
59. Phillips WT, Klipper RW, Awasthi VD, et al (1999) Poly(ethylene glycol)-modified liposome-encapsulated hemoglobin: a long circulating red cell substitute. J Pharm Exp Ther 288:665–670
60. Singh M, Ferdous AJ, Jackson TL (1999) Stealth monensis liposomes as a potentiator of adriamycin in cancer treatment. J Controlled Release 59:43–53
61. Meyer O, Kirpotin D, Hong K, et al (1998) Cationic liposomes coated with polyethyle glycol as carriers for oligonucleotide. J Biol Chem 273:15621–15627
62. Sakai H, Tomiyama K, Sou K, et al (2000) Poly(ethylene glycol)-conjugation and deoxygenation enable long-term preservation of hemoglobin-vesicles as oxygen carriers in a liquid state Bioconjugate Chem 11:425–432
63. Fletcher JR, Ramwell PW (1980) The effects of prostacyclin on endotoxin shock and endotoxin-induced platelet aggregation in dogs. Circ Shock 7:299–308
64. Shibayama Y, Asaka S, Nakata K (1991) Endotoxin hepatotoxicity augmented by alcohol. Exp Mol Pathol 55:196–202
65. U.S. Department of Health and Human Services Public Health Service, Food and Drug Administration (1987) Guideline on validation of the limulus amebocyte lysate test as an end-product endotoxin test for human and animal parenteral drugs, biological products, and medical devices
66. Levin J, Bang FB (1964) The role of endotoxin in the extracellulalr coagulation of limulus blood. Bull Johns Hopkins Hospital 115:265–274
67. Fujiwara H, Ishida S, Shimazaki Y, et al (1990) Measurement of endotoxin in blood products using an endotoxin specific Limulus test reagent and its relation to pyrogenic activities in rabbit. Yakugaku Zasshi 110:332–340 (in Japanese)
68. Carr C Jr, Morrison DC (1984) Lipopolysaccharide interaction with rabbit erythrocyte membranes. Infect Immun 43:600–606
69. Kaca W, Roth RI, Levin J (1994) Hemoglobin, a newly recognized lipopolysaccharide (LPS)-binding protein that enhances LPS biological activity. J Biol Chem 269:25078–25084
70. Roth RI, Levin J, Chapman KW, et al (1993) Production of modified crosslinked cell-free hemoglobin for human use: the role of quantitative determination of endotoxin contamination. Transfusion 33:919–924
71. Yin ET, Galanos C, Kinsky S, et al (1972) Picogram-sensitive assay for endotoxin: Gelation of Limulus polyphemus blood cell lysate induced by purified lipopolysaccharides and lipid A from gram-negative bacteria. Biochim Biophys Acta 261:284–289
72. Richardson EC, Banerji B, Seid RC Jr, et al (1983) Interactions of lipid A and liposome-associated lipid A with Limulus polyphemus amoebocytes. Infect Immun 39:1385–1391
73. Sakai H, Hisamoto S, Fukutomi I, et al (2004) Detection of lipopolysaccharide in hemoglobin-vesicles by Limulus amebocyte lysate test with kinetic-turbidimetric gel clotting analysis and pretreatment of surfactant. J Pharm Sci 93:310–321
74. Jurgens G, Muller M, Koch MHJ, et al (2001) Interaction of hemoglobin with enterobacterial lipopolysaccharide and lipid A. Eur J Biochem 268:4233–4242
75. Cliff RO, Kwasiborski V, Rudolph AS (1995) A comparative study of the accurate measurement of endotoxin in liposome encapsulated hemoglobin. Artif Cells Blood Substitutes Immobil Biotechnol 23:331–336. Links
76. Harmon P, Cabral-Lilly D, Reed RA, et al (1997) The release and detection of endotoxin from liposomes. Anal Biochem 250:139–146

77. Piluso LG, Martinez MY (1999) Resolving liposomal inhibition of quantitative LAL methods. PDA J Pharm Sci Technol 53:260–263
78. Minobe S, Nawata M, Watanabe T, et al (1991) Specific assay for endotoxin using immobilized histidine and Limulus amebocyte lysate. Anal Biochem 198:292–297
79. Alayash AI (1999) Hemoglobin-based blood substitutes: oxygen carriers, pressor agents, or oxidants? Nat Biotechnol 17:545–549
80. Yamamoto Y, Brodsky MH, Baker JC, et al (1987) Detection and characterization of lipid hydroperoxides at picomole levels by high-performance liquid chromatography. Anal Biochem 160:7–13
81. Grisham MB, Gaginell TS, Von Ritter C, et al (1990) Effects of neutrophil-derived oxidants on intestinal permeability, electrolyte transport, and epithelial cell viability. Inflammation 14:531–542
82. Nagababu E, Rifkind JM (2000) Reaction of hydrogen peroxide with ferrylhemoglobin: superoxide production and heme degradation. Biochemistry 39:12503–12511
83. Gunther MR, Sampath V, Caughey WS (1999) Potential roles of myoglobin autoxidation in myocardial ischemia-reperfusion injury. Free Radic Biol Med 26:1388–1395
84. Svistunenko DA, Patel RP, Voloshchenko SV, et al (1997) The globin-based free radical of ferryl hemoglobin is detected in normal human blood. J Biol Chem 272:7114–7121
85. Clark MR (1988) Senescence of red blood cells: progress and problems. Physiol Rev 68:503–554
86. Mcleod LL, Alayash AI (1999) Detection of a ferrylhemoglobin intermediate in an endothelial cell model after hypoxia-reoxygenation. Am J Physiol Heart Circ Physiol 277:H92–H99
87. Goldman DW, Breyer RJ III, Yeh D, et al (1998) Acellular hemoglobin-mediated oxidative stress toward endothelium: a role for ferryl iron. Am J Physiol Heart Circ Physiol 275:H1046–H1053
88. D'Agnillo F, Alayash AI (2000) Interactions of hemoglobin with hydrogen peroxide alters thiol levels and course of endothelial cell death. Am J Physiol Heart Circ Physiol 279:H1880–H1889
89. Takeoka S, Teramura Y, Atoji T, et al (2002) Effect of Hb-encapsulation with vesicles on H_2O_2 reaction and lipid peroxidation. Bioconjugate Chem 13:1302–1308
90. Glick MR, Ryder KW (1993) Double trouble: hemolysis and stabilized hemoglobins (so you think you're seeing red now?). Clin Chem 39:1761–1763
91. Ma Z, Monk TG, Goodnough LT, et al (1997) Effect of hemoglobin- and perflubron-based oxygen carriers on common clinical laboratory tests. Clin Chem 43:1732–1737
92. Chance JJ, Norris EJ, Kroll MH (2000) Mechanism of interference of a polymerized hemoglobin blood substitutes in an alkaline phosphatase method. Clin Chem 46:1331–1337
93. Kazmierczak SC, Catrou PG, Best AE, et al (1999) Multiple regression analysis of interference effects from a hemoglobin-based oxygen carrier solution. Clin Chem Lab Med 37:453–464
94. Kazmierczak SC, Catrou PG, Boudreau D (1998) Simplified interpretative format for assessing test interference: studies with hemoglobin-based oxygen carrier solutions. Clin Chem 44:2347–2352
95. Sakai H, Tomiyama K, Masada Y, et al (2003) Pretreatment of serum containing Hb-vesicles (oxygen carriers) to avoid their interference in laboratory tests. Clin Chem Lab Med 41:222–231
96. Nolte D, Pickelmann S, Lang M, et al (2000) Compatibility of different colloid plasma expanders with Peflubron emulsion. Anesthesiology 93:1261–1270

97. Yoshizu A, Yamahata T, Izumi Y, et al (1997) The oxygen transporting capability of hemoglobin vesicle, an artificial oxygen carrier, evaluated in a rat hemorrhagic shock model. Artif Blood 5:18–22
98. Yoshizu A, Izumi Y, Park SI, et al (2004) Hemorrhagic shock resuscitation with an artificial oxygen carrier Hemoglobin Vesicle (HbV) maintains intestinal perfusion and suppresses the increase in plasma necrosis factor alpha (TNF α). ASAIO J (submitted)
99. Sakai H, Takeoka S, Wettstein R, et al (2002) Systemic and Microvascular responses to the hemorrhagic shock and resuscitation with Hb-vesicles. Am J Physiol Heart Circ Physiol 283:H1191–H1199
100. Sakai H, Horinouchi H, Masada Y, et al (2004) Hemoglobin-vesicles suspended in recombinant human serum albumin for resuscitation from hemorrhagic shock in anesthetized rats. Crit Care Med 32:539–545
101. Izumi Y, Sakai H, Hamada K, et al (1996) Physiologic responses to exchange transfusion with Hemoglobin Vesicles as an artificial oxygen carrier in anesthetized rats: changes in mean arterial pressure and renal cortical oxygen tension. Crit Care Med 24:1869–1873
102. Sakai H, Izumi Y, Yamahata T, et al (1995) Evaluation of oxygen transport of hemoglobin vesicles by exchange transfusion into rats. Artif Blood 3:81–86
103. Kobayashi K, Izumi Y, Yoshizu A, et al (1997) The oxygen carrying capability of hemoglobin vesicles evaluated in rat exchange transfusion models. Artif Cells Blood Substitues Immobil Biotechnol 25:357–366
104. Izumi Y, Sakai H, Takeoka S, et al (1997) Evaluation of the capabilities of a hemoglobin vesicle as an artificial oxygen carrier in a rat exchange transfusion model. ASAIO J 43:289–297
105. Sakai H, Tsai AG, Rohlfs RJ, et al (1999) Microvascular responses to hemodilution with Hb-vesicles as red cell substitutes: Influences of O_2 affinity. Am J Physiol Heart Circ. Physiol 276:H553–H562
106. Erni D, Wettstein R, Schramm S, et al (2003) Normovolemic hemodilution with hemoglobin-vesicle solution attenuates hypoxia in ischemic hamster flap tissue. Am J Physiol Heart Circ Physiol 284:H1702–H1709
107. Contaldo C, Schramm S, Wettstein R, et al (2003) Improved oxygenation in ischemic hamster flap tissue is correlated with increasing hemodilution with Hb vesicles and their O_2 affinity. Am J Physiol Heart Circ Physiol 285:H1140–H1147
108. Tsai AG, Intaglietta M (2001) High viscosity plasma expanders: Volume restitution fluid for lowering the perfusion trigger. Biorheology 38:229–237
109. Sakai H, Suzuki Y, Kinoshita M, et al (2003) O_2 release from Hb vesicles evaluated using an artificial, narrow O_2-permaeble tube: comparison with RBCs and acellular Hbs. Am J Physiol Heart Circ Physiol 285:H2543–H2551
110. Page TC, Light WR, McKay CB, et al (1998) Oxygen transport by erythrocyte/ hemoglobin solution mixtures in an in vitro capillary as a model of hemoglobin-based oxygen carrier performance. Microvasc Res 55:54–66
111. Baines AD, Adamson G, Wojciechowski P, et al (1998) Effect of modifying O_2 diffusivity and delivery on glomerular and tubular function in hypoxic perfused kidney. Am J Physiol Renal Physiol 274:F744–F752
112. Rohlfs RJ, Bruner E, Chiu A, et al (1998) Arterial blood pressure responses to cell-free hemoglobin solutions and the reaction with nitric oxide. J Biol Chem 273:12128–12134
113. Tsai AG, Kerger H, Intaglietta M (1995) Microcirculatory consequences of blood substitution with $\alpha\alpha$-hemoglobin. In: Winslow RM, Vandegriff K, Intaglietta M (eds)

Blood substitutes: physiological basis of efficacy. Birkhauser, Boston, pp 155–174

114. Rabinovici R, Rudolph AS, Yue TL, et al (1990) Biological responses to liposome-encapsulated hemoglobin (LEH) are improved by a PAF antagonist. Circ Shock 31:431–445
115. Loughrey HC, Bally MB, Reinish LW, et al (1990) The binding of phosphatidylglycerol liposomes to rat platelets is mediated by complement. Thromb Haemost 64:172–176
116. Doerschuk CM, Gie RP, Bally MB, et al (1989) Platelet distribution in rabbits following infusion of liposomes. Thromb Haemost 61:392–396
117. Wakamoto S, Fujihara M, Abe H, et al (2001) Effects of poly(ethyleneglycol)-modified hemoglobin vesicles on agonist-induced platelet aggregation and RANTES release in vitro. Artif Cells Blood Substit Immobil Biotechnol 29:191–201
118. Hatipoglu U, Gao X, Verral S, et al (1998) Sterically stabilized phospholipids attenuate human neutrophils chemotaxis in vitro. Life Sci 63:693–699
119. Ito T, Fujihara M, Abe H, et al (2001) Effects of poly(ethyleneglycol)-modified hemoglobin vesicles on N-formyl-methionyl-leucyl-phenylalanine-induced responses of polymorphonuclear neutrophils in vitro. Artif Cells Blood Substit Immobil Biotechnol 29:427–437
120. Abassi Z, Kotob S, Pieruzzi F, et al (1997) Effect of polymerization on the hypertensive action of diaspirin cross-linked hemoglobin in rats. J Lab Clin Med 129:603–610
121. Gardiner SM, Compton AM, Bennett T, et al (1990) Control of regional blood flow by endothelium-derived nitric oxide. Hypertension 15:486–492
122. Doherty, DH, Doyle MP, et al (1988) Rate of reaction with nitric oxide determines the hypertensive effect of cell-free hemoglobin. Nat Biotechnol 16:672–676
123. Moncada, S, Palmer RMJ, Higgs EA (1991) Nitric oxide: physiology, pathophysiology, and pharmacology. Pharmacol Rev 43:109–131
124. Rioux, F, Drapeau G, Marceau F (1995) Recombinant human hemoglobin (rHb1.1) selectively inhibits vasorelaxation elicted by nitric oxide donors in rabbit isolated aortic rings. J Cardiovasc Pharmacol 25:587–594
125. Nakai, K, Ohta T, Sakuma I, et al (1996) Inhibition of endothelium-dependent relaxation by hemoglobin in rabbit aortic strips: comparison between acellular hemoglobin derivatives and cellular hemoglobins. J Cardiovasc Pharmacol 28:115–123
126. Sakai, H, Hara H, Tsai AG, et al (1999) Changes in resistance vessels during hemorrhagic shock and resuscitation in conscious hamster model. Am J Physiol Heart Circ Physiol 276:H563–H571
127. Sakai H, Hara H, Tsai AG, et al (2000) Constriction of resistance arteries determines L-NAME-induced hypertension in a conscious hamster model. Microvasc Res 60:21–27
128. Sakai H, Hara H, Yuasa M, et al (2000) Molecular dimensions of Hb-based O_2 carriers determine constriction of resistance arteries and hypertension. Am J Physiol Heart Circ Physiol 279:H908–H915
129. Makino N, Suematsu M, Sugiura Y, et al (2001) Altered expression of heme oxygenase-1 in the livers of patients with portal hypertensive diseases.Hepatology 33:32–42
130. Goda N, Suzuki K, Naito M, et al (1998) Distribution of heme oxygenase isoforms in rat liver. Topographic basis for carbon monoxide-mediated microvascular relaxation. J Clin Invest 101:604–612
131. Rudolph AS, Klipper RW, Goins B, et al (1991) In vivo biodistribution of a radiolabeled blood substitute: ^{99m}Tc-labeled liposome-encapsulated hemoglobin in an anesthetized rabbit. Proc Natl Acad Sci USA 88:10976–10980

132. Sou K, Klipper R, Goins B, et al (2003) Pharmacokinetics of the hemoglobin-vesicles (HbV) in rats. Artif Blood 11:117 (Abstract)
133. Sakai H, Horinouchi H, Tomiyama K, et al (2001) Hemoglobin-vesicles as oxygen carriers: influence on phagocytic activity and histopathological changes in reticuloendothelial system. Am J Pathol 159:1079–1088
134. Sakai H, Horinouchi H, Masada Y, et al (2004) Metabolism of hemoglobin-vesicles (artificial oxygen carriers) and their influence on organ functions in a rat model. Biomaterials 25:4317–4325
135. Sakai H, Masada Y, Horinouchi H, et al (2003) Daily repeated infusion of Hb-vesicels (HbV) into Wistar rats for two weeks: A preliminary safety study. Artif Blood 11:72 (Abstract)

Successful Ex Vivo Normothermic Liver Perfusion with Purely Artificial Products Using Artificial Blood

Tadashi Katsuramaki, Akihiro Nui, Hitoshi Kikuchi, Kazuma Kukita, Minoru Nagayama, Makoto Meguro, Hitoshi Kimura, Masato Isobe, and Koichi Hirata

Summary. We tried to make an ex vivo functioning liver with an artificial perfusate that consisted of artificial blood in the pig liver. A liver graft from a female pig weighing 20 kg was harvested in the usual manner. The perfusion solution consisted of artificial blood, L-15 medium, distilled water, bovine serum albumin, NaHCO3, NaOH, KCl, human regular insulin, 50% glucose solution, and dexamethasone. The isolated liver was perfused with this oxygenated perfusate through the portal vein at a rate of 300 ml/min for 9 h. Seven livers were perfused for 9 h in this system. Five of the livers showed mean oxygen consumption of over 8 ml-O2/min during perfusion. Histological findings showed that the hepatic architecture was almost completely preserved and numerous hepatocytes exhibited PAS-positive cytoplasmic glycogen deposits in these livers. These observations indicated that we succeeded in developing an ex vivo functioning liver with an artificial perfusate employing artificial blood.

Key words. Liver, Normothermic perfusion, Artificial blood, Extracorporeal perfusion

Introduction

Previously, some investigators reported normothermic extracorporeal liver perfusion circuits [1,2], which were used as bioartificial liver for support of hepatic failure [3–5], or as a preservation method for liver grafts in transplantation [6,7]. However, these were not true artificial perfusion systems because their perfusates used organ blood as the oxygen carrier.

First Department of Surgery, Sapporo Medical University, School of Medicine, South-1, West-16, Chuo-ku, Sapporo 060-8543, Japan

We have been studying a normothermic perfusion system that consists of artificial products using artificial blood in the pig liver. We succeeded in developing an ex vivo functioning liver with an artificial perfusate using artificial blood.

Materials and Methods

Animals

This study was performed in accordance with the Guidelines of Sapporo Medical University for Animal Experimentation. A female hybrid pig (hypor) weighing 20 kg was used after overnight fasting. After intratracheal intubation, the pig was mechanically ventilated with a respirator and underwent general anesthesia.

Operative Procedures

The liver graft was harvested in the usual manner. The common bile duct, the portal vein and the hepatic artery were isolated, and then a 12 Fr cannula was inserted into the portal vein via the splenic vein. The gall bladder was removed, and a plastic tube was placed in the common bile duct to collect bile juice. After preparation was completed, heparin sodium (500 units/kg, i.v.) was administered. After 5 min heparin administration, the liver was flushed out in situ with 2000 ml of lactate Ringer solution (Lactec, Otsuka Pharmaceutical, Tokyo, Japan) containing heparin sodium (5 IU/ml) via the portal vein. The liver graft was taken out and then placed in the perfusion system. The suprahepatic inferior vena cava was ligated, and a 12 Fr canula for outflow was inserted into the infrahepatic inferior vena cava.

Perfusion Solution

The Neo Red Cell (NRC) was used as artificial blood in this experiment which was offered by Termo (Tokyo, Japan). NRC contains hemoglobuliin with a concentration of 6.0 g/dl. The perfusion solution consisted of NRC, 600 ml; L-15 medium (Sigma Chemical, St. Louis, MO, USA), 40 ml; distilled water, 240 ml; bovine serum albumin (Sigma), 27 g; NaHCO3, 2.2 g; NaOH, 90 mg; KCl, 3.6 ml; human regular insulin, 24 IU; 50% glucose solution, 2 ml; and dexamethasone, 4 mg. The total amount of the perfusion solution was 900 ml. The hemoglobin concentration was 3.7 g/dl.

Perfusion System

The perfusion system consisted of an oxygenator including a heat exchanger (CAPIOX, Termo), a Bio pump (Bio Medics, Minneapolis, MN, USA), and a reserver (Fig. 1). The liver was placed in air in a special sterile basin. This system required 500 ml of perfusion solution for priming of the circuit. The isolated liver was perfused with an oxygenated perfusate at a rate of 300 ml/min through the portal vein for 9 h (Fig. 1). Outflow of the perfusate was collected from the infrahepatic vena cava. The perfusate solution was continuously warmed in the heat exchanger to maintain the temperature at 37°C.

Gas Analysis of Perfusion Solution

Samples of the perfusate were collected from the inflow and outflow circuit every 1 h during perfusion. Samples were analyzed for PaO2, PaCO2, pH

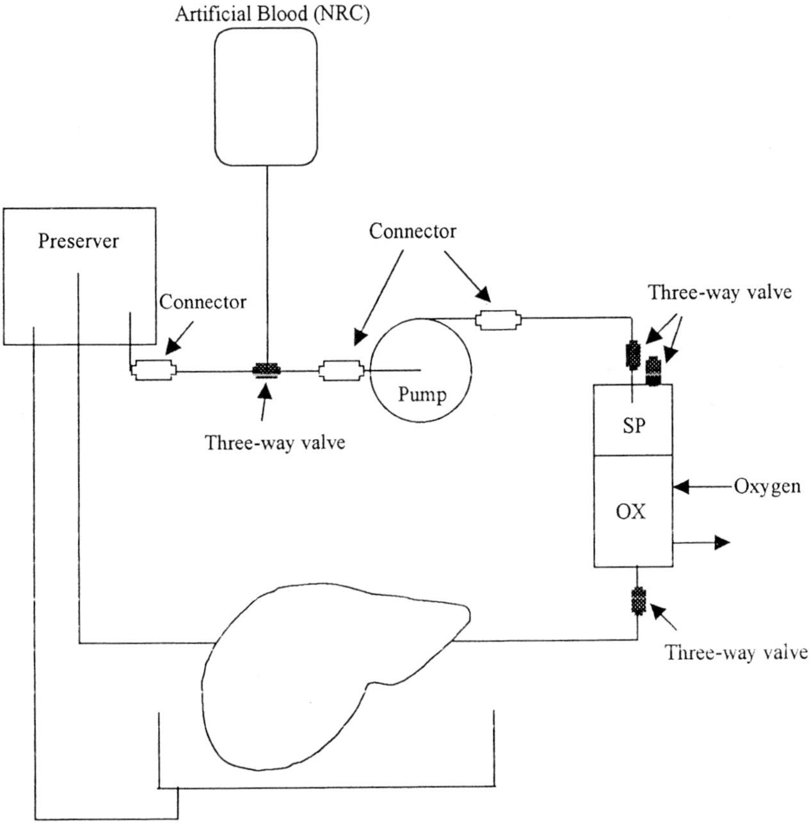

Fig. 1. Diagram of the ex vivo liver perfusion circuit. The perfusion system consists of an oxygenator including a heat exchanger, a Bio pump, and a reserver. The isolated liver was perfused with oxygenated perfusate at a rate of 300 ml/min through the portal vein. Outflow of the perfusate was collected from the infrahepatic vena cava

and O2 saturation with an blood gas analyzer ABL 520 (Radiometer, USA).

Histology

Hepatic tissue was obtained from the right median lobe before ischemia at the end of the perfusion. It was fixed in 10% buffered formalin and 5 μm thick sections were stained with hematoxylin and eosin. For the determination of glycogenesis, PAS staining was performed.

Oxygen Consumption

The hepatic oxygen consumption was calculated by the following formula.

Oxygen consumption = [oxygen delivery from NRC + oxygen delivery from perfusion solution] × R × T / P × 1/10. Oxygen delivery from NRC (mmol/L) = [{oxygen saturation (pre-post) × (hemoglobin concentration (g/dL) – metohemoglobin (g/dL)) × 10}/64450] × 4 × 1000. Oxygen delivery from the perfusion solution (mmol/L) = (pO2)/(760 – saturated vapor pressure)/Henry coefficient × 1000. R:gas constant:R(l · atm/· mol), T:absolute temperature(K), P:oxygen partial pressure(torr/760:atm). All data were expressed as mean ± SE.

Results

Seven livers were perfused for 9 h in this system. During perfusion, every lobe of the liver was perfused well. Among these 7 livers, 5 had mean oxygen consumption of over 8 ml-O2/min during perfusion; however, 2 livers had low oxygen consumption of under 5 ml-O2/min (Table 1). The livers with high

TABLE 1. Summary of grafts

	Mean oxygen consumption ($ml\text{-}O^2/min$)	Oxygen saturation of outflow at 2 h after perfusion (%)	PAS stain
High oxygen consumption grafts			
1	10.2	29	+
2	12.1	42	+
3	8.7	56	+
4	13.6	45	+
5	9.8	9	+
Low oxygen consumption grafts			
6	3.6	90	–
7	4.3	80	–

PAS, periodic acid-Schiff.

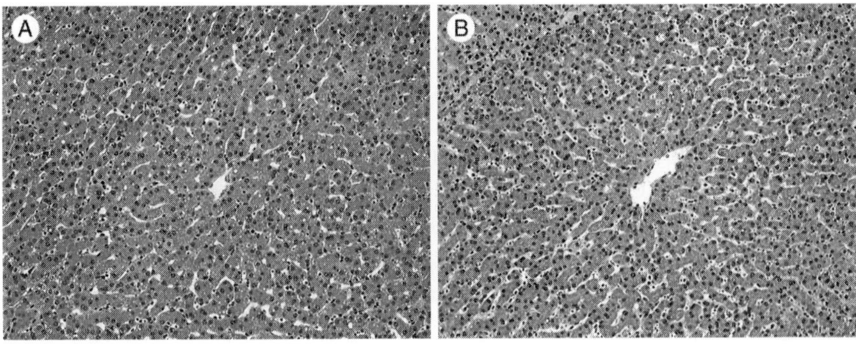

FIG. 2. Hepatic architecture was well preserved at 9 h after perfusion, and there was no difference between before (**A**) and after (**B**) perfusion. Hematoxylin-eosin stain, ×100

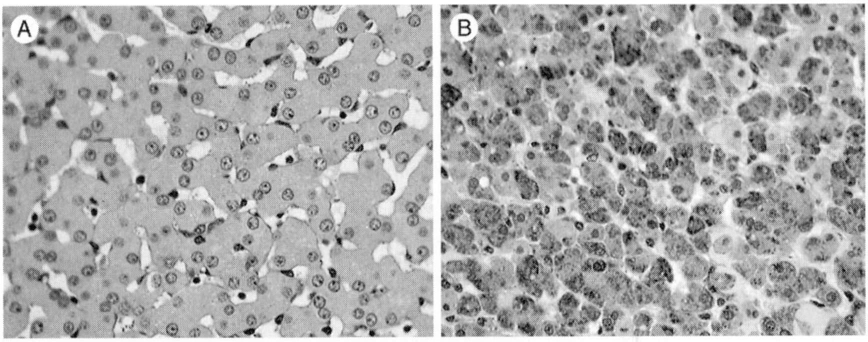

FIG. 3. Liver cells at just after laparotomy show absence of glycogen deposits by PAS staining (**A**). After 9 h of perfusion, numerous liver cells exhibit PAS-positive cytoplasmic glycogen deposits (**B**). PAS stain, ×200

oxygen consumption also showed oxygen saturation of outflow (hepatic vein) under 80% until the end of perfusion. However, the two livers with low oxygen consumption had oxygen saturation of outflow of over 80% during perfusion.

Histological findings showed that hepatic architecture was almost completely preserved at 9 h after perfusion in high oxygen consumption livers (Fig. 2). Liver cells at just after laparotomy showed the absence of glycogen deposits by PAS staining because of overnight fasting. However, numerous liver cells exhibited PAS-positive cytoplasmic glycogen deposits at 9 h after perfusion in high oxygen consumption livers (Fig. 3). These PAS-positive cytoplasmic glycogen deposits were not recognized in low consumption livers (Table 1).

Discussion

The aim of our study was the development of a normothermic perfusion system that employed artificial products. Our perfusion solution consisted of hepatocyte culture medium (L-15), distilled water, bovine serum albumin, NaHCO3, NaOH, KCl, human regular insulin, glucose, and dexamethasone. The most important part of the solution was Neo Red Cell as an oxygen carrier. By using this, we made a successful perfusion solution without biological blood. In this study, seven livers were perfused during 9 h. Five livers had high oxygen consumption and the other two livers had low oxygen consumption. In the histological examination, numerous liver cells exhibited PAS-positive cytoplasmic glycogen deposits in high oxygen consumption livers from 5 h after perfusion, although these findings were not recognized in low oxygen consumption livers. From these observations, we considered that we succeeded in the development of an ex vivo functioning liver without any use of physiological products such as biological blood. If we can achieve a longer perfusion period, ex vivo hepatic organ culture may be possible. However, several problems remain to be solved in our system. Among the 7 livers, 2 low oxygen consumption and these livers did not exhibit glycogenesis. Although the reason for this was unknown, we considered that some livers were not suitable for these artificial systems or that these livers were perhaps primary nonfunction livers due to some problems in our harvesting method. If these low oxygen consumption livers had primary nonfunction, it would still be possible to evaluate graft viability by use of this system because low oxygen consumption livers immediately exhibited high oxygen saturation of outflow (hepatic vein).

We performed only 9 h perfusion in this system. Further oimprovement of the system will be necessary for more prolonged perfusion.

In conclusion, we succeeded in developing a normothermic liver perfusion system consisting of artificial products such as artificial blood. Although several problems remain to be solved, this system has the potential to become an organ culture system, which is our final aim.

References

1. Rodriguez-Reynoso S, Portilla E, Garcia D, et al (2001) Blood flow rate and energy charge in the isolated perfused canine liver. J Surg Res 99:40–46
2. Foley DP, Vittimberga FJ, Quarfordt SH, et al (1999) Biliary secretion of extracorporeal porcine livers with single and dual vessel perfusion. Transplantation 68:362–368
3. Nakamura N, Kamiyama Y, Takai S, et al (1999) Ex vivo liver perfusion with arterial blood from a pig with ischemic liver failure. Artif Organs 23:153–160
4. Horslen SP, Hammel JM, Fristoe LW, et al (2000) Extracorporeal liver perfusion using human and pig livers for acute liver failure. Transplantation 70:1472–1478

5. Borie DC, Eyraud D, Boleslawski E, et al (2001) Functional metabolic characteristics of intact pig livers during prolonged extracorporeal perfusion: potential for a unique biological liver-assist device. Transplantation 72:393–405
6. Dutkowski P, Odermatt B, Heinrich T, et al (1998) Hypothermic oscillating liver perfusion stimulates ATP synthesis prior to transplantation. J Surg Res 80:365–372
7. Schön MR, Kollmar O, Wolf S, et al (2001) Liver transplantation after organ preservation with normothermic extracorporeal perfusion. Ann Surg 233:114–123

Effect of Hemoglobin-Based Blood Substitutes on Nitric Oxide Transport: Mathematical Models

Aleksander S. Popel, Mahendra Kavdia, and Nikolaos M. Tsoukias

Summary. Nitric oxide is potent vasodilator acting through activation of soluble guanylate cyclase in the smooth muscle cells. Scavenging of free nitric oxide (NO) by hemoglobin-based oxygen carriers (HBOCs) is considered a major cause of vasoconstriction following transfusion with HBOC used as blood substitutes. However, direct measurements of NO concentration in the microvessels are limited and they are not available in the presence of HBOC. To gain a quantitative understanding of the effects of NO, we formulated several mathematical models to systematically investigate the transport of NO around microvessels in the presence of HBOC and its dependence on such factors as free-Hb concentration, HBOC reactivity with NO, shear-stress dependent rate of NO release by endothelium and free-Hb extravasation. The calculations predict a strong effect of HBOC extravasation and reactivity, but only a moderate effect of wall shear stress. The predicted NO concentration falls several-fold from its physiological level when HBOC is introduced. We analyzed the transport resistance in and around the red blood cell since it is a determining factor on the luminal NO consumption. Using similar approach, we also investigated NO transport characteristics of phospholipid vesicles encapsulating Hb introduced recently as the next generation of blood substitutes.

Key words. Hemoglobin-based oxygen carrier, NO scavenging, Extravasation, Vasoconstriction

---

Department of Biomedical Engineering, The Johns Hopkins University, School of Medicine, 720 Rutland Avenue, Baltimore, MD 21205, USA

Introduction

Nitric oxide is a simple diatomic molecule that exhibits a wide range of important physiological and pathophysiological activities, including regulation of vascular tone, cell adhesion, and vascular permeability; inhibition of platelet aggregation and leukocyte adhesion; neurotransmission; and, host defense response. Excessive production of NO depletes antioxidant stores, induces lipid peroxidation and promotes DNA damage. Effects of NO are implicated in numerous diseases such as septic shock, hypertension, diabetes mellitus, thrombosis, and neurodegenerative diseases. NO is produced by a number of cells, including endothelial cells, through the enzymatic degradation of L-arginine by several isoforms of the enzyme nitric oxide synthase (NOS). Hemoglobin (Hb) is known to be an NO scavenger and transfusions with free-Hb solutions frequently result in vasoconstriction and elevated blood pressure. In addition, there is a potential for affecting other NO functions. Present developments of hemoglobin-based oxygen carriers (HBOC) to be used as blood substitutes include human and bovine cross-linked and polymerized Hb, recombinant Hb, hemoglobin conjugated with macromolecules such as polyethylene glycol (PEG), vesicles- and nanoparticles-encapsulated Hb, and polynitroxylated polymerized Hb [1–3]. A number of these artificial oxygen carriers are in clinical trials. However, many fundamental aspects of molecular interactions, hemodynamics and molecular transport in the presence of HBOCs remain poorly understood and more basic research is necessary to better understand their effects under different in vivo conditions [4,5]. Therefore, a quantitative assessment of NO level in the tissue in the presence of HBOC would be very important for designing HBOCs and their clinical applications.

With these goals in mind, we have started systematic development of mathematical and computational models for oxygen and nitric oxide transport in the presence of HBOCs. To this end, we have analyzed transport of oxygen in single capillaries, organs, and whole organism [6–8]. In all these studies we paid attention to the effect of Hb-O_2 affinity and cooperativity on the efficiency of oxygen delivery by HBOC. Compared to studies of oxygen transport, mathematical modeling of NO diffusion in tissue under physiological conditions started only recently, less than a decade ago [9]. We have formulated reaction-diffusion equations describing transport of NO in the presence of HBOCs and applied them to the following problems: NO transport around red blood cells [10] and Hb-encapsulated vesicles (unpublished results), NO transport around individual capillaries [11] and arterioles [12,13]. We briefly review the models and results of computer simulations.

Results

NO Transport Around Red Blood Cells in the Presence of HBOC and Around Vesicles Encapsulating Hb

It has been well established experimentally that the reaction rate of NO with free-Hb is 2–3 orders of magnitude faster than the reaction rate with red blood cells (RBCs) containing equivalent amount of Hb. Two hypotheses were put forward to explain the difference: diffusion resistance in the "unstirred" plasma layer surrounding RBC, and resistance of the RBC membrane, primarily attributed to the cytoskeleton and adsorbed metHb molecules [14,15]. We analyzed NO diffusion into the RBC [10] and showed that the observed reaction rate can be predicted with a combination of the extracellular diffusion resistance and a Hb-NO reaction rate consistent with the experimental data for low hematocrits; data for physiological levels of hematocrit are not available. The reaction-diffusion model makes predictions for the reaction rate at higher hematocrits. The results for the reaction rate, k_{NO}, as a function of heme concentration are shown in Fig. 1 for free-Hb and RBC-encapsulated Hb. A very significant difference between the two cases should be noted; the difference has significant implications for bioavailability of NO in the smooth muscle in the presence of free-Hb in the lumen and, in case of Hb extravasation, outside the lumen.

Recent advances in biotechnology make it possible to encapsulate Hb into microscopic liposome vesicles [16]. We used the model of NO transport to predict the NO reaction rate in vesicle solutions. Results from representative simulations are presented in Fig. 1. k_{NO} is plotted as a function the total heme concentration in solution for vesicles of two different sizes (0.2 and 1 μm diameter). The heme concentration inside the vesicles was –20 mM). The rate of NO uptake by Hb vesicles falls between the uptake by free-Hb and RBCs.

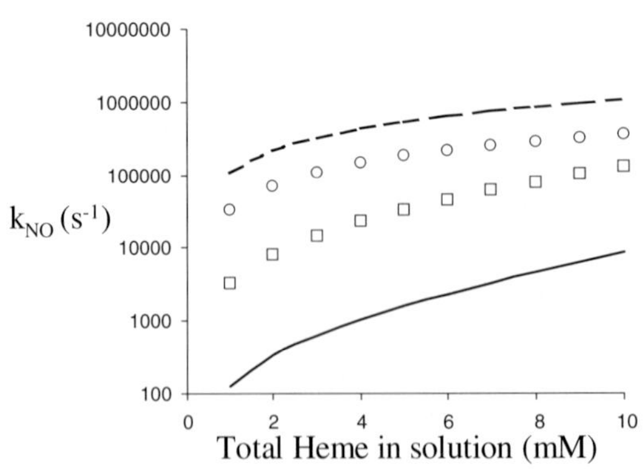

FIG. 1. NO consumption rate constant as a function of total heme concentration in solution for RBC-encapsulated Hb (*solid line*), free-Hb (*dashed line*), or Hb inside liposome vesicles (*symbols*). Vesicles with a diameter of 0.2 μm (*circles*) and 1 μm (*squares*) were examined. Hb concentration in the vesicles was 20 mM

For example, for a total heme concentration of 2 mM, which corresponds to a Hct of 10%, predicted NO reaction rate constants were: $2.2 \times 10^5\,s^{-1}$ for free-Hb, $340\,s^{-1}$ for RBCs, $6.9 \times 10^4\,s^{-1}$ for Hb-vesicles with 0.2 µm diameter and $8.2 \times 10^3\,s^{-1}$ for Hb-vesicles with 1 µm diameter. The NO reaction rate is a non-linear function of the total heme concentration in the solution. Solutions of vesicles highly concentrated with Hb have a smaller NO reactivity for the same amount of total heme present in solution. The effect of such a decrease in NO reactivity is more pronounced for vesicles with larger diameter. These predictions should be useful in designing vesicles for encapsulating Hb.

Models of NO Transport Around Arterioles

One of the major problems associated with transfusion of free-Hb solutions is scavenging of NO by Hb inside the vascular lumen and in the interstitium, in case of Hb extravasation. The resulting vasoconstriction and increase in vascular resistance limits blood flow and oxygen delivery, counter to the intended increase of oxygen delivery by HBOC. To quantitatively assess the distribution of NO in and around arterioles in the presence of HBOC, we formulated a model of an arteriole surrounded by capillary-perfused tissue and considered a wide range of physiologically important parameters that may affect the NO distribution [12,13].

Figure 2 presents the geometry of the model showing a cross section perpendicular to the arteriolar axis with sub regions including luminal region of cell-rich region (CR), cell-free region (CF) and glycocalyx (G). Nitric oxide produced by endothelial cells (E) can diffuse either to the lumen or through interstitial space (IS) to smooth muscle (SM) and then to parenchyma. In each of the regions, the transport of NO is described by the reaction-diffusion equation:

$$D_{NO}\frac{1}{r}\frac{\partial}{\partial r}\left(r\frac{\partial C_{NO}}{\partial r}\right)+q_{NO}-R_{NO}=0$$

where C_{NO} is the local NO concentration, q_{NO} is the production rate, and R_{NO} is the net rate of NO consumption. The consumption rate is expressed as $R_{NO} = k_i C_{NO}^n C_i$, where k_i is the reaction rate constant, n is the order of the reaction rate, and C_i is the concentration of the species reacting with NO in the region. The reactive species are Hb in the RBCs and free-Hb in the arteriolar lumen and in the capillaries surrounding the arteriole, free-Hb in the interstitial space between the endothelial and smooth muscle cells when extravasation occurs, dissolved oxygen in all the regions, and soluble guanylate cyclase (sGC) in the smooth muscle cells. Most of the anatomical and biophysical parameters can be estimated for different vessels and tissues based on published experimental data. There remains uncertainty in one of the key param-

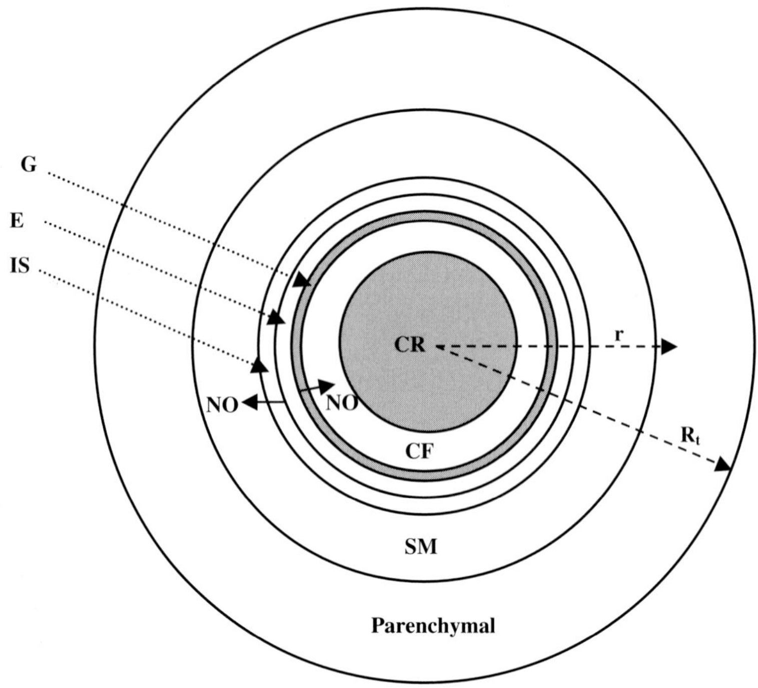

FIG. 2. Cross section of the model's geometry. *CR*, cell-rich region; *CF*, cell-free region; *G*, glycocalyx; *E*, endothelial cells; *IS*, interstitial space and *SM*, smooth muscle

eters, NO production rate by endothelial cells, which is estimated either from in vitro experiments [17] or with the help of a mathematical model [18] where the rate is selected so as to predict the NO concentration measured in the aorta wall [19]. The NO concentrations predicted by our model are proportional to the selected value of NO production by endothelial cells; even if the absolute values reflect the uncertainty in the NO production values, the relative changes of NO concentration demonstrate the effect of HBOC.

Figure 3 shows NO concentration profiles in and around a 50 μm diameter arteriole at Hct = 22.5 and 45%. The results show the concentration in the smooth muscle of the order of 100 nM, the magnitude decreasing with increasing hematocrit due to Hb scavenging of NO. The concentration sharply decreases in the lumen, even with the presence of RBC-free layer adjacent to the endothelium.

Figure 4a shows the effect of HBOC with different reaction rates of NO binding: $k_{Hb} = 58 \times 10^6 M^{-1} s^{-1}$ (per heme basis) is similar to wild-type Hb, while $k_{Hb} = 24 \times 10^6 M^{-1} s^{-1}$ and $2 \times 10^6 M^{-1} s^{-1}$ is for Hb molecules with reduced

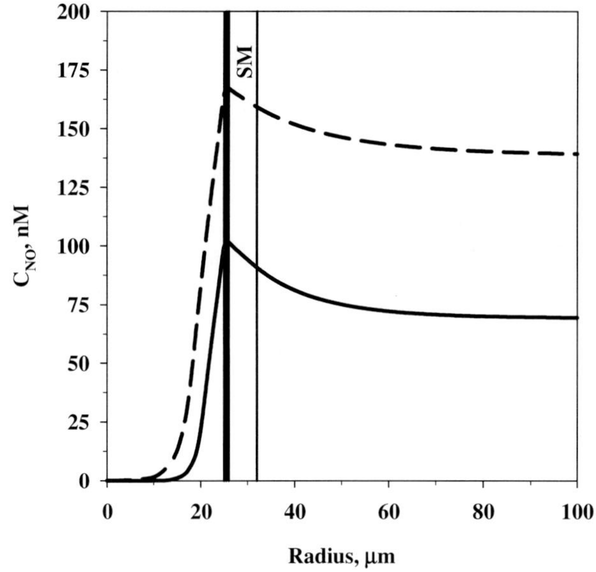

FIG. 3. NO concentration profiles in a 50 μm diameter arteriole; Hct 22.5% (*dashed line*) and 45% (*solid line*); no HBOC present

NO binding rates. The results demonstrate a strong effect of NO scavenging by HBOC; for Hb with a wild-type kinetics, the smooth muscle NO concentration decreases by an order of magnitude for Hct = 22.5%, from approximately 167 nM to 12 nM. Even for a 29-fold decrease in the reaction rate, the decrease is still significant: from 167 to 28 nM. Thus, the model suggests that the presence of intraluminal free-Hb strongly decreases NO concentration in the smooth muscle and parenchymal regions.

To understand the significance of our predictions of the impact of NO concentrations on vascular tone, we need to know the concentration of NO that activates hemoprotein sGC. NO functions as a signaling molecule for activating sGC: NO binds to the heme of sGC, and its activation results in catalyzing the conversion of guanosine triphosphate (GTP) to cyclic guanosine monophosphate (cGMP), thus relaxing smooth muscle cells. Experimental studies put NO concentration required for sGC activation at around 250 nM or less, with recent studies reporting a lower range of 5–100 nM, with a half maximal activation at 23 nM [20]. Note that the concentration values predicted by the model fall into this range. Does this mean that NO bioavailability is retained in the presence of HBOC? This important question needs to be answered by further in vivo experimental studies, preferably using direct measurements of NO concentration in the presence of HBOC.

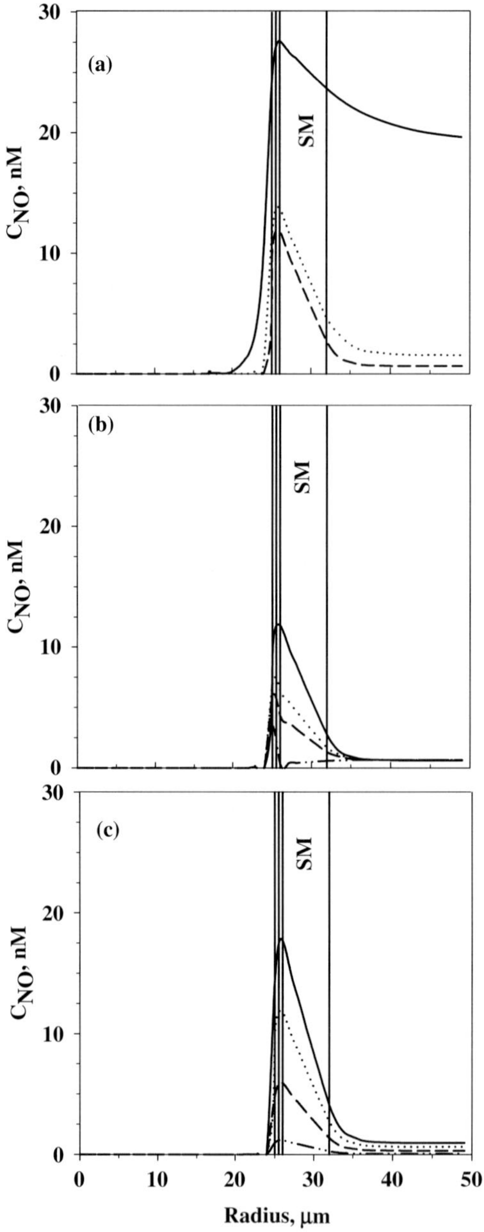

FIG. 4a–c. NO concentration profiles at Hct 22.5% with HBOC present. **a** varying HBOC-NO reactivity; 2×10^6 (*solid line*), 24×10^6 (*dotted line*) and 58×10^6 (*dashed line*) $M^{-1} s^{-1}$. **b** different degrees of extravasation; 0% (*solid line*), 5% (*dotted line*), 10% (*dashed line*), and 100% (*dotted-dashed line*). **c** different levels of wall shear stress; 36 (*solid line*), 24 (*dotted line*), 12 (*dashed line*), and 2.4 dyn/cm^2 (*dotted-dashed line*)

It is known that HBOCs can extravasate, with the rate of extravasation decreasing with increasing molecular weight/size. Deleterious vasoconstriction and pressor response associated with HBOC transfusion are often attributed to HBOC extravasation because vasoconstriction is reduced or disappears when larger, polymerized Hb molecules are used. We simulated HBOC extravasation in the model by varying the concentration of free-Hb in the interstitial space between the arteriolar endothelium and smooth muscle (a thin space 0.5 μm thick was assumed in the calculations). The results are illustrated in Fig. 4b for wild-type Hb with different Hb concentration in the interstitial space shown as % of luminal concentration. A 5% extravasation reduces the NO concentration in the smooth muscle in half; a 100% extravasation reduces the concentration to ~1 nM. Thus, the simulation shows that NO concentration is sensitive to Hb extravasation, even to small amounts, but the main decrease of C_{NO} results from free-Hb presence in the lumen.

NO production by endothelial cells is affected by wall shear stress, with approximately proportional increase in average production rate with shear stress. Since HBOC transfusion may result in changes in the wall shear stress, due to a combination of changes in the blood viscosity, blood flow, and vessel diameter, we investigated the effect of shear stress on NO concentration. Figure 4c shows the changes of C_{NO} when the wall shear stress or endothelial cell NO production varies within a wide range between 10% and 150% of its original value. The resulting changes of the NO concentration are in the range 1–18 nM. In contrast, C_{NO} in the smooth muscle varies significantly, (20–240 nM), with shear stress for a volume expander (data not shown).

Conclusion

Using reaction-diffusion mathematical models of NO transport in microvessels in the presence of HBOC, we have shown that several factors have significant impact on NO concentration distribution. Most importantly, introducing free-Hb into the lumen should lead to a drastic decrease in the NO concentration. Decreasing the reaction rate between NO and free-Hb would mitigate this effect to some degree. Changes in the wall shear stress also affect NO level, but the variation is much more pronounced for non-Hb-containing volume expanders than for HBOC. These theoretical predictions raise important quantitative questions about NO bioavailability in the presence of HBOC and the physiological factors that affect this bioavailability. They also suggest experimental measurements that should be done to gain a better understanding of the complex mechanisms of interaction between HBOC and nitric oxide under different pathophysiological conditions.

References

1. Chang TM (1999) Future prospects for artificial blood. Trends Biotechnol 17(2):61–67
2. Goodnough LT, Shander A, Brecher ME (2003) Transfusion medicine: looking to the future. Lancet 361(9352):161–169
3. Stowell CP, Levin J, Spiess BD, et al (2001) Progress in the development of RBC substitutes. Transfusion 41(2):287–299
4. Alayash AI (2000) Hemoglobin-based blood substitutes and the hazards of blood radicals. Free Radic Res 33(4):341–348
5. Bucci E (2001) Hemoglobin based oxygen carriers at a cross road: the old paradigms must be abandoned and much more basic science investigation is necessary. Artif Cells Blood Substit Immobil Biotechnol 29(4):vii–x
6. Vadapalli A, Goldman D, Popel AS (2002) Calculations of oxygen transport by red blood cells and hemoglobin solutions in capillaries. Artif Cells Blood Substit Immobil Biotechnol 30(3):157–188
7. Sharan M, Popel AS (2002) A compartmental model for oxygen transport in brain microcirculation in the presence of blood substitutes. J Theor Biol 216(4):479–500
8. Kavdia M, Pittman RN, Popel AS (2002) Theoretical analysis of effects of blood substitute affinity and cooperativity on organ oxygen transport. J Appl Physiol 93(6): 2122–2128
9. Buerk DG (2001) Can we model nitric oxide biotransport? A survey of mathematical models for a simple diatomic molecule with surprisingly complex biological activities. Annu Rev Biomed Eng 3:109–143
10. Tsoukias NM, Popel AS (2002) Erythrocyte consumption of nitric oxide in presence and absence of plasma-based hemoglobin. Am J Physiol Heart Circ Physiol 282(6):H2265–H2277
11. Tsoukias NM, Popel AS (2003) A model of nitric oxide capillary exchange. Microcirculation 10(6):479–495
12. Kavdia M, Tsoukias NM, Popel AS (2002) Model of nitric oxide diffusion in an arteriole: impact of hemoglobin- based blood substitutes. Am J Physiol Heart Circ Physiol 282(6):H2245–H2253
13. Kavdia M, Popel AS (2003) Wall shear stress differentially affects NO level in arterioles for volume expanders & Hb-based O2 carriers. Microvasc Res 66(1):49–58
14. Liu X, Samouilov A, Lancaster JR, Jr., et al (2002) Nitric oxide uptake by erythrocytes is primarily limited by extracellular diffusion not membrane resistance. J Biol Chem 277(29):26194–26199
15. Huang KT, Han TH, Hyduke DR, et al (2001) Modulation of nitric oxide bioavailability by erythrocytes. Proc Natl Acad Sci U S A 98(20):11771–11776
16. Erni D, Wettstein R, Schramm S, et al (2003) Normovolemic hemodilution with Hb vesicle solution attenuates hypoxia in ischemic hamster flap tissue. Am J Physiol Heart Circ Physiol 9:9
17. Kuchan MJ, Frangos JA (1994) Role of calcium and calmodulin in flow-induced nitric oxide production in endothelial cells. Am J Physiol 266(3 Pt 1):C628–C636
18. Vaughn MW, Kuo L, Liao JC (1998) Estimation of nitric oxide production and reaction rates in tissue by use of a mathematical model. Am J Physiol 274(6 Pt 2):H2163–H2176
19. Malinski T, Taha Z, Grunfeld S, et al (1993) Diffusion of nitric oxide in the aorta wall monitored in situ by porphyrinic microsensors. Biochem Biophys Res Commun 193(3):1076–1082

20. Condorelli P, George SC (2001) In vivo control of soluble guanylate cyclase activation by nitric oxide: a kinetic analysis. Biophys J 80(5):2110–2119
21. Brunori M (2001) Nitric oxide moves myoglobin centre stage. Trends Biochem Sci 26(4):209–210
22. Flogel U, Merx MW, Godecke A, et al (2001) Myoglobin: A scavenger of bioactive NO. Proc Natl Acad Sci USA 98(2):735–740

New Strategy for the Preparation of NO-Treated Red Blood Cells as a Blood Substitute

ANTONIO TSUNESHIGE and TAKASHI YONETANI

Summary. Our previous studies on the α-nitrosyl derivative of human adult hemoglobin (HbA), tetrameric Hb in which only the two α-subunits are ligated with nitric oxide (NO) [Yonetani et al., (1998) J Biol Chem 273: 20323], have shown that the α-nitrosyl HbA is a cooperative, low-affinity oxygen carrier. We have developed a simple method to convert all the intra-human red blood cells (RBCs) to a 50% saturation of hemes with NO exclusively bound to the α-subunits. Oxygen equilibrium measurements showed that the α-NO RBCs also exhibit reduced oxygen affinity (increased P_{50}) and diminished Bohr effect (i.e., the pH dependence of P_{50}). Despite the fact that its oxygen-carrying capacity is reduced by 50%, since two α-subunits are already ligated with NO, and only two β-subunits are capable of oxygen binding, α-NO RBCs can efficiently deliver oxygen to tissues under normal physiological conditions, making this material an excellent candidate for blood transfusion. Crucial steps in our protocol for the preparation of α-NO Hb-containing RBCs were revised and technical adjustments were made in order to improve the quality and integrity of RBCs during and after treatment, while avoiding the use of potentially noxious chemicals that could entail harmful effects. We were also able to reduce the preparation time. All of which will make viable an increased production volume of quality NO-treated RBCs for practical use.

Key words. Hemoglobin, Nitrosyl hemoglobin, Red blood cells, Blood substitute, Rejuvenation, Erythrocytes

---

Department of Biochemistry and Biophysics and the Johnson Foundation, University of Pennsylvania Medical Center, Philadelphia, PA 19104-6059, USA

Introduction

The main component in human red blood cells (RBCs) is hemoglobin (Hb), a tetrameric heme protein composed of two heterodimers of the form αβ. Its major physiological function is the transport of oxygen from lungs to peripheral tissues, and carbon dioxide from tissues to lungs. Each subunit of the tetramer has a heme group to which oxygen binds reversibly and altogether in a cooperative manner. However, Hb as such cannot perform its physiological function as its oxygen affinity is rather high, thus hampering the release of oxygen at tissue levels.

The major metabolic process carried out in RBCs is glycolysis. Among the metabolites produced inside RBCs from the consumption of glucose is 2,3-diphosphoglycerate (DPG). This compound is the principal functional modulator of Hb in vivo. When DPG interacts with Hb, the oxygen affinity for oxygen is lowered to optimal levels so that gas transport can be accomplished effectively within the reduced gradient in partial pressures of oxygen between lungs and tissues.

Despite all the efforts aimed at designing alternative blood substitutes, and all the potential risks of infection the use of blood for transfusion entails if pathogens remain undetected, stored blood is the only reasonable and feasible alternative for transfusion available to date. However, great improvements have been accomplished recently on detecting infectious threats present in stored blood, all of which ensure a relatively safer use of this blood for transfusions.

One of the main problems with stored blood is that intracellular levels of DPG decay with time as glycolytic activity ceases in the absence of nutrients. As a consequence, the oxygen affinity of stored RBCs increases with time, hampering the optimal delivery of oxygen from lungs to tissues, and making it less suitable for transfusion. On the other hand, DPG cannot be infused into RBCs to restore the optimal levels found in fresh RBCs. This fact imposes a limit to the shelf lifetime of stored blood for practical use. This period can vary from 3 to 5 weeks, depending on the country. The amount of expired blood that is discarded from blood banks constitutes from 5 to 20% of the total volume of collected blood; a number that is far from insignificant.

Our previous studies on the α-nitrosyl derivative of Hb, that is, a tetrameric Hb in which only the heme groups in the α-subunits are ligated with nitric oxide (NO), have demonstrated that under acidic conditions and/or the presence of allosteric effectors, such as DPG, this derivative shows strikingly reduced affinity for oxygen in the β-subunits while exhibiting cooperativity, despite the fact that both the α-subunits are already ligated [1]. Based on this observation, we attempted to produce this derivative within intact RBCs [2–4] and the results were extremely promising. For the present study, we tried to optimize previous pilot preparation protocols in order to make the entire process applicable to large scale production, while reducing dramatically the preparation time without compromising the quality of the final product. At the same time, we concentrated on avoiding the use of reagents that can be potentially noxious, and replaced them with reagents similar in functionality but exerting protective action over the integrity of RBCs. We also discuss the requirements blood substitutes should meet to make them suitable for practical use in transfusion.

Material and Methods

Expired packed RBCs were obtained from the local branch of the American Red Cross and were processed as previously described [4] with modifications. RBCs were washed three times with 0.15 M sodium phosphate buffer, pH 5.5, containing 2 mM adenine, 45 mM glucose, and 29 mM mannitol (Sigma Aldrich, St. Louis, MO USA), which is a modification of the SAGM solution (sodium, adenine, glucose, mannitol), by repeated resuspension and centrifugation at 3,000 rpm for 10 min. RBCs were then suspended in a 4-fold volume of the same buffer. Deoxygenation was achieved at room temperature by gently bubbling washed pure Ar into the suspension at room temperature in the presence of egg yolk lecithin (Sigma Aldrich) to prevent foam formation.

Nitric oxide was provided in two alternative ways. In the first method, we used an NO donor, FK409 (Fujisawa Pharmaceuticals, Osaka, Japan), also knows as NOR-3. This compound was dissolved in a minimal amount of dimethyl sulfoxide and added to a thoroughly deoxygenated RBC suspension. The amount of NO spontaneously released was detected by EPR as nitrosyl heme, at determined time intervals. No reducing agent was added in the collected samples. The total NO releasing capacity was determined by EPR spectroscopy in the presence of sodium dithionite for the complete release of NO and its quenching by binding to the hemes, by a titration similar to that done with glutathione-SNO (GSNO), as previously described [4]. The second method was carried out with GSNO as NO donor. However, different from our previous protocols, NO was released by spontaneous decomposition of the reagent, rather by reduction in the presence of sodium dithionite.

Results and Discussion

In the present work, special care was taken to improving the previous pilot preparation protocols towards the accomplishment of three main goals: (i) feasibility to upscale the production, (ii) reduction of preparation time while improving the quality of the final product, and (iii) avoidance of potentially noxious chemicals that might compromise biocompatibility.

From earlier experience, it was noted that prolonged shaking of RBC suspensions during the deoxygenation process resulted in a considerable breakage of cells, likely due to mechanical sheer forces created between the vessel wall surface and the cells. Cell membrane fragility to mechanical stress can be improved by the presence of mannitol [5] and adenine [6]. Our modified formulation of the RBC suspension solution containing these two components fulfilled several objectives, one of them being the preservation of integrity if the RBC membranes after extensive nitrogen gas bubbling into the suspension at room temperature. The complete removal of oxygen from the RBC suspension is crucial before the addition of the NO releasing agent in order to prevent the formation of harmful nitrogen oxides that might oxidize Hb and damage the RBC membrane. Oxygen removal was accomplished in a much shorter period of time (3–4 h) by direct bubbling of nitrogen into the suspension at room temperature. We also noticed that despite the exposure of RBCs to physical stress and NO, a reduced degree of hemolysis was produced when compared to our previous protocols. It seems indeed that the presence of adenine and mannitol in the suspension solution helped to preserve the integrity of the RBC membrane along the rejuvenation treatment. Moreover, with the complete removal of oxygen, the presence of sodium dithionite was not necessary and with this, the addition of this potentially noxious agent was prevented.

One of the difficulties encountered in our earlier preparations was the tuning of the rate at which NO was administered into the RBC suspension. As NO is added in small quantities, the chances of one NO molecule to bind to either α- or β-subunits on a deoxyHb tetramer are equal. This distinct process does not trigger the transition from a low to a high affinity conformation as long as most of the other binding sites in the Hb tetramer remain unoccupied. When NO binds to an α-subunit, the axial coordination of the heme iron with the proximal histidine is prone to break and by doing so the NO molecule remains attached to the α-heme, converting the Hb tetramer into a species with extremely low affinity for ligands [1]. On the other hand, binding of NO to a β-subunit is a reversible process and does not convert the tetramer into a high affinity species as long as the saturation level of the other subunits remains low. Subsequently, NO is released and continues redistributing among other binding sites with a preferential binding to the α-subunits. However, when NO is added in bulk amounts, the chances to saturate all hemes at once in a tetramer are high. A fully NO-ligated Hb exhibits high affinity and as a result the release of NO from the β-subunits is hindered, and so is truncated the redistribution of NO that leads to the enrichment of Hb molecules containing NO-ligated α-hemes.

In this work, we studied the use of two substances that release NO over time. As shown in Fig. 1, FK409 displays a half-life time of NO release of 70 min, at 15°C, pH 7.4, following a first order reaction scheme. This rate is slow enough to prevent the "choking" of hemes with NO within a Hb tetramer and allows the redistribution of NO. This observation led us to consider GSNO as an NO donor. Figure 2 shows the time profile of NO-Hb formation within RBCs, carried out at room temperature. It can be noticed that the rate of NO release is much faster than that for FK409, even after temperature corrections from 22°C to 15°C are made. Nevertheless, as revealed in the inset, the NO released binds preferentially to the α-subunits, as detected by the formation of the characteristic hyperfine structure around g ~ 2, which originates from a 5-coordinated nitrosyl-heme. It is clear that the complete deoxygenation of RBCs can be achieved in 3–4 h at room temperature, and that the redistribution of NO after addition of the NO donor is completed in about 3 h.

With the present improvements, it was feasible to carry out the preparation of NO-treated RBCs at room temperature and in large volumes. Using a

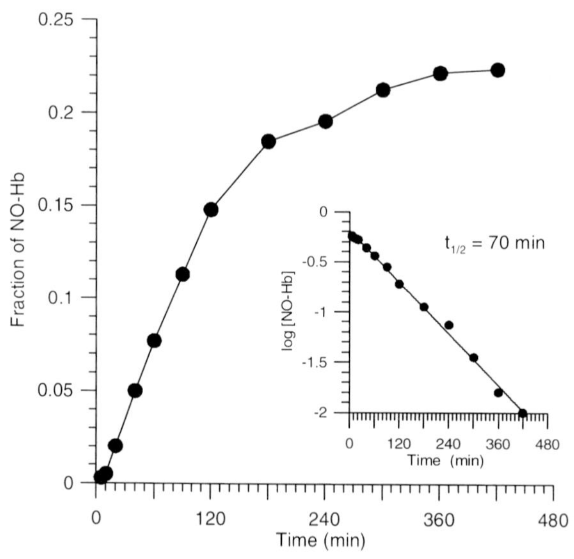

FIG. 1. Time profile of NO-Hb formation within deoxygenated RBCs after incubation with FK409 at 15°C, pH 7.4. A suspension of 10% RBCs in the modified SAGM solution was thoroughly deoxygenated with argon. Then an undersaturating amount over hemes of FK409 dissolved in a minimum amount of dimethyl sulfoxide was added into the suspension. Aliquots were taken anaerobically at discrete times, placed inside EPR tubes and frozen in liquid nitrogen. The concentration of nitrosyl heme was determined by EPR spectroscopy as previously described [2–4]. The *inset* shows the kinetic behavior of the decomposition of FK409, following a first order reaction with a half lifetime of 70 min

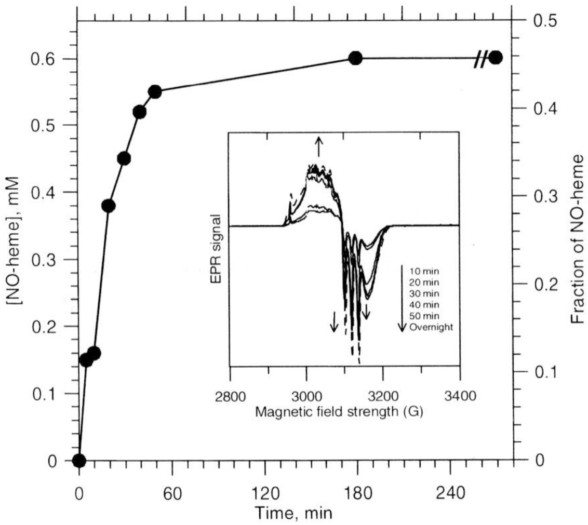

FIG. 2. Time profile of NO-Hb formation within deoxygenated RBCs after incubation with GSNO at room temperature, pH 5.5. The final concentration corresponds approximately to an amount of 50% over heme concentration. Packed RBCs were suspended in a volume about 30 times of the modified SAGM solution. The figure in the *inset* shows the gradual formation of NO-Hb as detected over time by EPR. Most of the formation of NO-Hb within RBCs was completed after 3 h and did not vary after overnight incubation at 4°C

modified suspension solution and the bubbling of argon into the suspension, complete removal of oxygen from RBCs was achieved without the use of sodium dithionite in a relatively short period of time, while preserving the integrity of cell membranes. The spontaneous and gradual release of NO from NO donors (FK409 or GSNO) facilitated the redistribution of NO with preferential binding to the α-subunits, and avoided the problems involved with the bulk addition of NO into the RBC suspension. Subsequent studies will focus on the control of NO release from several NO donors and the effect temperature exerts on the redistribution of NO throughout vacant hemes. Knowing these parameters, it should be possible to predict the distribution of NO inside RBCs without the need for EPR monitoring.

Acknowledgments. We thank Dr. Makoto Suematsu, Keio University Medical School, Tokyo, Japan, and Dr. Toshiro Inubushi, Shiga University of Medical Science, Ohtsu, Japan, for their continuous support and invaluable critical input to these studies. We also thank Dr. Yoshihiko Oyanagui, Fujisawa Pharmaceuticals, Osaka, Japan, for kindly providing the NO donor FK409 used in the present study. This study was supported by NIH grant HL 14508.

References

1. Yonetani T, Tsuneshige A, Zhou X-s, et al (1998) Electron paramagnetic resonance and oxygen binding studies of α-nitrosyl hemoglobin. J Biol Chem 273:20323–20333
2. Yonetani T, Tsuneshige A (2000) USA Patent 6,087,087, 11 July 2000
3. Tsuneshige A, Yonetani T (2001) Art cells. Blood Subs and Immob Biotech 29:347–357
4. Tsuneshige A, Yonetani I (2001) In: S Evans, J Biaglow, DF Wilson (eds) Advanced Experimental Medical Biology. Kluwer Academic, pp 1–6
5. Heaton A, Miripol J, Aster R, et al (1984) Use of adsol preservation solution for prolonged storage of low viscosity AS-1 red blood cells. Brit J Haematol 57:467–478
6. Hong TV, Wuilleret B (1984) Effects of rejuvenation of blood on 2,3-diphosphoglycerate and adenosine triphosphate and mechanical resistance of red blood cells. Vox Sanguinis 29:306–310

Oxygen-Carrying Plasma Hemoprotein Including Synthetic Heme

TERUYUKI KOMATSU and EISHUN TSUCHIDA

Summary. Recombinant human serum albumin (rHSA) incorporating tetraphenylporphyrinatoiron(II) derivative with four pivaloylamino substituents (FepivP), albumin-heme, is an entirely synthetic hemoprotein that can reversibly bind and release O_2 under physiological conditions. We have recently found that replacing the substituent groups of FepivP with more hydrophobic 1-methylcyclohexanoylamino groups, affording FecycP, substantially stabilizes the formed O_2–adduct complex. The O_2- and CO-binding abilities and blood compatibility of this new rHSA-heme hybrid (rHSA-FecycP) have been investigated by spectroscopy. The maximum number of FecycP binding to one albumin was determined to be eight. Because the isoelectric point and circular dichroism (CD) spectral pattern were identical to those of rHSA itself, the two-dimensional structure of the host albumin could be unchanged after the incorporation of FecycP. Laser-flash photolysis experiments gave the association and dissociation rate constants for O_2 and CO (k_{on}, k_{off}). The rebinding kinetics of these gaseous ligands consists of multiple exponentials. We conjectured that the O_2- and CO-binding reactions are affected by the molecular environment around each of the active heme sites. rHSA-FecycP showed almost the same O_2-binding affinity($P_{1/2}^{O_2}$ 34 torr at 37°C) and thermodynamic parameters (ΔH, ΔS) for the oxygenation as rHSA-FepivP. In contrast, the half-life of the O_2-adduct complex (9 h, 37°C) became significantly longer than that of rHSA-FepivP (by a factor of 4.5), which is close to that of myoglobin. The obtained red solution was stable and demonstrated a long shelf life (>2 years) at room temperature. The equivalent mixture of rHSA-FecycP and whole blood exhibited no coagulation or precipitation, indicating its high blood compatibility.

Advanced Research Institute for Science and Engineering, Waseda University, 3-4-1 Okubo, Shinjuku-ku, Tokyo 169-8555, Japan

Key words. Human serum albumin, Albumin-heme, Synthetic hemoprotein, Oxygen-binding ability, Red blood cell substitute

Introduction

Human serum albumin (HSA) used for clinical treatment in Japan amounted to 1.9 million l (in terms of a blood source) in 2002 [1]. Most was administered to hemorrhagic shocked patients as a resuscitation fluid. If HSA can transport oxygen (O_2) like red blood cells, it could be of extreme medical importance not only as a blood replacement but also as an O_2 therapeutic agent.

In our circulatory system, free hemin, an iron(III) complex of protoporphyrin IX dissociated from methemoglobin, is potentially toxic because it may (1) intercalate phospholipid membranes, (2) be a major source of iron for bacterial pathogens, and (3) catalyze the formation of free radicals. Hemopexin has high affinity for binding protein with hemin, having the highest binding constant of any known protein ($K > 10^{12} M^{-1}$), but it releases it into liver cells via specific surface receptors [2]. Crystal structure analysis of the hemopexin-hemin complex revealed that the hemin is tightly bound by double histidine coordinations to the central ferric ion and multiple hydrogen bondings with the amino acid residues [3]. Nevertheless, the concentration of hemopexin in the plasma is rather low (<17 μM). HSA may also provide reserve binding capacity of hemin in various conditions (e.g., trauma, inflammation, hemolysis). In fact, HSA binds hemin with a relatively high affinity ($K = 10^8 M^{-1}$) [4]. We have determined the single crystal structure of the HSA-hemin-myristate complex with a resolution of 3.2 Å [5]. Hemin is accommodated into the narrow D-shaped pocket in subdomain IB; and proximal coordination with Tyr-161 and three hydrogen bondings with basic amino acids contribute to maintaining the assembly. Addition of a sodium dithionate into this solution under an N_2 atmosphere reduced the central ferric ion to the ferrous state, although exposure to O_2 gas immediately oxidized the iron(II) center (T. Komatsu, N. Ohmichi, E. Tsuchida, unpublished data, 2004).

We have found that tetraphenylporphyrinatoiron(II) derivative with four pivaloylamino substituents (FepivP) (Fig. 1) was also incorporated into HSA, and the obtained albumin-heme (HSA-FepivP) can reversibly bind and release O_2 under physiological conditions in the same manner as hemoglobin (Hb) and myoglobin (Mb) [6–12]. Because recombinant HSA (rHSA) was manufactured on a large scale by expression in *Pichia pastoris* [13], rHSA-heme hybrid has become entirely synthetic and absolutely free of infectious pathogens. Our animal experiments have also demonstrated that rHSA-heme works as an "oxygen-carrying plasma hemoprotein" in the bloodstream [14; T. Komatsu et al., unpublished data, 2004].

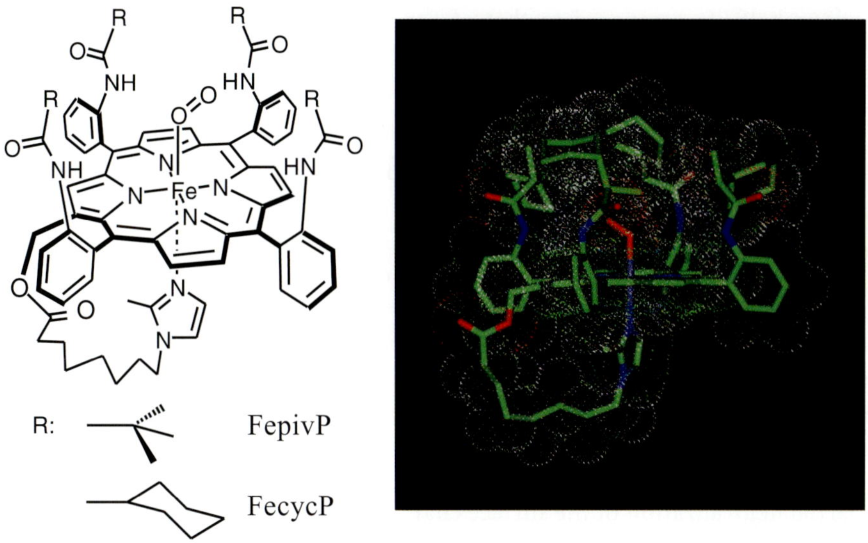

FIG. 1. Structures of the new tetraphenylporphyrinatoiron(II) derivative with more hydrophobic 1-methylcyclohexanoylamino groups on the porphyrin ring plane (FecycP) and pivaloylamino substituents (FepivP), and the simulated structure of oxygenated FecycP. The extensible systematic forcefield (ESFF) simulation was performed using an Insight II system (Molecular Simulations, San Diego, CA, USA). The structure was generated by alternative minimization and annealing dynamic calculations from 1000 K to 100 K. The dielectric constant was fixed at 2.38 D, corresponding to the toluene solution. The *dotted surface* represents the van der Waals radius

Half of the Hb-based O_2 carrier in advanced clinical trials still exhibited vasoconstriction, which increased blood pressure and decreased cardiac output [15–19]. The precise mechanism of this hypertension is controversial, but many investigators suspect that the Hb molecules penetrate the vascular endothelium and bind the endothelial-derived relaxing factor (EDRF), namely nitric oxide [20–27]. Others believe that excessive delivery of O_2 to arteriolar vascular walls induces autoregulatory vasoconstriction [28–33]. Interestingly, rHSA-heme does not induce such a vasopressor effect [34]. The electrostatic repulsion between the albumin surface and glomerular basement membrane around the endothelial cell retards rapid leakage of the rHSA-heme molecule and quick scavenging of NO. Albumin-heme is now recognized to be one of the most promising materials as a new class of red blood cell substitute.

To improve the O_2-binding ability of rHSA-FepivP, we have synthesized new tetraphenylporphyrinatoiron(II) derivative with more hydrophobic 1-methylcyclohexanoylamino groups on the porphyrin ring plane (FecycP) (Fig. 1) [35]. rHSA-FecycP forms a significantly stable O_2-adduct complex with a long half-life compared to that of FepivP (by a factor of 4.5). We herein report the O_2- and CO-binding abilities of this entirely synthetic albumin-based O_2 carrier.

Incorporation of Heme into rHSA

Based on quantitative analysis of the absorption intensity for the Soret band of aqueous rHSA-FecycP, the maximum number of FecycP binding to an rHSA was determined to be eight using a molar extinction coefficient [35]. FecycP is accommodated into certain domains of rHSA with binding constants of 10^6–$10^4\,M^{-1}$.

The isoelectric points (*p*I) of the obtained rHSA-FecycP hybrid (FecycP/rHSA = 1–8 mol/mol) were 4.8, exactly the same as those of rHSA. Fatty acid binding, for example, induced a reduction in the *p*I value due to partial neutralization of the surface charge. The FecycP molecule without any ionic side chain interacts nonspecifically with a hydrophobic subdomain of rHSA, so its surface charge distributions are unaltered. Consequently, the essential biological roles as serum albumin [i.e., control of colloid osmotic pressure (COP) and plasma expansion] are essentially sustained after the incorporation of FecycP.

The secondary and tertiary structures of rHSA and the deformation upon FecycP binding were measured by circular dichroism (CD) spectroscopy. The spectral pattern showed typical double-minimum negative peaks in the ultraviolet (UV) region independent of the number of FecycP molecular bound (Fig. 2). The estimated α-helix content was approximately 67%, suggesting that the FecycP association did not cause any high-ordered structural change in the host albumin. Moreover, rHSA-FecycP showed no induced CD in the Soret region (400–500 nm). The hemin binding to the serum albumin is accompanied by a rise in the extrinsic negative Cotton effect in the Soret region because it binds to albumin through axial coordination, allowing a large degree of immobilization [36,37]. We concluded that hydrophobic interaction is the major molecular force of FecycP binding, and its incorporation does not induce any changes in the highly ordered structure or in the surface net charges of rHSA.

O_2-Binding Property of rHSA-Heme

The UV-visible absorption spectrum of the aqueous rHSA hybrid that included carbonyl FecycP showed the formation of the typical CO-coordinated low-spin tetraphenylporphyrinatoiron(II) derivative (λ_{max}: 429, 545 nm). Light irradiation of this solution under an O_2 atmosphere led to

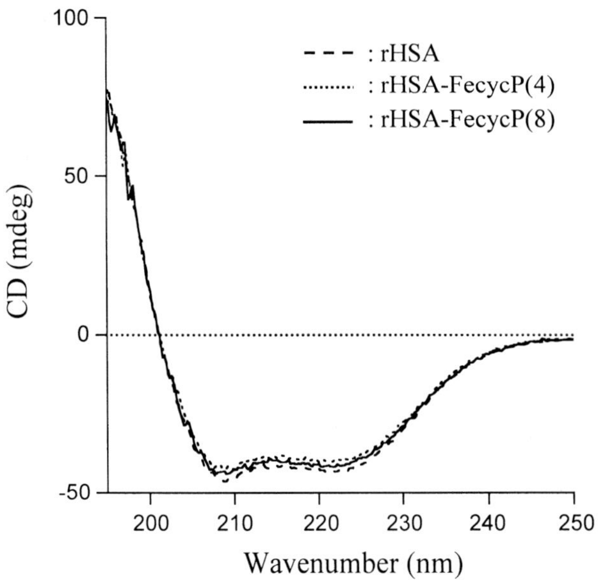

FIG. 2. Circular dichroism (*CD*) spectra of recombinant human serum albumin (*rHSA*) and rHSA-FecycP in water at 25°C

CO dissociation, giving the O_2-adduct complex (λ_{max}: 428, 555 nm). Upon exposure of the oxygenated rHSA-FecycP to N_2, the UV-visible absorption pattern changed to that of the five-*N*-coordinated high-spin iron(II) complex with an intramolecularly coordinated proximal imidazole (λ_{max}: 445, 543, 567 nm). This oxygenation was reversibly dependent on the O_2 partial pressure and sufficiently stable under physiological conditions (37°C, pH 7.4) (Fig. 3). The rate of irreversible oxidation is satisfactorily slow (vide infra).

The O_2 coordination to FecycP in human serum albumin is expressed by Eq. 1.

$$\mathrm{FeP} + \mathrm{O_2} \underset{k_{off}^{O_2}}{\overset{k_{on}^{O_2}}{\rightleftarrows}} \mathrm{FeP\text{-}O_2} \quad (1)$$

$$\left[P_{1/2}{}^{O_2} = \left(K^{O_2}\right)^{-1} = k_{on}{}^{O_2} / k_{off}{}^{O_2}\right]$$

The O_2 association and O_2-dissociation rate constants ($k_{on}{}^{O_2}$, $k_{off}{}^{O_2}$) were explored by laser flash photolysis (Table 1) [9,35,38–40]. The detailed kinetic evaluation of rHSA-FecycP gave the following results.

1. The absorption decays accompanying O_2 recombination were composed of three phases of first-order kinetics; the curves were fit by a triple-exponential equation [9]. The minor (<10%) and fastest component was

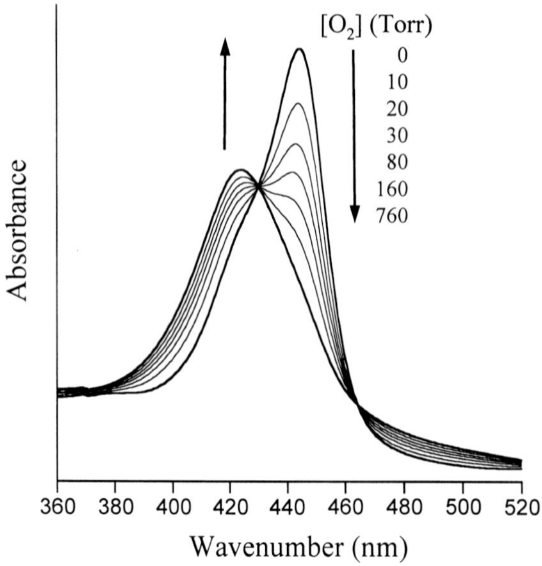

FIG. 3. Ultraviolet-visible. Absorption spectral changes of rHSA-FecycP(4) dependent on the O_2 partial pressure in phosphate-buffered solution (pH 7.3) at 37°C. The number in parenthesis is molar ratio of FecycP and rHSA

TABLE 1. O_2 association and dissociation rate constants for rHSA-FecycP in phosphate-buffered solution (pH 7.3) at 25°C

	$k_{on}[M^{-1}s^{-1}]$		$k_{off}[s^{-1}]$	
Substance	Fast	Slow	Fast	Slow
rHSA-FecycP(8)	4.6×10^7	7.3×10^6	9.8×10^2	1.6×10^2
rHSA-FepivP(8)[a]	3.4×10^7	9.5×10^6	7.5×10^2	2.0×10^2
Hb (T-state)α[b]	2.9×10^6		1.8×10^2	

rHSA, recombinant human serum albumin; FecycP, tetraphenylporphyrinatoiron(II) derivative with 1-methyl cyclohexanoylamino groups; FepivP, tetraphenyl porphyrinato-iron (II) with pivaloyamino substitute; Hb, hemoglobin.
[a] Ref. [9].
[b] pH 7, 20°C; Ref. [40].
The numbers in parenthesis is molar ratio of porphyrin and rHSA.

independent of the O_2 concentrations. It should be correlated with a base elimination [41].
2. Based on careful inspection of the two slower phases, the association rate constants for the fast and slow rebinding [k_{on}(fast) and k_{on}(slow)] of O_2 were calculated. The k_{on}(fast) values are four- to fivefold higher than the k_{on}(slow) volues.
3. The concentration ratios of the fast and slow reactions were 2:1 to 3:1.

Based on these findings, we can conclude that the O_2 association with FecycP in the hydrophobic domains of rHSA is influenced by the molecular

TABLE 2. O_2-binding equilibrium parameters and half-lifetime of rHSA-FecycP in phosphate-buffered solution (pH 7.3)

Substance	$P_{1/2}$(torr)[a]	ΔH[kJ mol^{-1}]	ΔS[J K^{-1}mol^{-1}]	$\tau_{1/2}$[h][a]
rHSA-FecycP(4)	34	−59	−108	9
rHSA-FecycP(8)	35	−59	−107	9
rHSA-FepivP(4)[b]	36	−60	−114	2
rHSA-FepivP(8)[b]	33	−60	−112	2
Red cells[c]	27			
Hbα	40[d]	−57 to −65[e]	−116 to −133[e]	35[f]
Mb[d]	40[d]	−57 to −65[e]	−116 to −133[e]	12[g]

[a] At 37°C.
[b] Ref. [8].
[c] pH 7.4; ref. [42].
[d] T-state, pH 7, 20°C; ref. [40].
[e] pH 7.4; ref. [43].
[f] At 37°C, pH 7.2; ref. [44].
[g] At 35°C, pH 7.0; ref. [45].
The number in parenthesis is molar ratio of porphyrin and rHSA.

microenvironment around each O_2 coordination site (e.g., steric hindrance of the amino acid residue and difference in polarity).

The O_2-binding affinity for such oxygenation could be directly determined. Adequate isosbestic behavior was maintained during the course of a spectrophotometric titration of O_2 (Fig. 3). According to the kinetic experiments, the $P_{1/2}$ values were divided into two components using our previously reported equation [9]. The calculated $P_{1/2}$ for the fast and slow phases were identical in each case (Table 2). The thermodynamic parameters (ΔH, ΔS) of oxygenation were also measured by the van't Hoff plots of the K^{O_2} values (Fig. 4) [8]. The $P_{1/2}{}^{O_2}$, ΔH, and ΔS values for oxygenation of rHSA-FecycP resembled those of Hb and Mb [8,40,42–45]. Moreover, we could not find significant differences in these parameters for rHSA-FepivP and rHSA-FecycP. This result indicates that the substituent structure on the porphyrin plane does not cause any substantial change in the O_2 equilibria and kinetics of rHSA-heme.

Stability of O_2-Adduct Complex of Albumin-Heme

Accompanying the autooxidation of the central iron(II), the absorption band (λ_{max} 555 nm) slowly disappeared at 37°C, leading to formation of the inactive ferric porphyrin. The effect of the heme structure on the half-life of the O_2-adduct complex against the ferric state ($\tau_{1/2}$) was marked. The rHSA-FecycP had a $\tau_{1/2}$ of 9 h, which is 4.5-fold longer than that of rHSA-FepivP and close to that of the Mb (12 h at 37°C) [46].

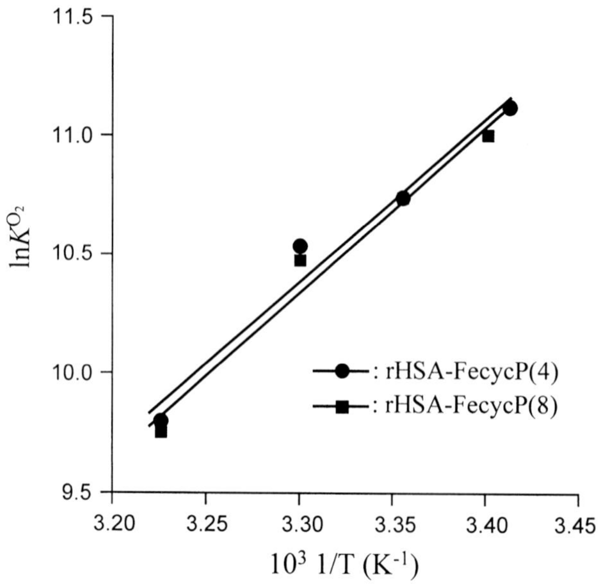

FIG. 4. Van't Hoff plots of O_2-binding affinity of rHSA-FecycP in phosphate-buffered solution (pH 7.3)

CO-Binding Property of rHSA-Heme

Upon addition of CO gas through the deoxy or oxy state of the rHSA-FecycP solution, the spectrum immediately exhibited formation of the carbonyl complex. The CO-binding affinity ($P_{1/2}^{CO}$) of rHSA-FecycP became 2.5-fold higher than that of rHSA-FepivP (Table 3) [9,47,48]. Kinetically, this is due to the low CO dissociation rate constant, k_{off}^{CO}. More recently, CO/O_2 discrimination of Hb and Mb has not been based mainly on distal steric constraints in the heme pocket; the emphasis has shifted to polar interactions in the binding pocket [49,50]. That is, a polar environment could favor the highly polarized coordinated Fe-O_2 unit over the apolar Fe-CO moiety. In FecycP, the hydrophobic cavity around the central ferrous ion probably contributes to the rise in CO-binding affinity. This interpretation is in good agreement with assumptions by other investigators.

Blood Compatibility

The red rHSA-FecycP solution showed a long shelf life (>2 years) at temperatures of 4°–37°C without any aggregation or precipitation. The solution properties also satisfied physiological requirements. The specific gravity was 1.013 (FecycP/rHSA = 1–8 mol/mol). The viscosity of 1.2 cP (at a high shear

TABLE 3. CO-binding parameters of rHSA-FecycP in phosphate-buffered solution (pH 7.3) at 25°C

Substance	$P_{1/2}^{CO}$(torr)	$k_{on}(M^{-1}s^{-1})$	
		Fast	Slow
rHSA-FecycP(8)	0.04	5.9×10^6	8.9×10^5
rHSA-FepivP(8)	0.10	4.9×10^6	6.7×10^5
Hb (T-state)α[a]	0.30	2.2×10^5	

[a] Aqueous, pH 7.0–7.4, 20°C; refs. [47, 48].
The number in parenthesis is molar ratio of porphyrin and rHSA.

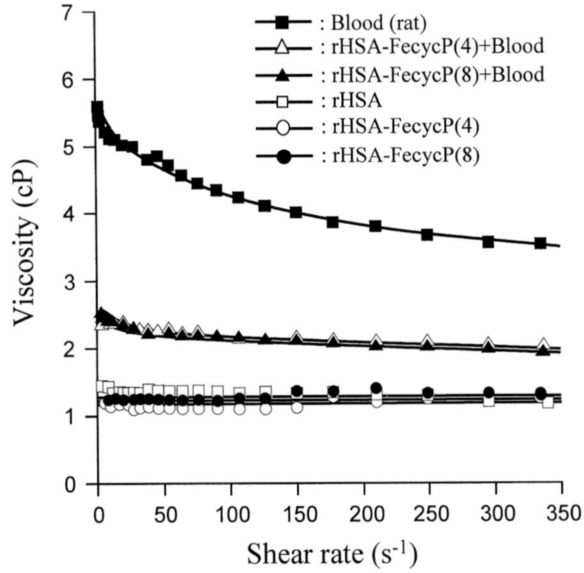

FIG. 5. Viscosity of rHSA-FecycP solution with whole blood at 37°C

rate of $230\,s^{-1}$) was much lower than that of whole blood (4.0 cP) and exhibited Newtonian-type shear rate dependence similar to that of rHSA itself (Fig. 5). Furthermore, the viscosity of the mixed dispersion with freshly drawn blood (1:1, v/v) showed 2.0 cP (at $230\,s^{-1}$), indicating that rHSA-FecycP had good compatibility with blood. Optical microscopic observations also revealed that the homogeneous morphology of the red blood cells was not affected by mixing with whole blood (not shown).

Conclusions

Human serum albumin incorporating synthetic heme formed an O_2-adduct complex under physiological conditions. In particular, oxygenated rHSA-FecycP showed high stability compared to the previous rHSA-FepivP, and its half-life reached a value similar to that of the native Mb. It has been also found that another rHSA-heme complex incorporating an FecycP analogue with a histidyl base at the porphyrin periphery had an extremely long half-life of the oxygenated complex (25 h) under the same conditions (in this case the O_2-binding affinity is quite high) [35]. rHSA–FecycP with a $P_{1/2}$ value (34 torr at 37°C) similar to that of red blood cells is now the most promising material to be used as an artificial O_2 carrier. Exchange transfusion with rHSA-FecycP into anesthetized beagles to evaluate its clinical safety and efficacy is now under investigation.

Acknowledgments. This work was partially supported by Health Science Research Grants from MHLW, Grant-in-Aid for Scientific Research (No. 16350093) from JSPS, and Grant-in-Aid for Exploratory Research (No. 16655049) from MEXT. The authors are grateful to NIPRO Corp. for their supporting the oxygen-infusion project. We also thank Mr. Seiji Ishihara (Waseda University) for his skilful physicochemical experiment.

References

1. Homepage of Ministry of Health, Labor, and Welfare, Japan (2003) (http://www.mhlw.go.jp/shingi/2003/06/s0627-12.html)
2. Tolosano E, Altruda F (2002) Hemopexin: structure, function, and regulation. DNA Cell Biol 21:297–306
3. Paoli M, Anderson BF, Baler HM, et al (1999) Crystal structure of hemopexin reveals a novel high-affinity heme site formed between two β-propeller domains. Nat Struct Biol 6:926–931
4. Adams PA, Berman MC (1980) Kinetics and mechanism of the interaction between human serum albumin and monomeric heamin. Biochem J 191:95–102
5. Zunszain PA, Ghuman J, Komatsu T, et al (2003) Crystal structural analysis of human serum albumin complexed with hemin and fatty acid. BMC Struct Biol 3:6
6. Komatsu T, Hamamatsu K, Wu J, et al (1999) Physicochemical properties and O_2-coordination structure of human serum albumin incorporating tetrakis(*o*-pivamido)phenylporphyrinatoiron(II) derivatives. Bioconjug Chem 10:82–86
7. Komatsu T, Hamamatsu K, Tsuchida E (1999) Cross-linked human serum albumin dimers incorporating sixteen (tetraphenylporphinato)iron(II) derivatives: synthesis, characterization, and O_2-binding property. Macromolecules 32:8388–8391
8. Tsuchida E, Komatsu T, Mastukawa, et al (1999) Human serum albumin incorporating tetrakis(*o*-pivalamido)phenylporphinato-iron(II) derivative as a totally synthetic O_2-carrying hemoprotein. Bioconjug Chem 10:797–802
9. Komatsu T, Matsukawa Y, Tsuchida E (2000) Kinetics of CO and O_2 binding to human serum albumin-heme hybrid. Bioconjug Chem 11:772–776
10. Komatsu T, Matsukawa Y, Tsuchida E (2001) Reaction of nitric oxide with synthetic hemoprotein, human serum albumin incorporating tetraphenylporphyrinatoiron(II) derivatives. Bioconjug Chem 12:71–75
11. Komatsu T, Okada T, Moritake M, et al (2001) O_2-binding properties of double-sided porphyrinatoiron(II)s with polar substituents and their human serum albumin hybrids. Bull Chem Soc Jpn 74:1695–1702

12. Huang Y, Komatsu T, Nakagawa A, et al (2003) Compatibility in vitro of albumin-heme (O_2 carrier) with blood cell components. J Biomed Mater Res 66A:292–297
13. Sumi A, Ohtani W, Kobayashi K, et al (1993) Purification and physicochemical properties of recombinant human serum albumin. Biotechnol Blood Proteins 227:293–298
14. Tsuchida E, Komatsu T, Hamamatsu K, et al (2000) Exchange transfusion of albumin-heme as an artificial O_2-infusion into anesthetized rats: physiological responses, O_2-delivery and reduction of the oxidized hemin sites by red blood cells. Bioconjug Chem 11:46–50
15. Chang TMS (1997) Recent and future developments in modified hemoglobin and microencapsulated hemoglobin as red blood cell substitutes. Artif Cells Blood Substit Immobil Biotechnol 25:1–24
16. Tsuchida E (1998) Perspectives of blood substitutes. In: Tsuchida E (ed) Blood substitutes: present and future perspectives. Elsevier Science, Lausanne, pp 1–14
17. Winslow RM (1998) The role of blood substitutes in emerging healthcare systems. In: Tsuchida E (ed) Blood substitutes: present and future perspectives. Elsevier Science, Lausanne, pp 15–32
18. Winslow RM (1999) New transfusion strategies: red cell substitutes. Annu Rev Med 50:337–353
19. Squires JE (2002) Artificial blood. Science 295:1002–1005
20. Keipert P, Chang T (1998) Pyridoxylated-polyhemoglobin solution: a low viscosity oxygen-delivery blood replacement fluid with normal oncotic pressure and long term storage feasibility. Biomater Artif Cells 16:185–196
21. Keipert PE, Gonzales A, Gomez CL, et al (1993) Acute changes in systemic blood pressure and urine output of conscious rats following exchange transfusion with diaspirin-crosslinked hemoglobin solution. Transfusion 33:701–708
22. Hess JR, MacDonald VW, Brinkley WW (1993) Synthetic and pulmonary hypertension after resuscitation with cell-free hemoglobin. J Appl Physiol 74:1769–1778
23. Schultz SC, Grady B, Cole F, et al (1993) A role for endothelin and nitric oxide in the pressor response to diaspirin cross-linked hemoglobin. J Lab Clin Med 122:301–308
24. Thompson A, McGarry AE, Valeri CR, et al (1994) Stroma-free hemoglobin increases blood pressure and GFR in the hypotensive rat: role of nitric oxide. J Appl Physiol 77:2348–2354
25. Sharma AC, Singh G, Gulati A (1995) Role of NO mechanism in cardiovascular effects of diaspirin cross-linked hemoglobin in anesthetized rats. Am J Physiol 269:H1379–H1399
26. Moisan S, Drapeau G, Burhop KE, et al (1998) Mechanism of the acute pressor effect and bradycardia elicited by disapirin crosslinked hemoglobin in anesthetized rats. Can J Physiol Pharmacol 76:434–442
27. Abassi Z, Kotob S, Pieruzzi F, et al (1997) Effects of polymerization on the hypertensive action of diaspirin cross-linked hemoglobin in rats. J Lab Clin Med 129:603–610
28. Guyton AC, Ross JM, Carrier O, et al (1964) Evidence for tissue oxygen demand as the major factor causing autoregulation. Circ Res 14:1–60
29. Johnson PC (1986) Autoregulation of blood flow. Circ Res 59:483–495
30. Vandegriff KD, Winslow RM (1995) A theoretical analysis of oxygen transport: a new strategy for the design of hemoglobin-based red cell substitutes. In: Winslow RM, Vandegriff KD, Intaglietta M (eds). Blood substitutes: physiological basis of efficiency. Birkhäuser, Boston, pp 143–154
31. Tsai AG, Kerger H, Intaglietta M (1995) Microcirculatory consequences of blood substitution with $\alpha\alpha$-hemoglobin. In: Winslow RM, Vandegriff KD, Intaglietta M (eds) Blood substitutes: physiological basis of efficiency. Birkhäuser, Boston, pp 155–174

32. Rohlfs RJ, Bruner E, Chiu A, et al (1998) Arterial blood pressure responses to cell-free hemoglobin solutions and the reaction with nitric oxide. J Biol Chem 273:12128–12134
33. Winslow RM (2000) αα-Crosslinked hemoglobin: was failure predicted by preclinical testing? Vox Sang 79:1–20
34. Tsuchida E, Komatsu T, Matsukawa Y, et al (2003) Human serum albumin incorporating synthetic heme: red blood cell substitute without hypertension by nitric oxide scavenging. J Biomed Mater Res 64A:257–261
35. Komatsu T, Matsukawa Y, Tsuchida E (2002) Effect of heme structure on O_2-binding properties of human serum albumin-heme hybrids: intramolecular histidine coordination provides a stable O_2-adduct complex. Bioconjug Chem 13:397–402
36. Beaven H, Chen CH, D'Albis A, et al (1974) A spectroscopic studies of the haemin-human-serum-albumin system. Eur J Biochem 41:539–546
37. Casella L, Gullotti M, Ploi S, et al (1993) Haem-protein interactions: the binding of haem complexes to serum albumin. Gazz Chim Itali 123:149–154
38. Traylor TG, Tsuchiya S, Campbell D, et al (1985) Anthracene heme cyclophanes: steric effects in CO, O_2, and RNC binding. J Am Chem Soc 107:604–614
39. Collman JP, Brauman JI, Iverson BL, et al (1983) O_2 and CO binding to iron(II) porphyrins: a comparison of the "picket fence" and "pocket" porphyrins. J Am Chem Soc 105:3052–3064
40. Sawicki CA, Gibson QH (1977) Properties of the T state of human oxyhemoglobin stideid by laser flash photolysis. J Biol Chem 252:7538–7547
41. Geibel J, Cannon J, Campbell D, et al (1978) Model compounds for R-state and T-state hemoglobins. J Am Chem Soc 100:3575–3585
42. Severinghaus JW (1966) Blood gas calculator. J Appl Physiol 21:1108–1116
43. Imai K, Yonetani T (1975) Thermodynamical studies of oxygen equilibrium of hemoglobin. J Biol Chem 250:7093–7098
44. Sugawara Y, Shikama K (1980) Autoxidation of native oxymyoglobin. Eur J Biochem 110:241–246
45. Mansouri A, Winterhalter H (1973) Nonequivalence of chains in hemoglobin oxidation. Biochemistry 12:4946–4949
46. Sugawara Y, Shikama K (1980) Autoxidation of native oxymyoglobin. Eur J Biochem 110:241–246
47. Steinmeier RC, Parkhurst LJ (1975) Kinetic studies on the five principle components of normal adult human hemoglobin. Biochemistry 14:1564–1573
48. Sharma VS, Schmidt MR, Ranney HM (1976) Dissociation of CO from carboxyhemoglobin. J Biol Chem 251:4267–4272
49. Springer BA, Sligar SG, Olson JS, et al (1994) Mechanism of ligand recognition in myoglobin. Chem Rev 94:699–714
50. Matsuura M, Tani F, Naruta Y (2002) Formation and characterization of carbon monoxide adducts of iron "twin coronet" porphyrins: extremely low CO affinity and a strong negative polar effect on bound CO. J Am Chem Soc 124:1941–1950

Micromechanical Properties of Newly Developed Polyelectrolyte Microcapsules (PEMC)

HANS BÄUMLER[1], CHRISTINA KELEMEN[2], RITA MITLÖHNER[1], RADOSTINA GEORGIEVA[3], ASTRID KRABI[2], SILKE SCHÄLING[1], GERHARD ARTMANN[2], and HOLGER KIESEWETTER[1]

Summary. Microcapsules fabricated from polyelectrolytes offer advantages in that they are permeable to polar molecules and are extremely stable against chemical and physical influences as compared with liposomes. Polyelectrolyte microcapsules (PEMC) were prepared by consecutive multiple adsorption of different polyanions and polycations on decomposable/dissolvable biological templates like red blood cells. Poly(styrene sulfonate) [PSS], dextransulfate and human serum albumin were adsorbed alternately with poly(allylamine hydrochloride) [PAH] onto glutardialdehyde treated red blood cells as template, which was decomposed after completing the coating by a hypochlorite solution. Deformability properties of PEMC were studied by means of micropipette technique and confocal laser scanning imaging. The morphological properties of the PEMC were characterised by atomic force microscopy, confocal laser scanning microscopy and electrophoretic mobility. Rheological properties were investigated by viscosimetry as well aggregometry (light backscattering). The detectable surface charge was always negative. The wall thickness as well as the bending modulus (BM) of the PEMC was dependent on the number of layers and the used polyelectrolytes. The thicknesses were in the range between 7 and 28 nm and the BM was 4 to 5 magnitudes larger than the BM of red blood cells, which results in a slightly increased apparent blood viscosity and an increased aggregation time of a mixture of PEMC and blood (1 : 1).

Key words. Microcapsules, Polyelectrolytes, Deformability, Electrophoresis

[1] Institute of Transfusion Medicine, Charité, Humboldt University of Berlin, D-10098 Berlin, Germany
[2] Department of Applied Biophysics, TFH Aachen, D-52428 Jülich, Germany
[3] Max Planck Institute of Colloids and Interfaces, D-14424 Potsdam-Golm, Germany

Introduction

Recently, micro- and nano-sized polyelectrolyte capsules have been fabricated applying the layer-by-layer adsorption technique on charged colloidal particles with subsequent decomposition and removal of the core [1–3]. The size of the capsules can be varied from 0.1 to tens of microns depending on the size of the template. The thickness of the capsule wall depends on the number of assembled polyelectrolyte layers and can be adjusted in the nanometer range [4]. A variety of colloidal particles, like melamine resin latexes (MRL) [1–3,5–7] or biological cells [3,8] have already been used as templates for the capsule preparation.

In the fabrication of the red blood cells (RBC) capsules a deproteinizer has been used resulting in an oxidation of both the biological template and the assembled polyelectrolyte layers. This causes a loss of amino groups in the film as well as a significant mass reduction. In addition, the oxidation and release of biological material lead to a transient osmotic expansion [7]. The reversibility of the expansion was explained by the elasticity of the shell wall representing a polymer net held together by bonds formed during oxidation.

The novel capsules may have applications in biology and medicine as micro-containers and micro-reactors for drugs, enzymes, DNA and other bioactive substances. Their size and shape, and their mechanical and chemical stability mimic that of the cells. Especially, microcapsules fabricated on RBC are very interesting for this purpose because their elastic properties and their shape largely match the original biological template [8].

A new polyelectrolyte combination of the biocompatible dextran sulphate and poly(allylamine hydrochloride) was used for capsule preparation. The micromechanical properties of these new capsules were compared with poly(styrene sulphonate)/poly(allyl amine hydrochloride) capsules.

Materials and Methods

Materials

The sources of chemicals were the following:

Polyelectrolytes: poly (styrene sulphonate, sodium salt) (PSS), Mw 70000, Aldrich (Steinheim, Germany); poly (allyl amine hydrochloride), (PAH), Mw 70000, Aldrich; dextran sulphate, ($DxSO_4$), Mw 500000, Pharmacia Fine Chemicals (Uppsala, Sweden), human serum albumin, (HSA), Mw ca. 65000, Sigma (St. Louis, MO, USA).

Labelled substances: fluorescein isothiocyanate labelled human serum albumin, (FITC-HSA), fluorescein isothiocyanate labelled dextran, (FITC-Dextran), Mw 77000; Sigma.

Other chemicals: glutaraldehyde (Grade I), Sigma-Aldrich (Schnelldorf, Germany); sodium hypochlorite (NaOCl), sodium chloride (NaCl) and phosphate buffer solution (PBS).

Capsule Preparation

Erythrocyte Fixation

Erythrocytes were obtained from fresh human blood anti-coagulated with ethylene diamine tetra-acetate (EDTA) by means of centrifugation and subsequently washed twice in buffered NaCl solution (140 mM NaCl, 5.6 mM KCl, 5.8 mM sodium phosphate buffer, pH 7.4). The cells were then stabilized with glutaraldehyde [9] at a final concentration of 2% for 60 min at 20°C. After fixation the cells were washed at least four times with distilled water and then resuspended in 154 mM NaCl solution.

Polyelectrolyte Film Assembly and Core Dissolution

The stepwise adsorption of oppositely charged polymers was performed using a filtration technique [3] and is schematically illustrated in Fig. 1. The polyelectrolyte assembly was performed either with PSS or $DxSO_4$ as the negatively charged polyelectrolytes followed by PAH as the positive polyelectrolyte. The coating was always started with the negative polymer. Fixed erythrocytes were suspended in buffer-free 1 mg/ml polyelectrolyte and 0.5 M NaCl with a final cell concentration of 10%(v/v). The pH values were 5.0 ± 0.1, 5.5 ± 0.1 and 6.0 ± 0.2 for the PAH, PSS and $DxSO_4$ solutions,

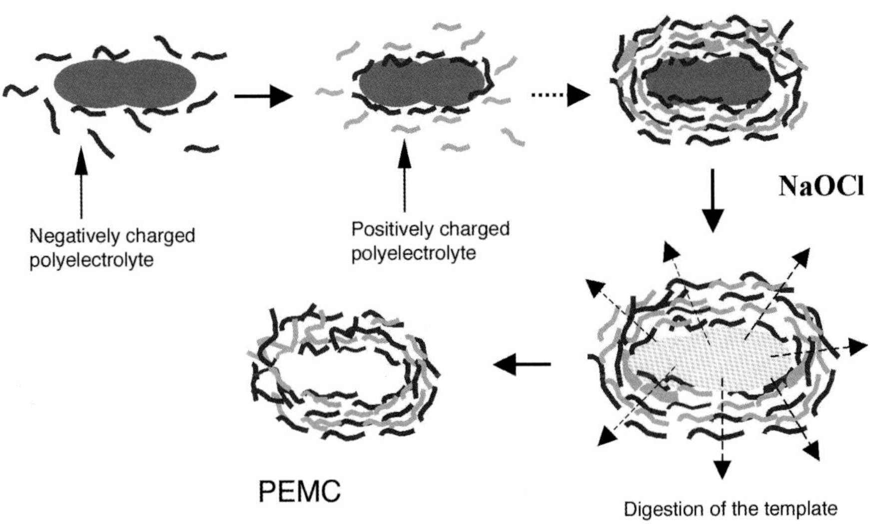

FIG. 1. Scheme of the layer-by-layer adsorption (LbL) of polyelectrolytes on a red blood cell template. *PEMC*, polyelectrolyte microcapsules

respectively. The cells were incubated under slight stirring for 15 min at room temperature. Washing the samples twice in a 100 mM NaCl (pH 6.5 ÷ 7.0) solution finished each step.

For the preparation of the microcapsules erythrocytes with five, seven or fifteen layers $(PSS/PAH)_2PSS$, $(PSS/PAH)_3PSS$, $(PSS/PAH)_7PSS$, or $(DxSO_4/PAH)_2DxSO_4$, $(DxSO_4/PAH)_3DxSO_4$, $(DxSO_4/PAH)_7DxSO_4$, respectively, were suspended in a solution of 140 mM NaCl and 1.2% NaOCl. Within 20 min of incubation at 20°C the cellular template was dissolved obtaining hollow polyelectrolyte capsules [8]. Afterwards the sample was washed three times with a 154 mM NaCl solution and additionally with distilled water until a supernatant conductivity of 0.5 mS/m was reached. Since the capsules are permeable for small ions rinsing with water does not induce any osmotic response.

Confocal Laser Scanning Microscopy

Confocal images were taken with a confocal laser-scanning system CLSM 510 META attached to an inverse microscope from Zeiss (Jena, Germany), equipped with a 100× oil immersion objective with a numerical aperture of 1.4.

Scanning Force Microscopy

Scanning Force Microscopy SFM images have been recorded in air at room temperature using a Nanoscope III Multimode SFM (Digital Instrument, Santa Barbara, CA, USA) in contact mode. Microlithographed tips on silicon nitride (Si_3N_4) cantilevers with a force constant of 0.58 N/m (Digital Instrument) have been used. Scanning Force Microscopy (SFM) images were processed by using the Nanoscope software. Samples have been prepared by applying a drop of the capsule solution onto a freshly cleaved mica substrate. After allowing the capsules to settle the substrate was extensively rinsed in water and then dried under a gentle stream of nitrogen [10].

Electrophoretic Mobility Measurements

The electrophoretic mobility of the polyelectrolyte covered erythrocytes as well as of the capsules was measured by means of an electrophoresis cell/particle analyser [11] (Electrophor, Hasotec, Rostock, Germany). The procedure has been described in detail elsewhere [12].

Micropipette Aspiration Technique

The deformability measurements were performed in distilled water under video-microscopic control by means of a micropipette aspiration technique

[13]. Cylindrical glass capillaries with an internal diameter of 2.5 μm and 4 μm and a negative (suction) pressure in the range between 0 and 450 Pa were applied.

Viscosimetric and Aggregation Measurements

The viscosities of whole blood (number of RBC 5×10^{12}/l) as well as of blood PEMC mixtures (1:1; PEMC and RBC concentration 5×10^{12}/l) were determined by means of a capillary viscometer (Fresenius, Bad Homburg, Germany) at a shear rate of $600\,s^{-1}$. The aggregation measurements of the same samples were performed by means of a light back scattering technique (Regulest, Nancy, France). The experimental set-up uses a rotational viscometer, which consists of two transparent coaxial cylinders with an annular gap between them of h = 1 mm (inner radius 10 mm and outer radius 11 mm) that can hold about 2 ml of red cell suspension. A Couette flow was established between the two cylinders. The shear rate γ is generated across the gap by rotating the outer cylinder $5\,s^{-1} \leq \gamma \leq 800\,s^{-1}$. The inner cylinder remains stationary to prevent the formation of Taylor vortices. The cell suspension was probed with a normally incident laser light (wavelength λ = 780 nm, beam diameter d = 1 mm, power 3 mW) that enters perpendicularly to the flow direction. The laser light flux multiply scattered either from red cells or aggregates was detected in the backward direction at small angles $160° < \phi < 170°$ by a photometric device. The analogue signal was digitized and processed by the computer [14–17].

Results and Discussion

After completing the adsorption cycles the template (i.e., the RBC core) was removed by digestion with the NaCl + NaOCl solution. This procedure dissolves the proteins and lipid membrane, thereby causing an increase of the capsule's internal osmotic pressure and a swelling of the microcapsule [8]. However, these osmotically active agents can diffuse through the polyelectrolyte layer; after equilibration of the osmotic forces, the elastic recoil properties of the microcapsule returns it to approximately the original RBC size. Figure 2 presents atomic force microscopy (AFM) images of polyelectrolyte shells prepared using discocytic and an echinocytic RBC as templates. Note that while the more ellipsoidal discocytic-based shells show only relatively few creases and folds, coating of crenated echinocytic RBC results in structured shells clearly showing the spikes of the original template. Subsequent washings of the microcapsules in NaCl solution permits separation of the remaining cellular components from the microcapsules. Figure 3 presents CLSM images of PEMCs on discocyte as well as echinocyte templates in water.

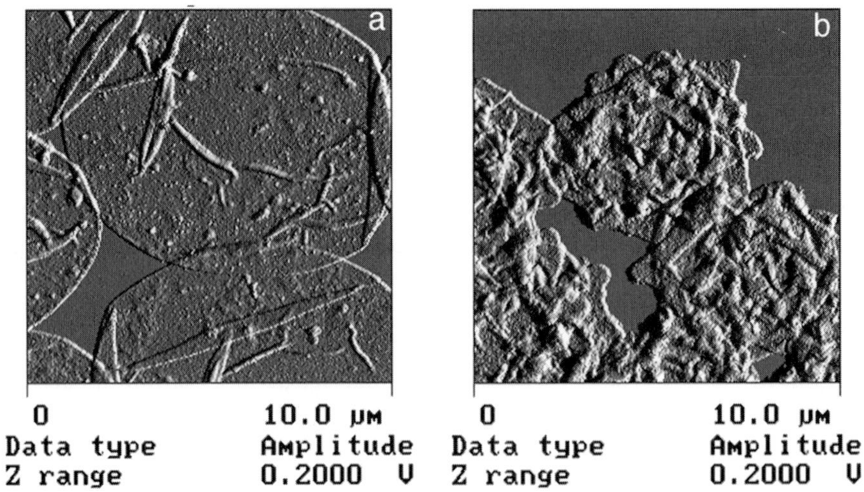

FIG. 2. Atomic force microscopy (AFM) images of PEMC using discocytic red blood cells (**a**) and echinocytes (**b**) as templates show the original shape of the used RBC templates

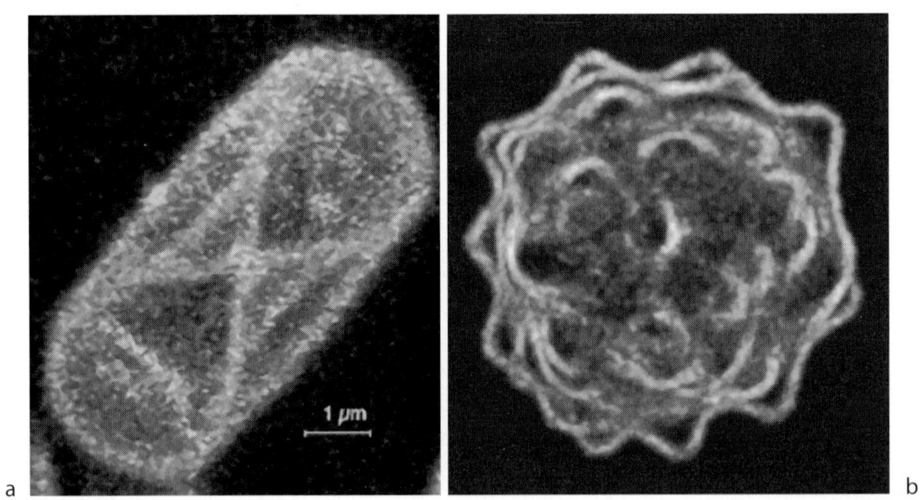

FIG. 3. 3-D confocal laser scanning images of PEMC using discocytic red blood cells (**a**) and echinocytes (**b**) as templates. The original shape of the RBC template is mimicked by the PEMC

The shells were labelled with FITC-HSA. The structure of the PEMC is clearly visible.

Subsequent washings of the microcapsules in NaCl solution permit separation of the remaining cellular components from the microcapsules.

The effects of the NaCl + NaOCl treatment on the surface charge of the polyelectrolyte layer were investigated by measuring the EPM of the microcapsules before and after digesting the template. The EPM of the PE covered RBC is about twice as high as for the control RBC. After the digestion of the template the EPM of the PE coated RBC is not significantly different compared to the PEMC (Fig. 4), which is independent of the used PE. The deproteinizer modifies the chemistry of the PE layer. The positive charges from the amino groups in PAH are lost, and PSS is partly released. This results in a structure that contains only negative charges.

The wall thickness of PEMC was determined by means of atomic force microscopic imaging. PEMC with 5, 9 and 15 polyelectrolyte layers using PAH/PSS, PAH/$DxSO_4$, and PAH/(PSS + HSA), respectively were analyzed. The wall thickness increases in dependence on the number of layers linearly in the investigated range. Additionally, the wall thickness depends on the polymer

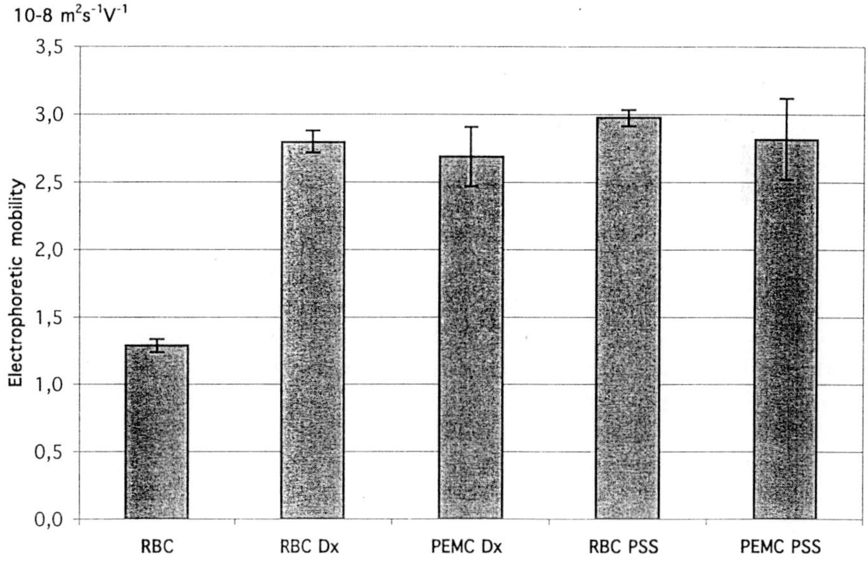

FIG. 4. Mean values and S.D. of the negative electrophoretic mobility of red blood cells (*RBC*), PAH/dextran sulphate coated RBC (*RBC Dx*), PAH/dextran sulphate PEMC (*Dx PEMC*), PAH/PSS coated RBC (*RBC PSS*), and PAH/PSS PEMC (*PEMC PSS*). The differences between the PE coated RBC and after dissolution of the template-PEMC-are not significant

TABLE 1. Wall thickness

Number of layers	Wall thickness (nm)					
	PSS/PAH		$DxSO_4$/PAH		PSS + HSA/PAH	
	Mean	SD	Mean	SD	Mean	SD
5	14,66	0,81	6,64	0,58	9,28	1,06
9	16,88	1,93	9,82	1,03	12,09	1,11
15	24,24	2,22	14,71	0,62	19,68	0,80

Wall thickness of PEMC of PPS poly (styrene sulphonate, sodium salt) (PSS), Mw 70000 and poly (allyl amine hydrochloride), (PAH), Mw 70000: PSS/PAH; dextran sulphate, ($DxSO_4$), Mw 500000 and PAH: $DxSO_4$/PAH and a mixture of human serum albumin, (HSA), Mw ca. 65000 and PSS (1:1) and PAH: (PSS + HSA)/PAH, respectively in dependence on the number of polyelectrolyte layers in the dry state determined by means of AFM imaging.

TABLE 2. Buckling pressure and calculated bending modulus using the model of Evans [19] for RBC and PEMC of different PE

Type of particle	Buckling pressure [cm H_2O]	Bending modulus [Nm]
RBC [19]		1.8×10^{-19}
$(PSS/PAH)_2/PSS$	320 ± 45	1.8×10^{-14}
$(DxSO_4/PAH)_2/DxSO_4$	120 ± 18	
$[(PSS + HSA)/PAH]_2/(PSS + HSA)$	80 ± 12	3.5×10^{-15}

The buckling pressure was determined applying a suction pressure on a capillary of a diameter of 2.5 µm. (T = 22°C).

used (Table 1). The polyelectrolyte combination of PAH and PSS shows the thickest wall compared to that of PAH and $DxSO_4$. Since the diameter of the PEMC depends on the number of layers the density of the PEMC wall is highest for 5 PE layer and decreases with increasing number of PE-layer [18], which has consequences for the permeability of macromolecules.

The buckling of PEMC as a measure of bsending properties of PEMC was determined by means of a micropipette aspiration technique. The buckling pressure was dependent on the number of PE layers (wall thickness) as well as on the used PE. The buckling pressure of the investigated PEMC is much larger than the pressure necessary to buckle the membrane of RBC, which results in a bending modulus of 4 magnitudes larger than the bending modulus of RBC [19] (Table 2). But it has to be considered that the PEMC wall is very permeable for small molecules as well as macromolecules [12]. Consequently, water flows rapidly through the PEMC wall and in reality a much weaker pressure difference is applied to the PEMC wall than in the case of the lipid membrane of the RBC. Therefore the measured pressure, which has to be applied on the PEMC can only be used as an rough estimate for the calculation of the bending modulus. Without doubt it can be stated that the investigated PEMC are deformable in contrast to the PEMC fabricated on melamin particles [7].

The influence of the PEMC on flow properties of blood suspensions was determined by means of viscometric measurements as well as by means of a light back scattering technique, which allows to determine the aggregation behaviour of blood. Figure 5 presents a CLSM image of a PEMC-blood mixture. It is obvious that the RBC do not interact with the yellow-green fluorescent PEMC, but form rouleaux with each other. The primary aggregation time t_A, which characterises the time of rouleau formation, is shorter for the

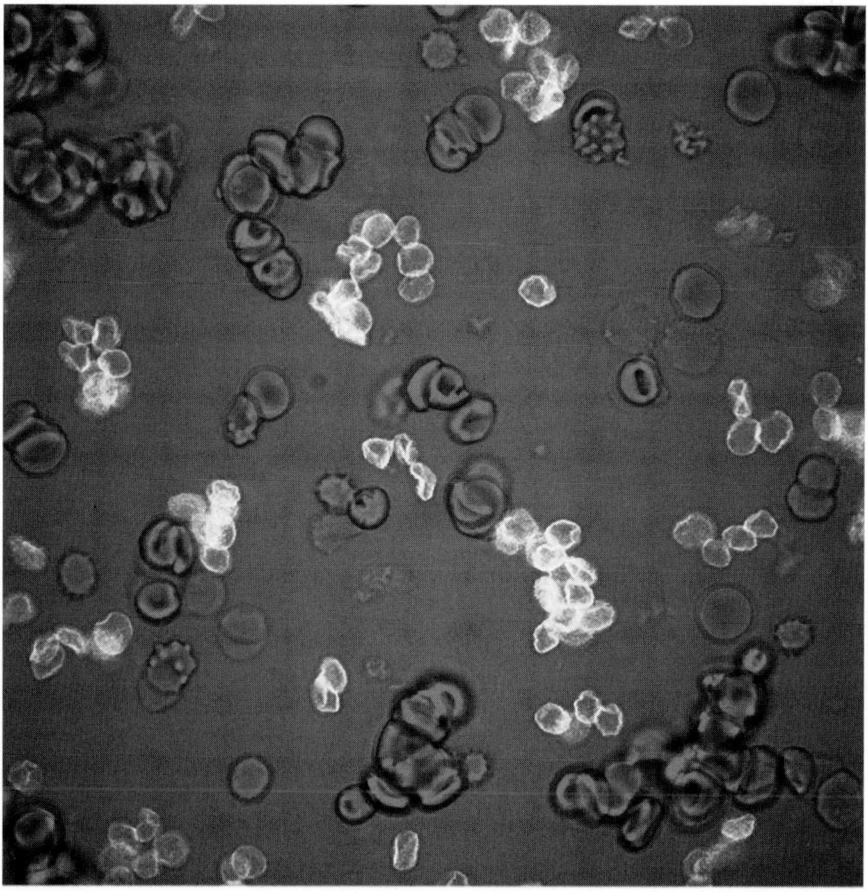

FIG. 5. Color laser scanning microscopy (CLSM) image of a mixture (1 : 1) of blood and fluorescein isothiocyanate (FITC) labelled PEMC in salt solution show that the RBC do not interact with the PEMC. ×1000

PEMC-blood mixture than for the pure blood with the same particle concentration (Fig. 6). The final aggregation time t_F representative of the 3 D time rouleau formation is in case of the PEMC-blood mixture only half of the values of blood. This clearly confirms the result of the CLSM image that the presence of PEMC reduces the number of RBC aggregates as well as the number of RBC per aggregate.

The PEMC also influence the overall rheological properties of blood characterised by the apparent viscosity at high shear rates. The apparent viscosity is significantly higher for the PEMC-blood mixture than for blood (Fig. 7). The reason seems to be that the PEMC do not completely disaggregate like the RBC. This assumption is consistent with the finding of a higher shear stress necessary to disaggregate the RBC-PEMC mixture compared to blood.

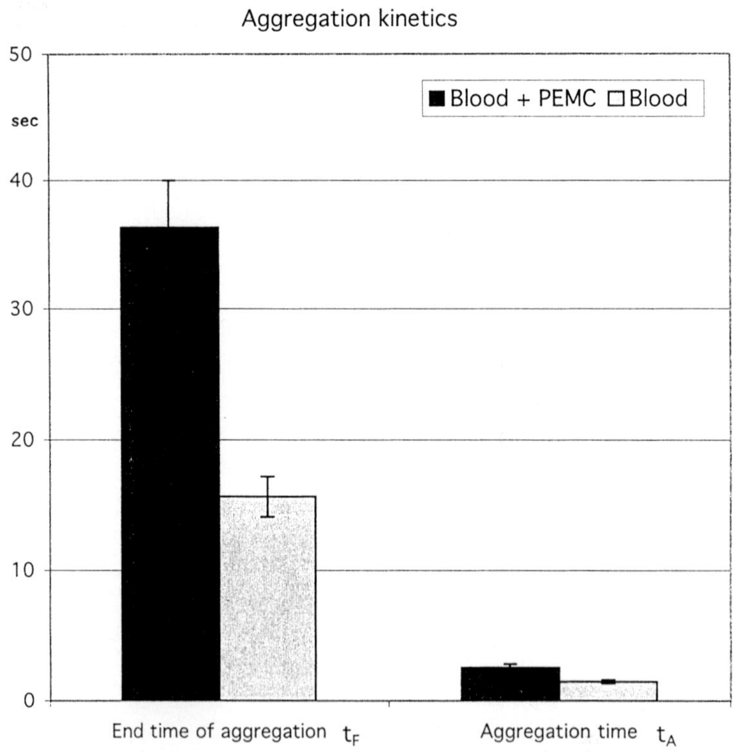

FIG. 6. The primary aggregation time t_A, which characterises the time of rouleau formation for the PEMC blood mixture and the pure blood with the same particle concentration (T = 37°C, PEMC and RBC concentration 5×10^{12}/l, 1:1 mixture) and the final aggregation time t_F representative of the 3-D time rouleau formation show that the presence of PEMC reduces the RBC aggregation

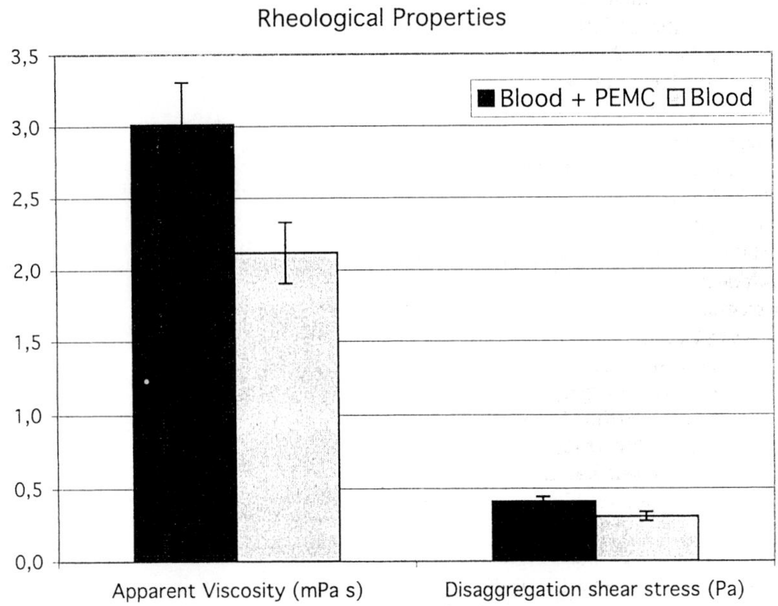

FIG. 7. Rheological properties of blood with and without PEMC characterised by the apparent viscosity at high shear rates and the disaggregation shear stress (T = 37°C, PEMC and RBC concentration 5×10^{12}/l, 1:1 mixture)

Conclusion

The newly developed PEMC with the shape of red blood cells are negatively charged, which is advantageous in respect of their interaction with the endothelium. The deformability of the PEMC is not as high as RBC, but exceeds that of other particles. The PEMC are permeable for charged as well as non charged macromolecules. This enables the filling of PEMC with oxygen transporting molecules.

Acknowledgments. The authors acknowledge the gift of the aggregometer by Jacques Dufaux (University Paris 7). This work was supported by grant 01K0-31P2813 of the Federal Ministry of Research and Technology of Germany.

References

1. Donath E, Sukhorukov GB, Caruso F, Davis S, Möwald H (1998) Neuartige Polymerhohlkörper durch Selbstorganisation von Polyelektrolyten auf kolloidalen Templaten. Angew Chemie 110:2323–2327
2. Sukhorukov GB, Brumen M, Donath E, Möhwald H (1999) Hollow polyelectrolyte shells: exclusion of polymers and donnan equilibrium. J Phys Chem B 103:6464–6440

3. Voigt A, Lichtenfeld H, Sukhorukov GB, Zastrow H, Donath E, Bäumler H, Möhwald H (1999) Membrane filtration for microencapsulation and microcapsules fabrication by layer-by-layer polyelectrolyte adsorption. Ind Eng Chem Res 38:4037–4043
4. Caruso F, Lichtenfeld H, Donath E, Möhwald H (1999) Investigation of electrostatic interactions in polyelectrolyte multilayer films: binding of anionic fluorescent probes to layers assembled onto colloids. Macromolecules 32:2317–2328
5. Radtchenko IL, Sukhorukov GB, Leporatti S, Khomutov GB, Donath E, Möhwald H (2000) Assembly of alternated multivalent ion/polyelectrolyte layers on colloidal particles. Stability of the multilayers and encapsulation of macromolecules into polyelectrolyte capsules. J Colloid Interface Sci 230:272–280
6. Sukhorukov GB, Antipov AA, Voigt A, Donath E, Möhwald H (2001) pH-controlled macromolecule encapsulation in and release from polyelectrolyte multilayer nanocapsules. Macromol Rapid Commun 22:44–46
7. Bäumler H, Artmann G, Voigt A, Mitlöhner R, Neu B, Kiesewetter H (2000) Plastic behavoir of polyelectrolyte microcapsules derived from colloid templates. J Microencapsulation 17:651–655
8. Neu B, Voigt A, Mitlöhner R, Leporatti S, Gao CY, Donath E, Kiesewetter H, Möhwald H, Meiselman HJ, Bäumler H (2001) Biological cells as templates for hollow microcapsules. J Microencapsul 18:385–395
9. Bäumler H, Djenev I, Iovchev S, Petrova R, Lerche D (1988) Polarizability of human red blood cells and conformational state of glycolcalyx. Stud Biophys 125:45–51
10. Georgieva R, Moya S, Hin M, Mitlöhner R, Donath E, Kiesewetter H, Möhwald H, Bäumler H (2002) Permeation of macromolecules into polyelectrolyte microcapsules. Biomacromolecules 3:517–524
11. Grümmer G, Knippel E, Budde A, Brockmann H, Treichler J (1995) An electrophoretic instrumentation for the multi-parameter analysis of cells and particles. Instr Sci Techn 23:265–276
12. Bäumler H, Donath E, Krabi A, Knippel W, Budde A, Kiesewetter H (1996) Electrophoresis of human red blood cells and platelets. Evidence for depletion of dextran. Biorheology 33:333–351
13. Artmann G, Sung K-LP, Horn T, Whittemore D, Norwich G, Chien S (1997) Micropipette aspiration of human erythrocytes induces echinocytes via membrane phospholipid translocation. Biophysical J 72:1434–1441
14. Snabre P (1988) Rhéologie des suspensions concentrées et agrégées de particles déformables. Thèse d'état (université Paris VII)
15. Snabre P, Mills P (1996) Rheology of weakly flocculated suspension of rigid particles. J Phys III France 6:1811–1834
16. Snabre P, Bitbol M, Mills P (1987) Cell disaggregation behavior in shear flow. Biophys J 51:95–807
17. Siadat M (1989) Conception et réalisation d'un agrégamètre érythrocytaire automatisé et informatisé, thèse de doctorat, (université Paris VII)
18. Mitlöhner R (2003) Design und Charakterisierung von Polyelektrolytkapseln. Diplomarbeit, TU Berlin
19. Evans EA (1989) Structure and deformation properties of red blood cells: concepts and quantitative methods. Methods Enzymol 173:3–35

Intravascular Microbubbles: An Ultra-Effective Means of Transporting Oxygen

Claes E.G. Lundgren, Guri W. Bergoe, and Ingvald M. Tyssebotn

Summary. Intravascular microbubbles generated by the intravenous injection of very small doses of a 2% emulsion of dodecafluoropentane were demonstrated to be able to transport physiologically significant amounts of oxygen in animal experiments. Thus, the treatment sustained life in rats and pigs with potentially fatal erythrocytopenia caused by hemorrhage and hemodilution, and adequate oxygenation was preserved in severe right-to-left circulatory shunts caused by partial airway blockage in pigs.

Key words. Erythrocyte substitutes, Anemia, Hemorrhage, Microbubbles, Oxygen transport

Introduction

Based on computer modeling of the behavior of subcapillay sized intravascular micro-bubbles Burkhard and Van Liew [1] have suggested that such bubbles may effectively support gas transport between the lungs and tissues. However, since the gas pressure in the bubbles is primarily determined by Laplace's relationship they would tend to rapidly loose the gas and collapse. Consequently, for the bubbles to be useful in oxygen transport, they need to be volume stabilized. This stabilization has been achieved by generating micro-bubbles from a 2% dodecafluoropentane (DDFP) emulsion originally designed for use as an ultrasound contrast medium (Sonus Pharmaceuticals Bothell, WA, USA). The bubbles are formed when the emulsion of DDFP (boiling temperature 29°C) is injected intravenously and warmed to body

Center for Research and Education in Special Environments and Department of Physiology and Biophysics, 124 Sherman Hall, School of Medicine and Biomedical Sciences, State University of New York at Buffalo, Buffalo, NY, USA

temperature. Expanding about 150 times, the DDFP particles in the emulsion evolve into bubbles, initially composed of DDFP gas. They will then equilibrate with O_2 and CO_2 tensions in surrounding tissues and blood. Thus, according to theory, O_2 is transported from the lungs to the tissues and CO_2 from the tissues to the lungs [1].

This chapter presents an overview of a series of different experimental animal studies aiming to demonstrate the feasibility of the aforementioned hypothesis, namely that DDFP derived intravascular micro-bubbles can transport physiologically significant amounts of oxygen.

Treatment of Potentially Fatal Erythrocyte Depletion in Oxygen-Breathing Rats [2,3]

Anesthetized rats (n = 24) breathing 70% oxygen were bled while circulatory volume was maintained by simultaneous infusion of an iso-osmotic albumin-Ringer's solution. Of the group, 8 animals (Controls) received preparation vehicle (0.7 ml/kg bwt). They showed a steadily falling arterial blood pressure and died when the hemoglobin had fallen to 2.8 ± 0.1 g/100 ml, about 80 min after the start of bleeding. The treatment animals (n = 16) received 0.7 ml/kg of a 2% DDFP emulsion, intravenously. They were bled to a hemoglobin concentration of 1.4–1.6 g/100 ml. After that, one group (n = 8) with a hemoglobin concentration of 1.4 ± 0.2 g/100 ml of the DDFP treated animals was kept under anesthesia and observed for 2–3 h. Their arterial blood pressures remained within normal range until euthanasia. The other treatment group (n = 8), with the hemoglobin concentration at 1.6 ± 0.2 g/100 ml, was allowed to wake up from anesthesia after completed DDFP treatment. At that time the inspired oxygen concentration was increased to 100%. These rats behaved normally, ate, drank and groomed. After 2 h of observation these animals were given an autologous blood transfusion to a hemoglobin level of about 7 g/100 ml and returned to air breathing. Multi-organ histology after euthanasia 21 days later showed no abnormalities.

Boosting of Oxygen Transport in Normal Rats

Two groups of anesthetized rats were instrumented for recording of oxygen tensions on the surface of an abdominal muscle. Oxygen tensions during air breathing were 50 ± 5 mmHg in control animals (n = 5) and 49 ± 8 mmHg in treatment animals (n = 5). Oxygen breathing and infusion of lactated Ringer's solution raised the values to 120 ± 11 and 121 ± 3 mmHg respectively. In the controls, which received vehicle iv, the oxygen tension remained essentially stable during 3 h of observation. By contrast, during infusion of 1.0 ml/kg of a 2% DDFP emulsion in the experimental group the muscle oxygen tension increased to levels 40–100% higher than in the controls. About 1.5 hours after the treatment infusion the oxygen tension began to decline and reached the control level about 50 min later.

Treatment of Experimental Right-to-Left Circulatory Shunts in Pigs[1]

Right-to-left circulatory shunting was induced in anesthetized pigs ($n = 9$) by adding steal or glass beads (about 1 mm diameter) to the inhaled air until shunt fractions of between 0.3 and 0.5 had been established. Arterial oxygen tensions had then fallen from about 80 mmHg to 30 mmHg but stabilized at about 70 mmHg, after initiation of oxygen breathing. Intravenous administration of a 2% DDFP emulsion was then made at 0.1 ml/kg over a 20 min period. The arterial oxygen rose in response, the average level ranging between 125 and 190 mmHg. This increase lasted for about 2.5 h after which seven of the animals (two having been euthanized) received a repeat dose that increased the average arterial oxygen tension to between 135 and 200 mmHg, the increase lasting for about 3 h. A third repeat dose in five of the animals showed an even further strengthened effect, oxygen tensions rising to 200 to 260 mmHg and lasting for 4 h. After the treatments blood pressure and heart rate remained normal and the muscle oxygen and carbon dioxide tensions appropriately reflected the changes in arterial gas tensions. Complement activation and platelet changes occurred when the shunt was applied but did not progress during infusion of the DDFP preparation.

Treatment of Potentially Fatal Erythrocyte Depletion in Pigs with Normal Arterial Oxygen Tensions [4]

This study explored whether potentially fatal erythrocyte depletion in normo-volemic pigs can be successfully treated with DDFP emulsion during air breathing. Anesthetized pigs were bled while given volume replacement with 6% dextran in lactated Ringer's solution. Arterial oxygen tensions were monitored every 15 min. Artificial ventilation and, if needed, oxygen admixture (not exceeding 5%) to the breathing air was given so that arterial oxygen tension was maintained in the normoxic range (90–100 mmHg). Control animals ($n = 6$) received emulsion vehicle in addition to the plasma expander. They died at a hemoglobin level of 3.0 ± 0.1 g/100 ml 260 min after the beginning of the hemodilution. The treatment animals had a final hemoglobin level

[1] In addition to the present authors, Drs. A. Olszowka and G. Logue of the State University of New York contributed as investigators to this study.

of 2.1 ± 0.1 g/100 ml. They received 0.7 ml of DDFP emulsion iv /kg. They were all observed for at least 100 min past the end of hemodilution. At that time, their mean arterial pressure had slowly declined from an average of 115 to 70 mmHg. At this point, two animals were euthanized while four were switched to spontaneous air breathing and observed for an additional period of up to 1 h and 45 min, mean arterial pressures remaining stable at about 70–75 mmHg up to the moment of euthanasia.

Conclusion

The efficiency of the DDFP-derived microbubbles for O_2 transport is underscored by the range of doses of DDFP in these studies which was only 0.002–0.014 ml/kg body weight. Extrapolation from these observations indicates that, during oxygen breathing, less than one ml of DDFP, in emulsion form, can provide for the resting metabolic oxygen consumption of an adult person. No significant side effects or histological abnormalities have been observed in the experiments described. In this context it is also noteworthy that a 2% DDFP emulsion, similar to the one used in these experiments, has been administered to over 2200 healthy volunteers and patients in bolus doses of 0.001–0.0024 ml/kg and has demonstrated an excellent safety profile (Personal communication from M. Low Sonus Pharmaceuticals, 2003).

Acknowledgments. The studies reviewed above were partially supported by Sonus Pharmaceuticals Inc. and partially by US Army Medical Research Acquisition Activity Grant (ID: DAMD170110778).

References

1. Burkard ME, Van Liew HD (1994) Oxygen transport to tissue by persistent bubbles: theory and simulations. J Appl Physiol 77(6):2874–2878
2. Tyssebotn I, Lundgren C, Bergoe G, Van Liew H, Goldinger J (1999) Stabilized microbubbles as a blood substitute. Undersea & Hyperbar Med 26: suppl., abstract 96
3. Tyssebotn I, Bergoe G, Goldinger J, Lundgren C (1999) Dodecafluoropentane (DDFP) stabilized microbubbles support life without blood in awake rats 26: abstract 97
4. Tyssebotn I, Bergoe GW, Lundgren CEG (2001) Volume-stabilized intravascular microbubbles provide vital oxygenation in hemoglobin depleted pigs during "air breathing". Undersea & Hyperbar Med 28, suppl., abstract E30

Oxygen-Dependent and Oxygen-Independent Effects of Perftoran

Eugene Maevsky and Genrih Ivanitsky

Summary. A brief review of the main properties of the low-concentrated emulsion Perftoran which contains perfluorodecalin and perfluoromethylcyclohexylpiperidine rapidly and slowly eliminated from the organism respectively. Perftoran carries an expected small volume of oxygen, but improves the oxygen regime in tissues and organisms due to kinetic acceleration of the oxygen flow and facilitates functions of the remaining erythrocytes. Activation of Adenosine triphosphate (ATP) synthesis in rat liver mitochondria after massive blood replacement and an improvement of the energy state and the survival of kidney grafts isolated during a severe hemorrhagic shock served as good indexes of the sufficient oxygen delivery by Perftoran. It has relatively low reactogenicity of Perftoran due to a small average particle size of emulsion of about 0.07 μm. The allowed threshold in particles size is smaller than 0.14 μm for Perftoran. The main oxygen-independent properties of Perftoran are the following: a decrease in rigidity of heart muscle during cardioplegia due to a reversible inhibition of Ca-current and a decrease in its sensitivity to epinephrine; immunosuppressive effect is connected with the inhibition of hyperactivated macrophages and primed neutrophils; de novo synthesis of the phenobarbital isoforms of P450 in liver is induced by perfluorodecalin.

Key words. Perfluorochemicals, Energy metabolism, Cardioplegia, Cytochrome P450

It was a great honor to present a paper devoted to Perftoran in Japan, where the pioneer studies in creating the first commercial standard perfluoro-

---

Institute of Theoretical and Experimental Biophysics of RAS, 142290, Pushchino, Institutskaya, 3, Moscow Region, Russia chemial (PFC) emulsions Fluosol 43 and Fluosol DA were done. This brief review elucidates some oxygen-dependent and oxygen-independent properties of Perftoran that is a low-concentrated emulsion of two types of PFCs: rapidly and slowly eliminated from the organism perfluorodecalin (PFD) and perfluoro-methylcyclohexylpiperidine (PFMCP). Perftoran contains 10 volume percent of PFCs emulsion stabilized by surfactant Proxanol which is similar to Pluronic F68. Water-salt solution in Perftoran is biocompatible and does not contain any plasma expander. An important peculiarity of Perftoran emulsion is a small average particles size of about 0.07 μm.

Perftoran capability to transfer oxygen is a trivial broadly described characteristics of PFC emulsion [1] but the oxygen-independent properties are due to unexpected biomedical effects connected with a modification of the cells and tissues functions after their biophysical relationships with PFC emulsion [2].

Oxygen-Dependent Properties of Perftoran

The main question arises as to whether the low-concentrated PFC emulsion can improve oxygen delivery. The biomedical and clinical studies such as the experiments on perfusion of the isolated heart, heart-lung complex and kidneys, partial and subtotal blood replacement in rats; substitution of a massive blood loss, treatment of hemorrhagic and traumatic shocks and heart infarcts have shown that Perftoran can maintain an oxygen regime in the organism and isolated organs on the satisfactory level, better than traditional protein-salt or polymer solutions [3–6].

Perftoran has all the well-known features of PFC emulsion to carry oxygen described in detail recently by J.G. Riess [1], among them: additional oxygen capacity of PFC emulsion, accelerated diffusion rate of oxygen and carbon dioxide in PFCs, enlarged diffusion surface for gas transfer, increased oxygen and carbon dioxide gradients between erythrocytes and tissues, and finally PFC particles can go through the occlusive and spastic vessels impermeable for erythrocytes because their size is 70 times larger than that of emulsion particles. In direct experiments [7] it was shown that the rate of oxygenation and deoxygenation in a mixture of blood with PFC emulsion was significantly higher than in the mixture of blood and water-salt solution. It is also necessary to take into account that PFD, one of the components of Perftoran, dissolves in the phospholipids of erythrocyte membranes [8]. This phenomenon is accompanied with an increase in lateral mobility of lipids in membranes and makes erythrocytes more elastic, improves their mechanical and chemical resistance.

Here we would like to emphasize that in most cases after a massive blood loss and hemodilution, the oxygen capacity of the remaining red blood cells

(RBC) is sufficient to transfer the necessary amount of oxygen. The problem lies not in the complete replacement of the lost RBC but in facilitating oxygen delivery to tissues together with the remaining RBC. Under these conditions oxygen delivery suffers from damaged kinetic characteristics and high affinity of Hb to O_2 in RBC, their increased rigidity and fusion, and also because of vasoconstriction which blockades the RBC penetration into the capillary blood stream. Due to its kinetics, diffusion and particle size advantages, Perftoran improved oxygen delivery from lungs to peripheric tissues together with the remaining RBCs. Apparently PFC droplets and red blood cells form the rapid and reversible gas-carrying conveyer.

To estimate oxygen-carrying efficiency of Perftoran we determined as the indexes of the sufficient oxygen delivery the functions of rat liver mitochondria (RLM) after massive blood replacement and the survival of kidney grafts isolated during severe hemorrhagic shock in dogs.

Saving of Oxidative Phosphorylation in RLM is Good Evidence of Perftoran Efficacy at Massive Blood Replacement

Changes in mitochondrial functions during hypoxia and ischemia play a crucial role in cell survival and in maintaining of tissue functions. After ischemia mitochondria lose respiratory control and decline adenosine triphosphate (ATP) synthesis [9] while after hypoxia they have an increased oxidative phosphorylation rate [10]. In our experiments [11] under promedol and ether anesthesia, the isovolemic blood replacement was carried out on male Wistar rats with Perftoran (supplemented by albumin to 3%) and with mixture of 3% albumin and salt solution, or with autoblood in control animals. During and after operation animals were placed in the chamber with high PO_2 of about 550–600 mm Hg. The hemoglobin content in rat blood decreased from 16.0 ± 1.4 to 5.0 ± 0.6, arterial PO_2 after 2 and 6 h reached 500 ± 12 and 480 ± 10 respectively. Venous pH before blood replacement (during anesthesia) was 7.22 ± 0.04 and after blood replacement with Perftoran it was 7.20 ± 0.04 and 7.15 ± 0.04 within 2 and 6 h respectively, while salt-albumin solution did not maintain venous pH higher than 7.10–7.12. RLM were isolated 6 h later after blood replacement and respiratory parameters were measured in thermostatic 1 ml cell with a Clark-type oxygen electrode [9,11].

Most animals survived in both groups almost identically (in the parallel experiments): 19 from 20 in the Perftoran group and 18 from 20 in the albumin group. But the price of life was different: 6 h after the blood replacement with salt-albumin solution the isolated RLM could not phosphorylate ATP. It was a symptom of deep ischemia. In contrast, after the blood replacement with Perftoran RLM phosphorylated ATP more actively than organelles

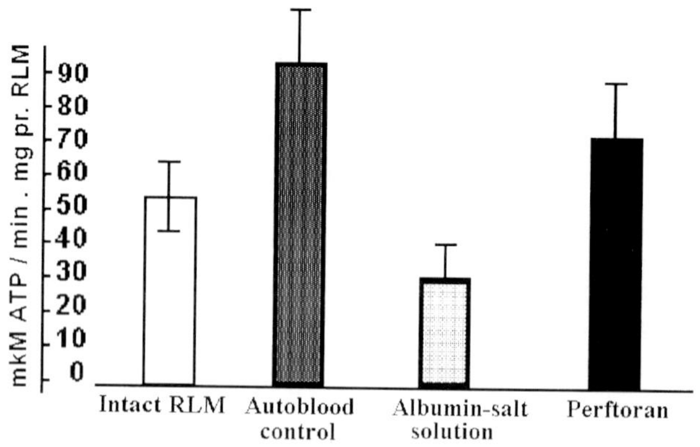

FIG. 1. Changes in the phosphorylation rate of ATP in rat liver mitochondria (RLM) isolated 6h later after 70% blood replacement with autoblood or albumin-salt solution, or Perftoran together with 3 % albumin

from the intact animals (Fig. 1). Such activation of oxidative phosphorylation in RLM is a good evidence of Perftoran efficiency and of the fact that the organ has undergone only acute hypoxia but not ischemia.

Survival of Dog Kidney Grafts Transplanted After Hemorrhagic Shock Is Evidence of Perftoran Efficacy [12]

Hemorrhagic shock was induced by acute blood loss of about 35 ml/kg until the arterial blood pressure decreased from 150/70 to 50/30 mm Hg, the kidney blood flow dropped from 2000 ± 120 ml/min kg to 800 ± 60 ml/min kg. One hour later the bleeding dogs were treated with infusions of dextran 60 or Perftoran in the volume of about 40 ml/kg together with breathing of oxygen-air mixture and injections of furosemid (to 1.5–2 mg/kg), droperidol (0.03–0.05 mg/kg), heparin (25000 U). After 2 h hemorrhagic shock kidneys were isolated. Survival of kidney grafts isolated from the "hemorrhagic" animals treated with Perftoran and transplanted into the dogs that were previously undergone nephtoectomy was much better than that with dextran. Perftoran in contrast to dextran enabled to keep ATP/ADP and lactate/pyruvate ratios in the dog kidney tissue (Fig. 2), prevented an increase in creatine and urea levels in the recipient blood, and prolonged kidney grafts life spans four- to five-fold.

Oxygen Delivery Is Impossible if There Is Anaphylactic Side Reaction

The obtained improvement of oxygen transfer would be impossible if Perftoran were an anaphylactic drug because of the anaphylactic reactions are accompanied by damages in microcirculation, by a drop of arterial pressure

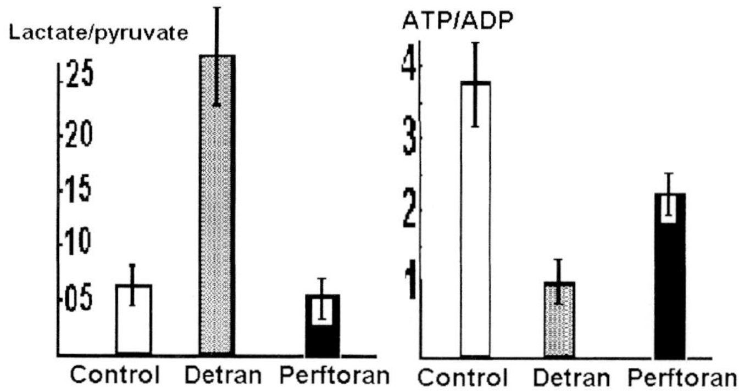

FIG. 2. Maintenance of ATP/ADP and lactate/pyruvate ratios in the dog kidney tissue isolated from the "hemorrhagic" dogs treated with Dextran 60 or Perftoran. *Control*, before blood losses. *Detran* and *Perftoran*, 2 h after blood losses and 1 h after infusions of Detran 60 or Perftoran

and by decrease in oxygen tension. A conventional point of view attributed these reactions of PFC emulsion to the presence of surfactant Pluronic F68 [13]. If the probability of anaphylactic side reactions is high, there is no other way but to exclude the use of such PFC emulsions. But the problem proves to be more complicated. Pyatovskaya [14] found that the neutropenic index which reflected reactogenicity was as a rule low after injection of Perftoran if the latter had particles with the size smaller than 0.1 μm after a short period of storage. Enlargement of the particle size owing to deviation in technology, temperature regime and storage time, conditions of transportation, and defrosting enhanced the danger of anaphylactic reactions development. The allowable threshold in particles size is of about 0.14 μm for Perftoran. Therefore the actual technology accepted in 1996 is focused on the average size of particles to be in the range of 0.07–0.08 μm, and it is prohibited to have particles with the size more than 0.16–0.18 μm. Thanks to that the average frequency of reactions decreased from 7% before 1996 (revealed on 912 patients) to 2 % (on 1824 patients).

Some Oxygen-Independent Properties of Perftoran

Relaxation and Preventing of Ca Overload Within Cardioplegia

Perftoran significantly increased the relaxation of heart muscle during cardioplegia [15–18]: ischemic contracture was much lower in the presence of PFC emulsion or proxanol solution in comparison with the usual hyperpotassium solution (Fig. 3). This phenomenon is due to the reversible inhibition of Ca-current through the cell membrane and a decrease in sensitivity

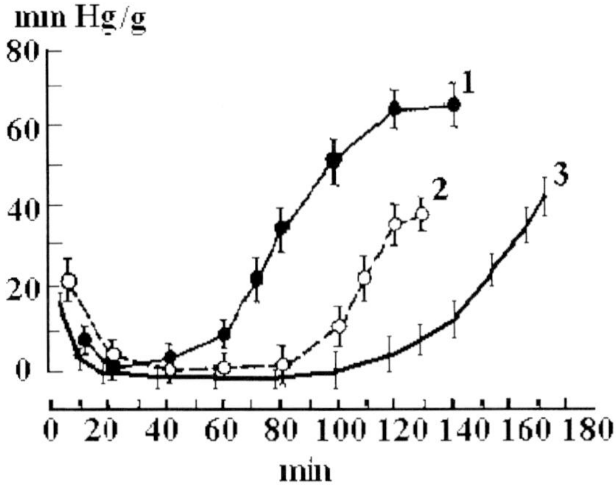

FIG. 3. Changes in the rest tensions of rat heart during cardioplegia at 17°C. *1*, hyperpotassium solution (71.8 mM NaCl, 29 mM KCl, 2.1 mM $MgCl_2$, 15 mM $NaHCO_3$, 1.4 mM NaH_2PO_4, 44 mM Mannitol, 28 mM Glucose, 1.2 mM Ca gluconate); *2*, hyperpotassium solution with 3% proxanol (surfactant from Perftoran); *3*, hyperpotassium solution with Perftoran. Rest tension in mm Hg per g heart weight

of Ca-channels to epinephrine caused by Perftoran independently on its saturation by oxygen. These mechanisms may be also responsible for diminishing of ischemic and reperfusion damages and for alleviating of resuscitation of heart electric activity and contractility after cardioplegia.

Immunosuppressive Effect of Perftoran

The immunosuppressive effect of Perftoran is apparently connected with the inhibition of hyperactivated macrophages and primed neutrophils after sorption and phagocytosis of emulsion droplets by these cells. In vitro, Obraszov et al. [19] showed that Perftoran inhibited the exaggerated production of reactive oxygen metabolites in neutrophils in responce to activating stimuli. In vivo we tested Perftoran inhibition of hyperactivated macrophages on the model of mice infected by retrovirus of Rausher erythroblast leukosis (study was performed by V. Buhman). The hyperactivation macrophages and production of virus particles by macrophages are accompanied by splenomegaly and formation of a great number of fused erythroblasts colonies in the spleen of infected mice. Intravenous or intraabdominal Perftoran infusions decreased the splenomegaly half and the formation of fusion colonies three- to five-fold. These results may bring us closer to the understanding why Perftoran can also have an antiinflammatory effect and decrease the frequency of graft rejections after organ transplantations.

Perftoran Infusion Induces De Novo Synthesis of Cytochrome P450 in Liver

Perftoran infusion induces de novo synthesis of cytochrome P450 in liver because of the substrate-enzyme complex formation between perfluorodecalin and cytochrome P450 [20,21]. Immune electrophoresis and substrate affinity evidenced that Perftoran induced noncancerogenic phenobarbital isoforms of P450. That induction resulted in accelerating xenobiotics hydroxylation, shortening phenobarbital sleep, inhibition of lipid peroxydation, and stimulation of the second phase of detoxycation. The duration of P450 induction is almost equal to the half-retention time of perfluorodecalin in liver.

Influence of Long Retention of PFMCP on the Tissues

A great number of investigators did not find any pathologic damage in the organs that accumulated PFMCP, which has the half-retention time of 90 days. Vasil'ev and Golubev [22] observed evaluation of histological picture of tissues which accumulated PFMCP. They found specific granulomas formed by macrophages containing PFCs. The granulomas went through several stages of development from macrophages' to epithelioids' and then to lymphatics' granulomas and after that disappeared without any trace. But parenchymal cells surrounding granulomas acquired an increased regeneration potential. Perhaps thanks to that Perftoran inhibited the connective tissue growth during hepatitis and cirrhosis [23].

Summing up, it would be necessary to emphasize that Perftoran carried the expected small volume of oxygen, but significantly improved the oxygen regime due to kinetic acceleration of the oxygen flow facilitating erythrocytes functions. Modification of some enzymes and membranes in the presence of Perftoran in the blood and PFCs in the tissues endows Perftoran with the unexpected properties which can determine its new field of applications in experimental and clinical practice.

References

1. Riess JG (2001) Oxygen carriers ("blood substitutes")—raison d'etre, chemistry, and some physiology. Chem Rev 101:2797–2919
2. Ivanitsky GR (2001) Biophysics at the turn of the millennium: perfluorocarbon media and gas-transporting blood substitutes. (translated from Russian) Biophysics 46(1):1–31
3. Islamov BI, Ladilov IV, Buevich VA, et al (1991) An emulsion of fluorocarbons as s protective agent against myocardial ischemia. (in Russian) Vestn Akad Med Nauk SSSR 3:39–43
4. Belojartsev FF, Ivanitsky GR, Islamov BI, et al (1983) Substitution of large amounts of blood with gas-transporting medium based on the perfluorocarbon emulsion. (in Russian) Dokl Physiol 270(2):487–491
5. Moroz VV, Krilov NL, Ivanitsky GR, et al (1999) Perftoran application in clinical medicine: Alternatives of blood substitution in surgery. (in Russian) Anesteziol Reanimatol. Suppl:126–135
6. Kligunenko EN, Gulega IE (1999) Optimization of medical treatment of patients at the middle-degrees critical blood loss. (in Russian) Meditsinskie Perspektivi 4(4): 44–47
7. Perevedentseva EV, Zaritskiy AR, Fok MV, et al (1998) Perfluorocarbon emulsions increase transfer of oxygen in plasma from erythrocyte to tissues. Artif Cells Blood Substit Immobil Biotechnol 26(2):223–229

8. Obraztsov VV, Kabal'nov AS, Sklifas AN, et al (1992) New model of the perluorocarbons elimination from the organism: dissolution of perfluorocarbons into the lipid components of blood. (in Russian) Biofizika 2:379–383
9. Schweiger H, Lutjen-Drecoll E, Arnold E, et al (1988) Ischemina-induced alterations in mitochondrial structure and function in brain, liver, and heart muscle of young and senescent rats. Biochem Med Metab Biol. 203:162–185
10. Mela L (1979) Mitochondrial function in cerebral ischemia and hypoxia: comparison of inhibitory and adaptive responses. Neurol Res 1(1):51–63
11. Maevsky EI, Brustovetsky NN, Grishina EV, et al (1999) Evaluation of gas-carrying properties of PFC emulsion with help of mitochondria reactions. (in Russian) In: Perfluoroorganic compounds in biology and medicine. Pushchino, pp 243–253
12. Onishenko NA, Sernjak PS, Kovalenko NB, et al (1990) Application of perfluorocarbon emulsion in kidney transplantation. (in Russian) Khirurgiia (Mosc) 6:90–102
13. Geyer RP (1988) Perfluorochemicals as oxygen transport vehicles. Biomat Art Cells Art Org 16(1–3):31–49
14. Piatovskaya NN, Sedova LA, Berkos MV, et al (1993) Comparative evaluation of reactoginicity of emulsions perfucol and perftoran. In: Perfluorocarbon active media for medicine and biology. New aspects of researches. (in Russian) Pushchino, pp 167–173
15. Belojartsev FF, Kaidash AN, Islamov BI, et al (1986) Assessment of possibilities of using fluorocarbon cardioplegia for antiischemic protection of the myocardium. (in Russian) Vestn Akad Med Nauk SSSR 6:37–43
16. Islamov BI, Mayevsky EI, Vorobyov SI, et al (1986) Effect of proxanols on electromechanical integration in the myocardium and their contribution against ischemia by using fluorocarbon emulsion. (in Russian) Vestn Akad Med Nauk SSSR 2:40–45
17. Islamov BI, Sakson ME, Pertsov AM, et al (1986) Features of electric-mechanic properties rehabilitation of isolated myocardium after fluorocarbon cardioplegia. (in Russian) Vestn Ross Akad Med Nauk 6:43–49
18. Kokoz YuM, Kobrinsky EM, Freidin AA, et al (1983) Influence of gas-carrying perfluorocarbon emulsion on myocardium (ion transport, contractile activity, and sensitivity to mediators). (in Russian) Dokl Akad Nauk SSSR 270(2):459–462
19. Obraztsov VV, Shekhtman DG, Sklifas AN, et al (1995) A perfluorocarbon emulsion inhibits neutrophil activation. (in Russian) Dokl Akad Nauk 342(6):819–822
20. Belojartsev FF, Ivanitsky GR, Maevsky EI, et al (1986) Chemically-inert fluorocarbons—inductors of enzymes of monooxygenase system in liver microsomes. (in Russian) Dokl Biochem Biophys (proceed Akad Nauk SSSR, translated from Russian) 286(3):729–732
21. Obraztsov VV, Shekhtman DG, Sklifas AN (1994) Uncoupling of the liver monooxygenase system by perfluorocarbons in vivo. (in Russian) Biochemistry (Mosc) 59(8):1175–1181
22. Vasiliev AE, Golubev AM (1984) Evolution of macrophage granulomas accumulating PFOC. (Russian) In: Fluorocarbon gas-carrying mediums. Pushchino, pp 130–134
23. Dalgatov GD, Medjidov RT (2000) Means for the treatment and prevention of the pathological growth of connective tissue in parenchymal organs. (in Russian) Patent RU 2146133 C1. 10.03.2000 Biull 7

State of the Art and Challenges in Blood Substitutes Research: A Case Study on Perfluorocarbon-Based Oxygen Carriers

Juan Carlos Briceño

Summary. In 1995 a research project on perfluorcarbon-based oxygen carriers (PFC-OCs) was started. Initial interest was prompted by reports of improved tissue oxygenation during cardiopulmonary bypass and by the advances of some formulations that were undergoing preclinical or clinical trials at that time. During Phase I of the project (1995–1999) knowledge of the manufacturing process of PFC-OCs was acquired and the PFC-OC Oxyfluor (HemaGen/PFC, St Louis, MO, USA) was tested in animal models of cardiopulmonary bypass and hemorrhagic shock. Phase II of the project (2000–2003) has led to the design and construction of a pilot plant for production of PFC–OCs, the procurement of the equipment and materials required for manufacturing sterile, injectable PFC emulsions, and the preparation of the first PFC-OCs. The completion of Phase II of the project allows the research team to manufacture new PFC-OCs and to evaluate them in the experimental models of suitable clinical procedures. A better knowledge of the physiological effects of the infusion of PFC-OCs is expected.

Key words. Blood substitutes, Oxygen carriers, Perfluorocarbon microemulsions

Introduction

In 1995 investigators initiated research on perfluorocarbon-based oxygen carriers (PFC-OCs) at the Fundación CardioInfantil (FCI) and the University of Los Andes (UA). Initial interest on the topic was prompted by the previous

Blood Substitutes Laboratory, Fundación CardioInfantil Calle 163A No. 28-60. PO Box 091479 and University of Los Andes, Bogotá, DC, Colombia
University of Los Andes, Carrera 1 No. 18A10, PO Box 4976, Bogotá, DC, Colombia

participation of the author in the development and evaluation of a hyperosmolar perfluorocarbon-based oxygen carrier (PFC-OC). This PFC-OC (perfluorodecalin, 20% w/v) was at that time tested for experimental cardiopulmonary bypass at the University of Texas [1]. These studies demonstrated that the PFC-OC increased cerebral blood flow, brain PO_2, P_vO_2, and reduced brain tissue hypercapnia. However, the PFC-OC did not prevent brain tissue acidosis, metabolic acidosis or anasarca. During the Phase I of the FCI-UA Blood Substitutes Project, Oxyfluor (HemaGen/PFC, St Louis, MO, USA), a 40% v/v perfluorodichlorooctane emulsion was evaluated in animal models of cardiopulmonary bypass and hemorrhagic shock. The objective of this chapter is to report the advances of Phase II of the project, regarding both the production and the evaluation of PFC-OCs.

The FCI-UA Blood Substitutes Project Phase I: 1995–1999

Research on the potential use of perfluorocarbon-based oxygen carriers (PFC-OCs) started at the Fundación CardioInfantil and the University of Los Andes in 1995 [2]. The oxygen-carrying properties of PFCs and the intense activity of companies with products undergoing preclinical or clinical trials drew the attention of the clinicians in the research group. Increasing the knowledge of the physiological effects of the infusion of PFC-OCs was also a source of interest. Accordingly, the Phase I of the FCI-UA Blood Substitutes Project was started. It was divided into three subprojects: production of PFC-OCs, evaluation of efficacy and evaluation of safety. A description of these subprojects is presented below.

Production of PFC-OCs

Objective

To study the feasibility of setting up the facilities for the experimental production of PFC-OCs.

Methodology

A feasibility study of local production of PFC-OCs was performed. This study included analysis of the methods of production of PFC-OCs, and the preliminary design of a laboratory facility for the production of PFC-OCs. In addition, procedures were established for the selection and procurement of the PFCs, emulsifiers, and surfactants most appropriate for clinical applications.

Results

From this activity the group acquired significant knowledge of the manufacturing process, materials, technology involved in producing PFC-OCs. It was realized the high costs of the equipment and materials required, and the need for external financial support for setting up the facilities for production of PFC-OCs.

Evaluation of the Efficacy of PFC-OCs on an Animal Model of Cardiopulmonary Bypass

Given the impossibility of producing PFC-OCs at that time, several companies with PFC-OCs products undergoing clinical and preclinical trials were contacted and asked for samples of PFC-OCs to be tested in experimental models of clinical procedures. One PFC-OC was thus obtained (Oxyfluor, 40% v/v perfluorodichlorooctane, HemaGen/PFC, St Louis, MO, USA).

Objective

To evaluate efficacy of use of PFC-OCs during experimental cardiopulmonary bypass.

Methodology

An animal model of cardiopulmonary bypass was implemented. In this model, 30-kg swine were subjected to 2 h of total normothermic nonpulsatile bypass from the right atrium to the ascending aorta. The extracorporeal circuit included a roller pump and a hollow fiber oxygenator. Mean arterial pressure was maintained at 50 mm Hg and flow rate at 80 $ml \cdot min^{-1} \cdot kg^{-1}$. Brain tissue pH, PO_2, and PCO_2, were measured using ion specific electrodes. Mixed venous, jugular venous and arterial blood gases, fluid balance, hematological and hemodynamical variables were also monitored before, during, and 30 min post bypass, after which the animals were killed. Whole body oxygen consumption was calculated. Tissue samples from brain, lungs, kidney, liver, spleen and muscle were taken for histological analysis. In the control group ($n = 8$), Ringer's lactate was used as priming solution and perfusate. In the study group Oxyfluor was used as priming solution.

Results

In these experiments Oxyfluor improved tissue oxygenation and total body oxygen consumption. Oxyfluor also reduced FCC_{RBC}, increasing oxygen transport reserve of the red blood cell phase. However, tissue fluid accumulation was not alleviated, and blood and brain acidosis were significantly aggravated by the use of Oxyfluor. It was also observed that the fractional contribution to oxygen consumption from the plasma phase (FCC_{PL}) in the Ringer's lactate group was similar to the fractional contribution to oxygen consumption from the PFC phase (FCC_{PFC}) in the Oxyfluor group. An interesting finding was that the secondary effects were not reduced by increasing tissue oxygenation and it was concluded that further research should be conducted to optimize the formulation of PFC-OCs for use in cardiopulmonary bypass and to reduce secondary effects [3].

Evaluation of the Safety of PFC-OCs on an Animal Model of Hemorrhagic Shock

Objective

To study hemodynamical, hematological and secondary effects of reinfusion with a PFC-OC in a model of hemorrhagic shock.

Methodology

1.0 kg rabbits were bled 60% of volemia at 1 ml/min through the femoral artery, and immediately the same volume was reinfused at 3 ml/min with Ringer's lactate ($n = 11$) or Oxyfluor ($n = 11$). Mean arterial pressure, ECG, and heart rate were monitored. Samples for blood gases, hematology and chemistry analysis were taken at the beginning of bleeding, halfway through bleeding, at end of bleeding, and at end of reinfusion. Animals were killed after one month, and tissue samples were taken for histological examination.

Results

During these experiments of hemorrhagic shock, PaO_2 increased and PvO_2 decreased, increasing oxygen extraction. Reinfusion with Oxyfluor did not cause negative changes in hemodynamics, hematology and blood gases of the animals. One-month survival rate was better in the Ringer's lactate group (6/11), than in the Oxyfluor group (1/11), due to low PO_2 of inspired air during and post, and probably to species sensitivity to PFC-induced increased pulmonary residual volume.

Conclusions of Phase I

From this initial phase of the project that lasted four years, the main conclusions were: an increased knowledge was acquired of the effects of PFC-OCs during experimental procedures, including the fact that despite improving tissue oxygenation on cardiopulmonary bypass, secondary effects were not alleviated; the need of further research to understand the physiological changes induced by PFC-OCs; the consolidation of a multidisciplinary group of anesthesiologists, cardiovascular surgeons, perfusionists and biomedical engineers working towards the identification and modification of clinical procedures on which PFC-OCs can be successfully used; and the need of external financial support for the construction of the laboratory for the production of PFC-OCs.

The FCI-UA Blood Substitutes Project Phase II: 2000–2003

A two-year grant from the National Science Foundation of Colombia (COLCIENCIAS) was awarded in April 2000. At that time, the objectives of the Phase II of the project were: to set up lab facilities and equipment for production of

PFC-OCs; to implement methodology for the formulation and manufacturing of PFC-OCs; to evaluate and optimize formulations of PFC-OCs in vitro and in animal models; to study the physiological changes induced by the infusion of PFC-OCs; to design the clinical trials for the PFC-OCs; and to transfer the technology of production and evaluation of PFC-OCs to the pharmaceutical industry. The project was divided into production and evaluation of PFC-OCs, which are presented next.

Production of PFC-OCs

The objective of this part was to manufacture PFC microemulsions that are stable, sterile, and able to transport significant amounts of oxygen when used as injectable oxygen carriers (PFC-OCs).

Methodology

Facilities

A clean-air pilot plant for preparation, emulsification and quality control of injectable PFC-OCs was designed and built.

Equipment and Materials

Equipment and materials for preparation, emulsification and quality control of injectable PFC-OCs were specified and purchased.

Human Resources

Personnel to design and supervise plant construction, equipment and materials purchasing, to operate the pilot plant and to manufacture PFC-OCs were recruited and trained.

Microemulsion Formulation and Preparation

PFC-OC microemulsions are being prepared with different combinations of PFCs and surfactants.

Results

Facilities

A 90-m^2 clean air pilot plant for manufacturing sterile, injectable solutions has been constructed at FCI. It started activities on December 2002.

Equipment and Materials

The PFC-OCs manufacturing equipment consists of a microfluidizer (model M110-Y, Microfluidics, Newton, MA, USA), a microdiffusor and an autoclave sterilizer. The PFC-OCs process control equipment includes a combined particle size and zeta potential analyzer (model 90Plus, Brookhaven Instruments, Holtsville, NY, USA). All basic materials for PFC-OCs production including the PFCs and surfactants have been purchased. The PFCs under evaluation are perfluorodecalin and perfluorooctyl bromide (F2 Chemicals, Preston,

UK), along with egg-yolk and soybean lecithin (Reference Epikuron 200, Ovothin 160 and Epikuron 170, Lucas Meyer, Hamburg, Germany).

Microemulsion Formulation and Preparation

The first microemulsions have been prepared. Stability and particle size appear to be within specifications.

Evaluation of PFC-OCs

The objective of this part was to evaluate the safety and efficacy of the PFC–OCs in vitro and in animal models of clinical procedures.

Methodology

In vitro evaluation consists of stability, biocompatibility and toxicity tests. In vivo studies include the evaluation of efficacy, safety (toxicity), and effect on microcirculation on animal models. After this evaluation, optimization of the formulation of the PFC-OCs is planned.

Results

These experiments are expected to begin once the stability evaluation is successfully completed.

Challenges

During Phase II of the project several challenges were faced which are discussed here. Regarding equipment and facilities the main difficulty was that the set up-costs of the pilot plant exceeded the provisions. The strict specifications of the plant resulted in increased costs of the facilities. Furthermore, as the production process was further detailed, additional equipment was required, even for small-scale output. These additional costs also resulted on a delay in the program of the project. Concerning the materials required for the project, the project budget was also strained by the high costs of the PFCs and the surfactants used in the formulations. Availability of PFCs is short, and data on their performance in biomedical use is scarce.

Challenges about human resources derived from the considerable effort that had to be dedicated to recruit the qualified personnel to design and supervise the construction of the pilot plant, to purchase the equipment and materials, to operate the pilot plant, and to manufacture the PFC–OCs. Another obstacle for the success of the entire project is the long-term sustainability of these essential personnel. In relation to microemulsion formulation and preparation, the most important challenge of the project at the present time is to consistently obtain microemulsions whose stability complies with the requirements for in vivo studies and for long-term storage.

Conclusions

When this project started in 1995 there was significant research and commercial interest in PFC-OCs. Products like Oxyfluor (HemaGen/PFC, St. Louis, MO, USA) and Oxygent (Alliance Pharmaceutical, San Diego, CA, USA) were undergoing clinical trials. Eight years later and despite reports that PFC-OCs increase tissue oxygenation in animal models of hemorrhagic shock [5], and cardiopulmonary bypass [3,6], no PFC-OC has yet been approved for clinical use by the FDA. During Phase I of this project, Oxyfluor™ (HemaGen/PFC) was tested in animal models of cardiopulmonary bypass and hemorrhagic shock. In Phase II of the project, a pilot plant for production of PFC–OCs has been designed and constructed. The equipment and materials required for manufacturing sterile, injectable PFC-OCs have been specified and purchased. The pilot plant started operations by the end of 2002. The first microemulsions have been produced and are currently being tested in vitro and in vivo. The research team has now the ability to design and produce new PFC-OCs, and to evaluate these PFC-OCs in animal models of suitable clinical procedures. Important challenges have been faced during this phase of the project, regarding facilities and equipment, materials, personnel and in the formulation and preparation of the microemulsions. These ongoing studies will contribute to understand the physiological changes and the secondary effects induced by the infusion of PFC–OCs.

Acknowledgments. The author wishes to acknowledge the assistance of his colleagues and students at the Fundación CardioInfantil and the University of Los Andes, and the financial support of these institutions and of COLCIENCIAS.

References

1. Briceño JC, Runge TM, Ottmers SE, et al (1997) Changes in brain pH, PO_2, PCO_2, cerebral blood flow and blood gases induced by a hyperosmolar oxyreplete hemosubstitute during cardiopulmonary bypass. ASAIO J 43:13–18
2. Briceño JC, Rincón IE, Vélez JF, et al (1997) Description of a project for the production and evaluation of oxygen-carrying hemosubstitutes. Artif Cells Blood Substit and Immobil Biotechnol 25:473–479
3. Briceño JC, Rincón IE, Vélez JF, et al (1999) Oxygen transport and consumption during experimental cardiopulmonary bypass using Oxyfluor. ASAIO J 45:322–327
4. Briceño JC, Rincón IE, García A, et al (1997) Effects of Ringer's Lactate and Oxyfluor as resuscitative fluids in a model of hemorrhagic shock in the rabbit. ASAIO Transactions 43:13

5. Goodin TH, Grossbard EB, Kaufman RJ, et al (1994) A perfluorochemical emulsion for prehospital resuscitation of experimental hemorrhagic shock: a prospective, randomized, controlled study. Crit Care Med 22:680–689
6. Holman WL, Spruell RD, Ferguson ER, et al (1995) Tissue oxygenation with graded dissolved oxygen delivery during cardiopulmonary bypass. J Thorac Cardiovasc Surg 110:774–785

Semifluorinated Alkanes as Stabilizing Agents of Fluorocarbon Emulsions

Sabina Marie Bertilla, Pascal Marie, and Marie Pierre Krafft

Summary. We obtained highly stable, small-sized, and narrowly dispersed perfluorooctyl bromide (PFOB) emulsions using combinations of phospholipids and semifluorinated alkanes $C_nF_{2n+1}C_mH_{2m+1}$ (FnHm diblocks) as the emulsifying system. For example, after 6 months at 25°C the average droplet diameter of an emulsion stabilized by F6H10 was only ~80 nm, compared to ~180 nm for the reference emulsion stabilized by phospholipids alone. In parallel, a co-surfactant effect has been demonstrated for F8H16 at the water–PFOB interface using pendant drop interfacial activity measurements, which supports the hypothesis that a fraction of the diblocks is located at the phospholipid interfacial film. We also established that the length of the hydrocarbon segment, Hm, must be comparable to that of the phospholipid's fatty chains to obtain the stabilization effect; a strong mismatch leads to rapid coalescence of droplets in the emulsion. For fluorocarbon emulsions, small droplet sizes translate into prolonged intravascular persistence and reduced side effects. FnHm diblocks thus provide a useful, versatile tool to improve the characteristics and stability of injectable fluorocarbon emulsions.

Key words. Fluorocarbon emulsion stabilization, Fluorocarbon/hydrocarbon diblock, Ostwald ripening, Molecular diffusion, Interfacial tension

Introduction

Exceptional biological inertness and gas-dissolving properties are the basis for the development of injectable fluorocarbon (FC)-in-water emulsions as temporary oxygen carriers for use during surgery [1]. Such synthetic "blood

Colloïdes et Interfaces, Institut Charles Sadron (CNRS), 6 rue Boussingault, 67083 Strasbourg Cedex, France substitutes" are devoid of the inherent complexity of hemoglobin solutions. Perfluorooctyl bromide ($C_8F_{17}Br$) (PFOB), emulsified with egg yolk phospholipids, has been investigated in Phase III clinical trials in Europe and the United States [2,3]. Further desirable progress in terms of emulsion characteristics includes improvement of the stability of the FC emulsion and reduction of droplet size to prolong intravascular persistence, reduce side effects, and facilitate oxygen diffusion. Our strategy with respect to achieving such improvements consists in reinforcing the interfacial film of the emulsion using nonpolar fluorophilic amphiphiles such as semifluorinated alkanes, $C_nF_{2n+1}C_mH_{2m+1}$ (FnHm diblocks).

Molecular diffusion (Ostwald ripening) has been determined to be the primary mechanism of coarsening in both dilute and concentrated FC-in-water emulsions over time [4–10]. An effective method for stabilizing PFOB emulsions against molecular diffusion is to add small amounts of perfluorodecyl bromide ($C_{10}F_{21}Br$, PFDB) to PFOB, which reduces the solubility and dispersibility of the dispersed FC phase, thereby reducing molecular diffusion [11]. An alternative means of stabilizing FC emulsions consists in the incorporation of FnHm diblocks in the phospholipid. Highly effective stabilization of egg yolk phospholipid (EYP)-based concentrated fluorocarbon emulsions has been obtained [12,13]. In the concept that underlies this procedure, the FnHm diblock molecules were expected to be located at the interface between the FC phase and the surrounding phospholipid film (Fig. 1). Whether the observed FC emulsion stabilization by FnHm diblocks is due to an interfacial effect (which supposes that the diblocks are, at least in part, located at the

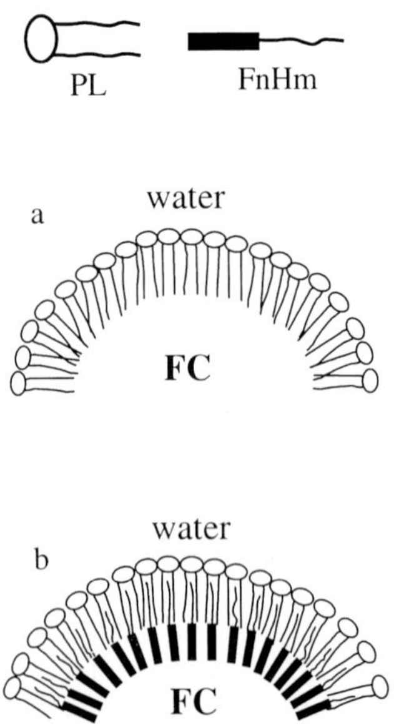

Fig. 1. Surface of a droplet of fluorocarbon (*FC*)-in-water emulsion stabilized by (**a**) a phospholipid (*PL*) alone or (**b**) a combination of PL and a semifluorinated diblock (*FnHm*). Owing to the amphiphilic character of the latter, it was hypothesized that the semifluorinated diblock would collect in part at the interface

interface) or solely to a reduction in solubility of the dispersed phase (as if the diblock molecules were dispersed uniformly within the FC droplets) has been a matter of debate [9,10,14].

Where biological aspects are concerned, some attention has been given to FnHm diblocks because of the multiple functions they can fulfill. In addition to their use for stabilization and precise control of particle size of FC-in-water emulsions, their use as a "surfactant" allows the preparation of hydrogenated oil-in-FC emulsions [15]. Incorporation of FnHm diblocks in the bilayer of vesicles can increase the vesicles' shelf stability, reduce their permeability [16,17], slow the kinetics of Ca^{2+}-induced fusion of dipalmitoylphosphatidylserine small unilamellar vesicles [18], and modify their behavior in a biological medium [19]. FnHm diblocks were demonstrated to form an internal, Teflon-like, fluorinated film within the bilayer of phospholipid vesicles [20].

The synthesis and purification of FnHm is straightforward [21,22]. Preliminary studies have indicated that diblocks do not perturb growth or viability of cell cultures [13]. No inhibition of carcinoma cell proliferation was noted with $C_6F_{13}C_{10}H_{21}$ (F6H10) [23]. The growth and survival of mice were not affected by the intraperitoneal administration of large doses (30 g/kg body weight) of $C_6F_{13}CH{=}CHC_{10}H_{21}$ (F6H10E) or F6H10 [13,24]. Even the iodinated mixed compound $C_6F_{13}CH{=}CIC_6H_{13}$ was tolerated intraperitoneally by mice at a dose of 45 g/kg body weight [25].

The half-life of F6H10E was evaluated to be 25 ± 5 days in the liver, the organ that had taken up most (70%) of the injected dose (3.6 g/kg) administered to rats in the form of a 25% w/v emulsion of pure diblock [13,24].

In the current study, we found that unusually fine, stable PFOB emulsions stabilized by combinations of natural phospholipids (PLs) and FnHm diblocks can be obtained. We also report a set of experiments designed to determine whether semifluorinated diblock molecules interact at the FC–water interface and elucidate the mechanism through which they stabilize FC emulsions. The interfacial tension between phospholipid solutions and PFOB containing various concentrations of F8H16 was measured using the pendant drop method. The particle growth in emulsions stabilized by phospholipid/diblock combinations was monitored using centrifugal photosedimentation or quasielastic light scattering.

Experimental

Materials

The diblocks F6H10 and F8H16 were synthesized according to Brace [21]. They were thoroughly purified by distillation (F6H10) or successive recrystallization from chloroform (F8H16). Their purity (>99%) was determined using gas chromatography, thin-layer chromatography, nuclear magnetic resonance, and elemental analysis. PFOB and PFDB were gifts from Alliance Pharmaceutical Corp. (San Diego, CA, USA). Perfluorohexadecane (PFHD) came from Fluorochem (Ugarit Chimie, Issy les Moulineaux, France), and EYP was kindly donated by Lipoid (Ludwigshafen, Germany). Dioctanoylphosphatidylcholine (PLC8), dilaurylphosphatidylcholine (DLPC), and dimyristoylphosphatidylcholine (DMPC) were purchased from Sigma (99% pure). Water was obtained from a MilliQ system (Millipore, Bedford, MA, USA).

Methods

Emulsion Preparation and Particle Size Measurement

A series of emulsions based on EYP, equimolar combinations of EYP and F6H10, and equimolar combinations of EYP and PFHD ($C_{16}F_{34}$) were prepared by high-pressure homogenization. These emulsions all contained 60% w/v PFOB and 3% w/v phospholipids. Their average droplet diameter and size distribution have been measured after preparation and monitored as a function of time using quasielastic light spectroscopy (Malvern Zeta Sizer 3000 HS; Malvern, Worcestershire, UK).

EYP-based Emulsions

EYP (3 g) was dispersed in water (100 ml) and homogenized with a low-energy mixer (Ultra-Turrax; Ika-Labortecknik, Staufen, Germany) for 15 min at 13 000 rpm at room temperature. PFOB (60 g) was added dropwise at 9000 rpm. The dispersion was stirred for 30 min at 13 000 rpm in a thermoregulated bath (5°–10°C). It was further homogenized under high pressure (1000 bars, 30 min) using a Microfluidizer (model 110; Microfluidics, Newton, MA, USA).

EYP/additive-based Emulsions

EYP (3 g) was dispersed in water (100 ml) and homogenized with a low-energy mixer for 5 min at 13 000 rpm at room temperature. An equimolar amount of the additive (F6H10 or PFHD) was then added. The dispersion was further homogenized at 13 000 rpm for 5 min in a thermoregulated bath (5°–10°C). PFOB addition (60 g), preemulsification, and high-pressure homogenization were achieved as described above. All the EYP-based emulsions were bottled in 10-ml vials. They were then heat-sterilized at 121°C for 15 min and stored at 25°C.

Other series of emulsions based on DMPC or PLC8, equimolar combinations of each of these phospholipids with F8H16, or equimolar combinations of these phospholipids with PFDB were prepared by high-pressure homogenization. Their average droplet diameter and size distribution were measured after preparation and monitored as a function of time using centrifugal photosedimentation (Horiba Capa 700; Horiba, Kyoto, Japan). The emulsions all contained PFOB (30% w/v) and phospholipids (4% w/v).

Reference Emulsions

DMPC (or PLC8) (1.2 g) was dispersed in water (25 ml) and homogenized with the Ultra-Turrax mixer for 15 min at 13 000 rpm at room temperature. PFOB (9 g) was added dropwise at 9000 rpm. The dispersion was stirred for 30 min at 13 000 rpm in a thermoregulated bath (5°–10°C). It was further homogenized under high pressure (1000 bars, 30 min) using the Microfluidizer.

Phospholipid/additive-based Emulsions

DMPC (or PLC8) (1.2 g) was dispersed in water (25 ml) and homogenized with a low-energy mixer for 5 min at 13 000 rpm at room temperature. An equimolar amount of the additive (F8H16 or PFDB) was then added. The dispersion was further homogenized at 13 000 rpm for 5 min, the temperature of the emulsion being maintained at 60°C (F8H16) or 25°C (PFDB) with thermoregulated baths. PFOB addition (9 g), preemulsification, and high-pressure homogenization were achieved as described above. The emulsions based on both DMPC or PLC8 were bottled in 10-ml vials. They were heat-sterilized at 121°C for 15 min and stored at 40°C.

Interfacial Tension Measurements

Preparation of the Samples

Because of low interfacial tension, it was impossible to form a PFOB droplet in a dispersion of phospholipid at concentrations higher than the phospholipid's critical micellar concentration (CMC). It was therefore necessary to prepare true phospholipid solutions rather than dispersions. The CMC of PLC8 has been measured experimentally (1×10^{-4} mol l^{-1} [9]), but the CMC of DMPC is not available. It can be approximated at 1×10^{-9} mol l^{-1}, however, knowing that the logarithm of the CMC decreases by about 1 unit per carbon atom added to the alkyl chain of the phospholipid. A DMPC solution (1.66×10^{-11} mol l^{-1}, 5 ml) was prepared by six subsequent 10-fold dilutions of a 1.66×10^{-5} mol l^{-1}-concentrated solution. The PLC8 solution (3.73×10^{-5} mol l^{-1}, 5 ml) was prepared by diluting 0.1 ml of a 1.86×10^{-3} mol l^{-1}-concentrated solution in 5 ml of water. Six solutions of F8H16 in PFOB (7.5, 5.0, 2.5, and

1.0×10^{-5} and 4 and 1×10^{-6} mol l^{-1}) were obtained by direct dilution of a 1×10^{-4} mol l^{-1}-concentrated F8H16 solution in PFOB.

Pendant-Drop Measurements

Interfacial tension measurements were made with a pendant-drop apparatus coupled with video digital image processing [26]. The PFOB pendant drop was formed at the tip of a glass capillary tube (internal diameter 1.1 mm) inside a quartz cell containing the phospholipid solution. The experimental setup was thermoregulated (25.0° ± 0.2°C). The drop was illuminated with a white-light source. The image recording system consisted of a microscope coupled to a video camera, a digital timer, and a microcomputer for image digitization. Digitized images were analyzed with Visilog Image Analysis Software (Noesis, Les Ulis, France) using filtering techniques, a morphological gradient method, mathematical morphology functions, and adaptive thresholding. Experimental drop profiles were analyzed with the axisymmetrical drop shape analysis profile algorithm [27]. A calculated Laplacian curve was compared with the experimental curve until an acceptable fit was reached. The interfacial tension was taken as the mean value of five measures. Each experiment was performed on one pendant drop; the profiles were recorded as a function of time. Standard deviations were estimated at 0.01 mN m^{-1}.

Results and Discussion

Obtaining Small-sized, Narrowly Dispersed PFOB Emulsions Based on Natural Phospholipids

The PFOB emulsions investigated contained a low concentration of EYPs (3% w/v) in line with formulations investigated for in vivo oxygen delivery. For the purpose of elucidating the stabilization mechanism we have compared three formulations (Table 1). In formulation 1, no stabilizing additive was used. In formulations 2 and 3, the diblock F6H10 or the heavy-fluorocarbon PFHD were used as the additive, respectively. PFHD was chosen because its boiling point is close to that of F6H10 (~252°C). Figure 2 depicts the aging curve (i.e., the variation of the average diameter as a function of time) of the PFOB emulsions at 25°C. It clearly shows that both PFHD and F6H10 stabilize the emulsion and that the emulsion stabilized by F6H10 is significantly more stable than that stabilized by PFHD. After 6 months at 25°C, the average droplet diameter in the emulsion stabilized by F6H10 is still only 80 nm compared to 120 nm for the emulsion stabilized by PFHD and 180 nm for the reference emulsion prepared with EYP alone (Fig. 3). The particle size

TABLE 1. Formulations of perfluorooctyl bromide emulsions

Perfluorooctyl bromide (PFOB; $C_8F_{17}Br$)	60 g (31 ml)
Egg yolk phospholipids (EYPs)	3 g
Stabilizing agents (equimolar/EggPC)	
Formulation 1	None
Formulation 2	$C_6F_{13}C_{10}H_{21}$ (F6H10 diblock)
Formulation 3	$C_{16}F_{34}$ (PFHD)
Other components	
$NaH_2PO_4 \cdot H_2O$	0.067 g
$Na_2HPO_4 \cdot 7H_2O$	0.458 g
NaCl	0.323 g
Water for injection: q.s. ad	100 ml

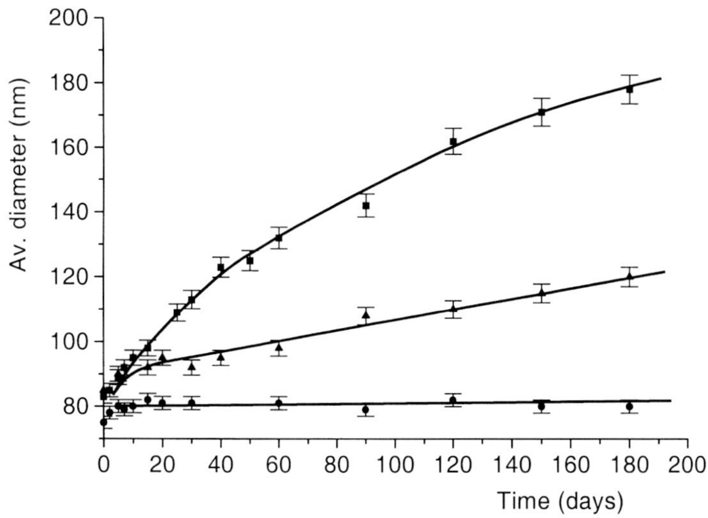

FIG. 2. Variation over time (at 25°C) of the average diameter of droplets in perfluorooctyl bromide (PFOB) emulsions stabilized by egg yolk phosphatidylcholine (EYP) alone (*squares*), an equimolar combination of EYP and perfluorohexadecane (PFHD) (*triangles*), or an equimolar combination of EYP and the diblock F6H10 (*circles*)

distribution of the emulsion stabilized by F6H10 is narrower than those of the emulsions stabilized by PFHD and obtained with EYP alone.

Molecular diffusion (Ostwald ripening) has been determined to be the primary mechanism of the droplet size increase over time in both dilute and concentrated FC-in-water emulsions [4–10]. Molecular diffusion originates from the difference in chemical potential that exists between differently sized droplets. According to the Kelvin equation, the chemical potential (and

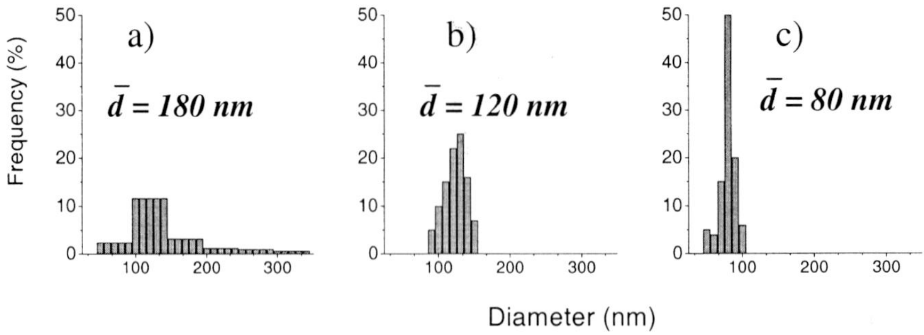

FIG. 3. Particle size distributions after 6 months at 25°C in PFOB emulsions stabilized by (**a**) EYP alone, (**b**) an equimolar combination of EYP and PFHD, or (**c**) an equimolar combination of EYP and F6H10. $\bar{d}$, average diameter

consequently the solubility of the dispersed phase in the continuous phase) depends on the droplet curvature radius. As a result of this difference in solubility, individual molecules tend to leave the smaller droplets and diffuse through the continuous phase to join larger ones, where the chemical potential is lower, resulting in progressive disappearance of the smaller droplets to the benefit of larger ones. According to the Lifshitz-Slesov-Wagner (LSW) theory [9,28], a system undergoing molecular diffusion is characterized by the following properties: (1) The cube of the droplet average radius ($\bar{r}^3$) increases linearly with time according to

$$\frac{d\bar{r}^3}{dt} = \omega = \frac{8VmCD\gamma_i}{9RT} f(\varphi) \qquad (1)$$

where ω is the Ostwald ripening rate; C and D are the solubility and diffusibility coefficients of the dispersed phase in the continuous phase, respectively; γ_i is the interfacial tension between the dispersed and continuous phases; Vm is the molar volume of the dispersed phase; R is the gas constant; T is the temperature; and $f(\varphi)$ is a factor that introduces the effect of the volume fraction of the dispersed phase on ω. (2) The distribution function of the droplet sizes $G(u)$, with $u = r/\bar{r}$ (droplet normalized radius), is time-invariant.

To limit Ostwald ripening in emulsions, it was proposed that a small amount of a second component be added that is soluble in the dispersed phase and practically insoluble in the continuous phase [29]. This additive diffuses much more slowly throughout the continuous phase than the major component of the dispersed phase. In a two-component system, an equilibrium state is reached when the difference in chemical potential (due to differences in the radius of the curvature) between droplets of different sizes is matched by the difference in chemical potential between droplets of different compositions.

It has been demonstrated that the aging of an emulsion with two components also obeys the LSW theory as reflected by a linear variation of the mean droplet volume with time and the time-invariance of the distribution function of the droplet sizes [5].

Figure 4 confirms the linear variation of the droplet volume over time characteristic of a molecular diffusion-controlled particle growth for the three emulsions investigated. The time-independence of the distribution functions, characteristic of molecular diffusion, was observed for all the EYP-based emulsifying systems investigated (Fig. 5).

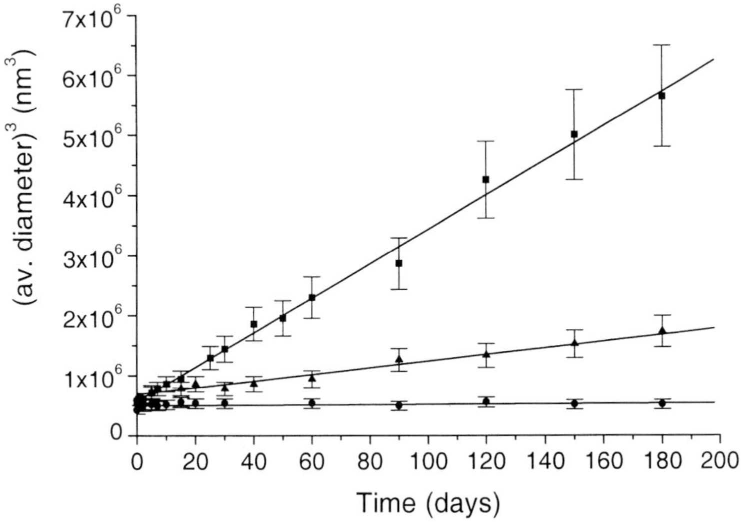

FIG. 4. Variation over time, at 25°C, of the cube of the average diameter of droplets in PFOB emulsions stabilized by EYP alone (*squares*), an equimolar combination of EYP and PFHD (*triangles*), or an equimolar combination of EYP and F6H10 (*circles*)

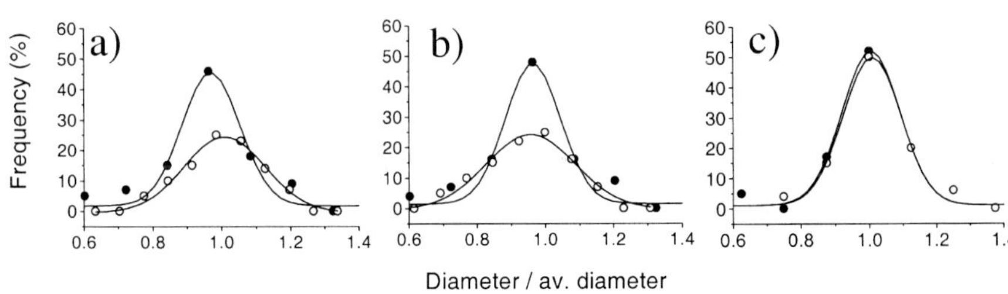

FIG. 5. Time invariance of the particle size distribution functions. The PFOB emulsions were stabilized by (**a**) EYP alone, (**b**) an equimolar combination of EYP and PFHD, or (**c**) an equimolar combination of EYP and F6H10. They were measured after preparation (*solid circles*) and after 90 days (*open circles*). Storage temperature 25°C

Diblock Activity at the Fluorocarbon/Phospholipid Solution Interface

We used the macroscopic model offered by the pendant-drop method to verify the hypothesis according to which the fluorocarbon/hydrocarbon diblock, owing to its amphiphilic character, would be at least partially present at the interface between the fluorocarbon and the phospholipid. Therefore, a drop of F8H16-containing PFOB was formed at the extremity of a capillary immersed in an aqueous dispersion of phospholipids. The analysis of the shape of the drop allowed us to determine the interfacial tension.

Figure 6 depicts the variations of the interfacial tension γ_i between solutions of DMPC, DLPC, and PCL8 and solutions of F8H16 in PFOB as obtained by the pendant-drop method. The curves display a typical shape in which, after the interface has been saturated with phospholipids, γ_i decreases more steeply and linearly owing to the change in the chemical potential of the solution. The leveling-off of the γ_i decrease that one would have expected by further increasing the F8H16 concentration was not observed, however, because γ_i became so low that the pendant FC drop fell, preventing further γ_i measurements.

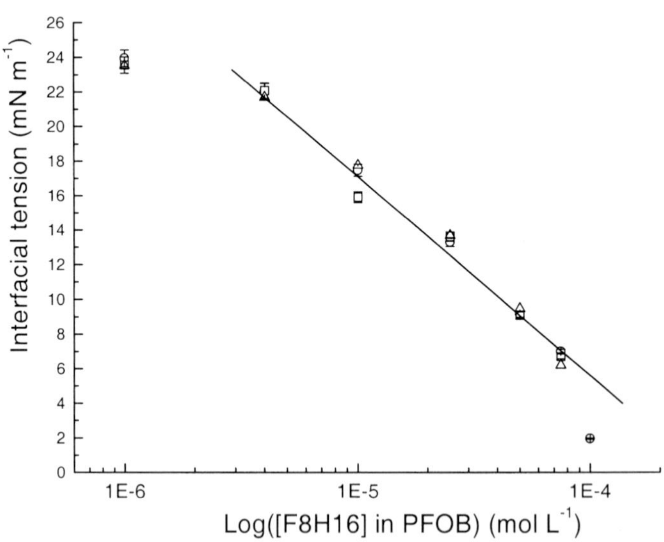

FIG. 6. Variation in the interfacial tension (γ_i) (pendant-drop method) between solutions of F8H16 in PFOB and aqueous phospholipid solutions, as a function of the logarithm of the F8H16 concentration in PFOB. The phospholipids investigated were dimyristoylphosphatidylcholine (DMPC) 1.66 × 10^{-11} mol l^{-1} (*triangles*), dilaurylphosphatidylcholine (DLPC) 1.25 × 10^{-9} mol l^{-1} (*squares*), and dioctanoylphosphatidylcholine (PLC8) 3.73 × 10^{-5} mol l^{-1} (*circles*)

The most important result of this study is the dramatic decrease in γ_i as a function of the logarithm of the F8H16 concentration. This result provides clear direct evidence that the F8H16 diblocks behave as a co-surfactant of phospholipids, which indicates that they are located, at least in part, at the PFOB–phospholipid interface.

Figure 6 also shows that the curves are similar for all the phospholipids investigated and that the slopes of the straight lines are essentially identical for all the phospholipids investigated. This means that the interfacial F8H16 concentration, which was calculated from the slopes of the γ_i variations to be ~1.3 molecules nm^{-2}, did not depend on the phospholipid's chain length. The F8H16 molecular area at the interface deduced from the interfacial concentrations is 0.8 nm^2. At the concentration of interface saturation ($4 \times 10^{-6} mol\,l^{-1}$), the percentage of F8H16 molecules that must be present at the interface should therefore be about 5% of the total F8H16.

Relation Between PFOB Emulsion Stabilization by FnHm Diblocks and the Relative Lengths of the Phospholipid's Fatty Acid Chains and the Diblock's Hydrocarbon Spacer

Figure 7 displays the variation of the cube of the average droplet diameters as a function of time at 40°C in emulsions stabilized with DMPC, DMPC/PFDB, or DMPC/F8H16 equimolar combinations. It confirms the linear variation of the droplet volume over time characteristic of molecular diffusion-controlled particle growth. It also shows that DMPC-based emulsions comprising either additive (F8H16 or PFDB) are more stable than emulsions stabilized by DMPC alone. It further shows that F8H16 is a more efficient stabilizer than PFDB. The time independence of the distribution functions (not shown) confirms that the mechanism of droplet coarsening is molecular diffusion for all three emulsifying systems investigated.

A strikingly different situation was found when the phospholipid was PLC8 (Fig. 8). Interestingly, it can be seen that PFDB still acts as a stabilizer for this lipid, whereas incorporation of F8H16 strongly destabilizes the emulsions. For the emulsions prepared with the pure lipid (PLC8) or stabilized by PLC8/PFDB combinations, the coarsening mechanism is still molecular diffusion, as assessed by the linear variations of the droplet volume over time and the time independence of the distribution functions. On the other hand, in the case of the emulsion formulated with PLC8/F8H16 combinations, the average droplet diameter increased exponentially over time, indicating that a coalescence-driven coarsening mechanism was at play.

The above results demonstrate that F8H16 behaves differently depending on the phospholipid's chain length. It stabilizes PFOB-in-water emulsions against Ostwald ripening when used in combination with a long-chain

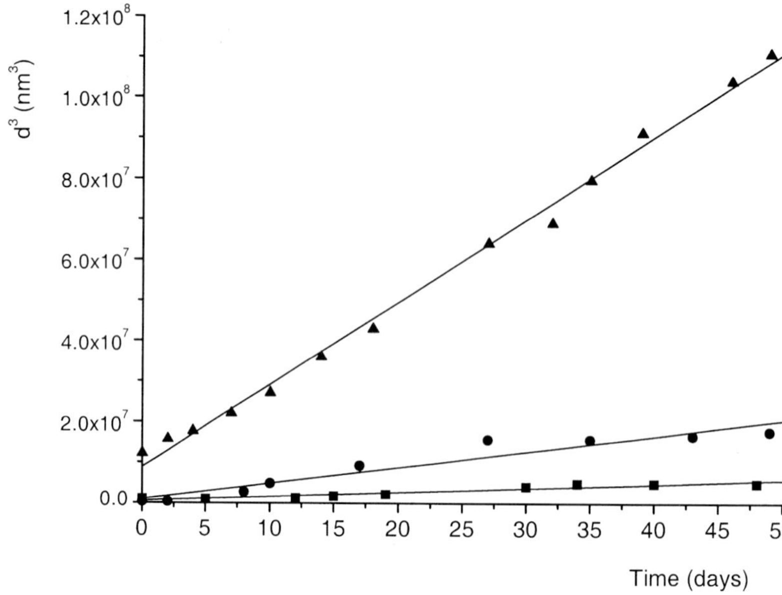

FIG. 7. Variation in the cube of the average droplet diameter (d^3) as a function of time at 40°C in PFOB-in-water emulsions prepared with DMPC alone (*triangles*), an equimolar mixture of DMPC and perfluorodecyl bromide (PFDB) (*circles*), or an equimolar mixture of DMPC and F8H16 (*squares*)

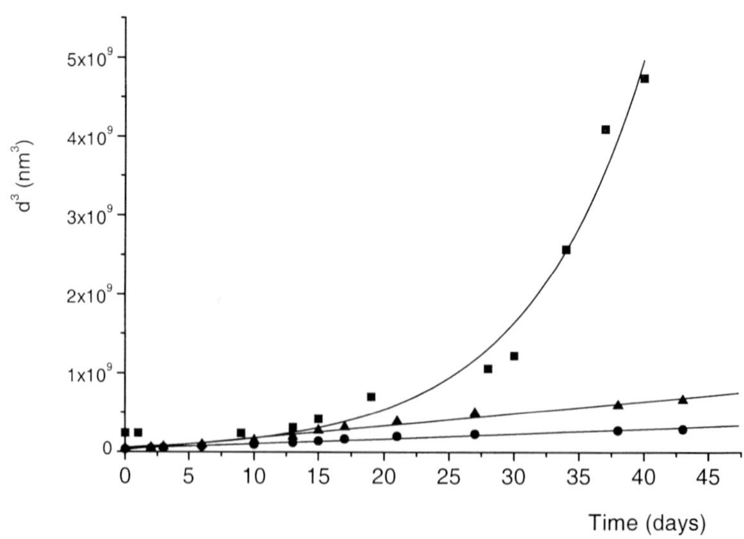

FIG. 8. Variation in the cube of the average droplet diameter (d^3) as a function of time at 40°C for PFOB-in-water emulsions prepared with PLC8 alone (*triangles*), an equimolar mixture of PLC8 and PFDB (*circles*), or an equimolar mixture of PLC8 and F8H16 (*squares*)

phospholipid (DMPC) but destabilizes emulsions prepared with a short-chain phospholipid (PLC8). Destabilization occurs, then, through droplet coalescence. In the latter case, a mismatch between the phospholipids' fatty acid chain length and the length of the hydrocarbon segment of F8H16 may account for the observed destabilization.

The fit between the fatty acid chains of DMPC, which are 14 carbon atoms long, and the H16 moiety of the diblock probably results in the formation of a better organized interfacial film, which accounts for the observed stabilization. The fact that the stabilization or destabilization effects are conditioned by the adequacy between the length of the Hm segment and that of the phospholipid's fatty chains further demonstrates the implication of the F8H16 diblock in the interfacial film. That PFDB stabilizes the emulsions whatever the phospholipid's chain length was expected, as it has been demonstrated that PFDB hinders molecular diffusion by lowering the solubility and diffusibility of the dispersed FC phase in the continuous aqueous phase. The difference in behavior of F8H16 and PFDB in this respect demonstrates a difference in the stabilization mechanism.

Conclusions

These studies showed that highly stable, small-sized FC-in-water emulsions can be obtained by incorporating a fluorocarbon/hydrocarbon diblock in the emulsifying system. Direct proof of the strong co-surfactant activity of the semifluorinated alkane F8H16 when present along with phospholipids at the water–PFOB interface is provided. It was also demonstrated that F8H16 stabilizes PFOB emulsions against Ostwald ripening more efficiently than a heavier, nonamphiphilic FC and, moreover, that the stabilization effect is dependent on the relative length of the phospholipid's fatty acid chains and that of the hydrogenated segment of the semifluorinated alkane. Therefore, we can conclude that the diblock molecule is involved in the interfacial film, and the decreased interfacial tension caused by the diblock must play a role in the stabilization mechanism.

Acknowledgments. We thank Prof. J.G. Riess (MRI Institute, University of California at San Diego) for fruitful discussions about the "dowel" effect. We also acknowledge Lipoid for the generous gift of phospholipids, Alliance Pharmaceutical Corp. for PFOB and PFDB, and AtoFina (Pierre Bénite, France) for fluorinated precursors. We are grateful to the Centre National de la Recherche Scientifique (CNRS) for financial support.

References

1. Riess JG (1998) Fluorocarbon-based oxygen delivery: basic principles and product development. In: Chang TMS (ed) Blood substitutes: methods, products and clinical trials. Karger Landes Systems, New York, pp 101–126
2. Riess JG (2001) Injectable oxygen carriers (blood substitutes): Raison d'être, chemistry, and some physiology. Chem Rev 101:2797–2919
3. Krafft MP, Chittofrati A, Riess JG (2003) Emulsions and microemulsions with a fluorocarbon phase. Curr Opin Colloid Interf Sci 8:251–258
4. Davis SS, Round HP, Purewal TS (1981) Ostwald ripening and the stability of emulsion systems: an explanation for the effect of an added third component. J Colloid Interf Sci 80:508–511
5. Kabalnov AS, Aprosin YD, Pavlova-Verevkina OB, Pertsov AV, Shchukin ED (1986) Influence of nature and composition of disperse phase in emulsions of perfluoroorganic compounds on the kinetics of the decrease in emulsion dispersity. Kolloidnyi Zhurnal 48:27–32
6. Varescon C, Arlen C, Le Blanc M, Riess JG (1989) An easy, convenient way of describing the stability of fluorocarbon emulsions. J Chim Phys 86:2111–2117
7. Kabalnov AS, Makarov KN, Shchukin ED (1992) Stability of perfluoroalkyl halide emulsions. Colloids Surf 62:101–104
8. Trevino L, Sole-Violan L, Daumur P, Devallez B, Postel M, Riess JG (1993) Molecular diffusion in concentrated fluorocarbon emulsions and its effect on emulsion stability. N J Chem 17:275–278
9. Weers JG (1998) Molecular diffusion in emulsion and emulsion mixture. In: Binks BP (ed) Modern aspects of emulsion science. Royal Society of Chemistry, Cambridge, pp 292–327
10. Krafft MP, Riess JG, Weers JG (1998) The design and engineering of oxygen-delivering fluorocarbon emulsions. In: Benita S (ed) Submicronic emulsions in drug targeting and delivery. Harwood Academic, Amsterdam, pp 235–333
11. Weers JG, Ni Y, Tarara TE, Pelura TJ, Arlauskas RA (1994) The effect of molecular diffusion on initial particle size distributions in phospholipid-stabilized fluorocarbon emulsions. Colloids Surf A 84:81–87
12. Riess JG, Sole-Violan L, Postel M (1992) A new concept for the stabilization of injectable fluorocarbon emulsions. J Dispos Sci Technol 13:349–355
13. Riess JG, Cornélus C, Follana R, Krafft MP, Mahé AM, Postel M, Zarif L (1994) Novel fluorocarbon-based injectable oxygen-carrying formulations with long-term room-temperature storage stability. Adv Exp Biol Med 345:227–234
14. Cornélus C, Krafft MP, Riess JG (1994) About the mechanism of stabilization of fluorocarbon emulsions by mixed fluorocarbon/hydrocarbon additives. J Colloid Interf Sci 163:391–394
15. Krafft MP, Dellamare L, Tarara T, Riess JG, Trevino L WO 97/21425. June 19, 1997
16. Trevino L, Frézard F, Rolland JP, Postel M, Riess JG (1994) Novel liposome systems based on the incorporation of (perfluoroalkyl)alkenes (FmHnE) into the bilayer of phospholipid liposomes. Colloids Surf 88:223–233
17. Trevino L, Frézard F, Postel M, Riess JG (1994) Incorporation of a perfluoroalkylalkane (R_FR_H) into the phospholipid bilayer of DMPC liposomes results in greater encapsulation stability. J Liposome Res 4:1017–1028
18. Ferro Y, Krafft MP (2002) Incorporation of semi-fluorinated alkanes in the bilayer of small unilamellar vesicles of phosphatidylserine: impact on fusion kinetics. Biochim Biophys Acta 1581:11–20

19. Privitera N, Naon R, Riess JG (1995) Hydrolysis of DMPC or DPPC by pancreatic phospholipase A_2 is slowed down when (perfluoroalkyl)alkanes are incorporated into the liposomal membrane. Biochim Biophys Acta 1254:1–6
20. Schmutz M, Michels B, Marie P, Krafft MP (2003) Fluorinated vesicles made from combinations of phospholipids and semifluorinated alkanes: direct experimental evidence of the location of the semifluorinated alkane within the bilayer. Langmuir 19: 4889–4894
21. Brace NO (1973) Free-radical addition of iodoperfluoroalkanes to terminal alkadienes: relative reactivity as a function of chain length and reaction conditions. J Org Chem 38:3167–3172
22. Rabolt JF, Russel TP, Tweig RT (1984) Structural studies of semifluorinated *n*-alkanes. 1. Synthesis and characterization of $F(CF_2)_n(CH_2)_mH$ in the solid state. Macromolecules 17:2786–2794
23. Meinert H, Knoblich A (1993) The use of semifluorinated alkanes in blood substitutes. Biomater Artif Cells Immob Biotechnol 21:583–595
24. Zarif L, Postel M, Septe B, Trevino L, Riess JG, Mahé A-M, Follana R (1994) Biodistribution of mixed fluorocarbon-hydrocarbon dowel molecules used as stabilizers of fluorocarbon emulsions: a quantitative study by fluorine nuclear magnetic resonance (NMR). Pharm Res 11:122–127
25. Sanchez V, Zarif L, Greiner J, Riess JG, Cippolini S, Bruneton JN (1994) Novel injectable fluorinated contrast agents with enhanced radiopacity. Artif Cells Blood Substit, Immob Biotechnol 22:1421–1428
26. Schreyeck G, Marie P (1999) Kinetics of the absorption of a PDMS-*g*-PEO copolymer at the PDMS/PEO interface. Langmuir 15:8212–8219
27. Rotenberg Y, Boruvka L, Neumann A (1983) Determination of surface tension and contact angle from the shapes of axisymmetric fluid interfaces. J Colloid Interf Sci 93:169–183
28. Kabalnov AS, Shchukin ED (1992) Ostwald ripening theory: applications to fluorocarbon emulsion stability. Adv Colloid Interf Sci 38:69–97
29. Higuchi WI, Misra J (1962) Physical degradation of emulsions via the molecular diffusion route and the possible prevention thereof. J Pharm Sci 51:459–466

Possible Role of Artificial Oxygen Carriers in Shock and Trauma

B. Thomas Kjellström

Summary. Trauma is the most common cause of death in young individuals in the industrialized world. One third of all trauma deaths take place within minutes to hours after injury. In this patient group, hemorrhage is a common cause of death. One important part of early treatment in trauma is i.v. administration of crystalloid and/or colloid resuscitation fluids to prevent the development of hemorrhagic/hypovolemic shock. While such fluids can restore blood volume, they cannot transport oxygen to the tissues. Ensuing tissue ischemia leads to anaerobic metabolism and to accumulation of toxic metabolites. This can, in turn, develop into irreversible shock and death. It would thus be advantageous if resuscitation fluids given on the scene not only restored loss of blood volume, but also could carry oxygen and deliver it to the tissues. In hospital blood for transfusion is not always readily available and typing and crossmatching can be time-consuming and costly. Consequently, in the hospital setting and during emergency surgery a resuscitation fluid that could deliver oxygen could be of value. Hemospan, a newly designed hemoglobin-based artificial oxygen carrier, has been tested in two different large animal hemorrhagic shock models. Normalization of hemodynamic as well as metabolic parameters was achieved without any signs of the detrimental vasoactivity seen with earlier hemoglobin-based products. Survival time also increased, even in comparison with autologous blood transfusions.

Key words. Artificial oxygen carriers, Shock, Trauma

Department of Defense Medicine, Retzius Väg 8, B1:5, FOI/Karolinska Institutet, SE-17177 Stockholm, Sweden

Introduction

In the industrialized world, trauma is the number one cause of death in age groups below 40–45 years of age [1,2]. Approximately half of all trauma deaths occur immediately after the accident; about 30% within a few hours after injury and the last 20% after days to weeks. In the first case, the cause of death is generally severe injuries to vital organs, e.g., the central nervous system, heart or major blood vessels. These patients die within minutes after trauma, and are most often not possible to save regardless of any therapeutic means. In the second group, hemorrhage is one common cause of death, while late complications, such as infection or multiple organ failure (MOF), cause the death of patients in the third group [3].

The loss of years of life due to trauma amounts to 36 years on an individual basis, which should be compared to the corresponding numbers relating to cancer, 15 years, and to cardiac disease, 12 years [4]. In the USA, about 21,000 individuals die annually due to trauma with a resulting annual loss of years of life of approximately 770,000 years. The resulting loss of productivity has been estimated to $6 billion. The annual hospital costs for trauma care in USA are estimated to be $10–15 billion, costs for disability and unemployment not included [5]. In Sweden, a country often considered to have a comparatively low trauma incidence, 10% of the population has to see a doctor every year after accidents, and approximately 1.5% of the population annually receives hospital care due to trauma [2].

Trauma care can be divided into three major phases: Phase I, the prehospital phase, which takes place on the scene of accident and/or during transport by ambulance or helicopter to the hospital. The transport time from scene to hospital can be quite variable, from minutes in a city to an hour or more in rural areas. Phase I trauma care will, depending on organization and circumstances, be delivered by paramedics, maybe under supervision of a registered nurse or a physician. Phase II, the hospital or in-hospital phase, by definition starts once the patient enters the hospital emergency room (ER) and is delivered by different members of the hospital staff. The IIIrd, or the late, phase is the rehabilitation phase, consisting of e.g. occupational therapy and physiotherapy, and will not be further dealt with in this paper.

The objectives of Phase I trauma care are to secure respiration, to stop overt hemorrhage and to counteract development of shock due to hypovolemia. In this context, development of hypovolemia and hypovolemic shock almost always is due to hemorrhage [3]. At a certain point, tissue perfusion in shock becomes inadequate for the oxygen need at the cellular level. Cellular hypoxia results in anaerobic metabolism, cellular acidosis, lactic acidosis, swelling of the microvascular endothelium and circulating white cells, blocking of the microcirculation and impaired organ function. Finally, if the patient survives the first hours to days, MOF may develop; a syndrome with a mortality of 50%–80% [3,6].

To counteract hypovolemia, resuscitation fluids are administered intravenously. Such fluids will restore circulating blood volume, but do not carry oxygen and will, consequently, not deliver any oxygen to the hypoxic cells even if the improved circulation per se may, at least transiently and to some extent, increase tissue oxygenation given an unimpaired respiration and microcirculation [6].

Resuscitation Fluids

Two major categories of i.v. resuscitation fluids have been used over the last decades in the treatment of hemorrhagic/hypovolemic shock, crystalloid or colloid solutions. The former, examples of which are normal saline and Ringer's lactate, are isotonic compared to blood, while the latter, dextran 70 and hydroxyethyl starch solutions (HES), are hypertonic [7].

In recent years, hypertonic-hyperoncotic resuscitation fluids have been advocated [8,9], registered for clinical use in some countries (for instance Rescue-Flow, Bio-Phausia, Uppsala, Sweden), but also questioned [10]. Crystalloids freely cross the capillary membrane and equilibrate with the whole extracellular fluid space. Large volumes (up to 5 times the volume deficit) have to be infused, and the intravasal retention is limited. Tissue edema may form [7]. Hypertonic solutions are characterized by high concentrations of e.g. crystalloids and one of their effects is a transient increase in plasma osmolality which, in turn, results in mobilization of intracellular fluid from the edematous endothelium and circulating white cells and thus increased blood volume [6]. By combining hypertonic solutions with solutions exerting high oncotic pressure, the increase in circulating volume will be preserved for several (4–8) hours [6].

What beneficial effects these different resuscitation fluids may have in restoring blood volume and supporting macro- and micro-circulation they cannot, however, fulfill one of the most important roles of blood itself, namely to deliver oxygen to tissues and cells.

Artificial Oxygen Carriers

There are, theoretically, three major advantages with artificial oxygen carriers (AOC) when compared with bank blood [11]:

Artificial oxygen carriers can be sterilized, which blood cannot—no risk of spreading infections like HIV or hepatitis.
Artificial oxygen carriers do not have any blood group antigens—no need for typing and cross-matching.
Artificial oxygen carriers could be stored for a long time, maybe as a stable, lyophilized powder—a great logistic advantage.

Two completely different categories of artificial oxygen carriers, or "artificial blood" exist today, namely hemoglobin-based oxygen carriers (HBOC) and products based on perfluorocarbons (PF) [11]. The latter have the advantage of being chemically manufactured and can thus be produced in large quantities, independently of biological sources. Perfluorocarbons are molecules similar to hydrocarbons, but with fluorine atoms instead of hydrogen atoms. Perfluorocarbons are excellent carriers of oxygen and carbon dioxide, which are dissolved in the PF liquid and easily extracted by the tissue [12]. At any given partial pressure of oxygen in equilibrium with PF, hemoglobin (Hb), however, binds more oxygen than is dissolved in the PF emulsion. This is one reason why patients in clinical trials with PF often have to breath 70–100% oxygen in order for the product to carry enough oxygen. Furthermore, complement activation, increased body temperature, decreasing platelet counts and prolonged bleeding time have been clinical problems with PF-based products undergoing clinical trials [12,13].

Hemoglobin-based oxygen carriers are based on Hb from different sources, such as outdated blood-bank blood or bovine blood but also human Hb produced by recombinant technology in microorganisms [14]. Hb exists within the red blood cells (RBC) in tetrameric form, but outside the cells each tetramer breaks down into two dimers. These dimers are known to be nephrotoxic, to exert a high oncotic pressure, to induce vasoactivity and to release oxygen at a low p_{50} [11,12,14]. These side effects have been known for decades and consequently much effort has been put down, trying to modify the Hb dimers to alleviate them [11,14]. Cross-linking of the Hb molecules prevent their break-down into dimers. Furthermore, the Hb molecule has been encapsulated, and also coated (conjugated) with compounds such as dextran and polyethylene glycol (PEG) [14].

Presently, several different AOC products, both HBOC and PF, of the first and second generation are undergoing clinical trials worldwide. Furthermore, PF based products are today in clinical use in Russia [15], but hitherto only one PF based product has been approved in the US for clinical use (in balloon angioplasty) [13] and one HBOC, in South Africa, for use in patients undergoing surgical procedures [16].

AOC in Shock and Trauma

Phase I and II trauma care aim at the reduction of trauma mortality and morbidity by resuscitation from hypovolemia/hypotension and by rapid restoration of oxygen delivery to the tissues [17]. From this point of view, it is evident that an ideal resuscitation fluid would be one that could fulfill both these criteria, restore circulation and organ perfusion as well as deliver oxygen. Bank blood is, of course, such a fluid, but can hardly be administered during Phase I, and is sometimes not as readily as one could expect during Phase II either [11]. Furthermore, the threat of donor blood shortage may very well become a reality in a not too distant future even in the developed part of the world, just as it already is in other, not so fortunate, areas [11]. Consequently, a lot of work has been dedicated to developing AOC suitable for treatment of traumatic hemorrhagic shock, and a large, randomized, multicenter study using a diaspirin cross-linked HBOC was conducted in 1997–1998. The study, unfortunately, had to be prematurely stopped, due to the fact that mortality was higher for the patients treated with this particular HBOC than for the controls receiving standard therapy. This untoward treatment effect was attributed to the vasopressor effect of the preparation [18,19].

In recent years, PEG-conjugated HBOC have been extensively tested in different animal models of exchange transfusion or hemorrhagic shock [20,21]. A novel product, Hemospan (Sangart, San Diego, CA, USA) based on the following design principles [22]:

High O_2 affinity
Viscosity close to the one of blood
Hyperonconicity
High molecular volume : mass ratio

has been tested in two different large animal models of hemorrhagic shock [23–25]. Hemospan was demonstrated to lack most of the negative vasoactivity effects mentioned above. Furthermore, survival time in a double insult model was longer with Hemospan than with standard hemorrhagic shock treatment (colloids) and even with autotransfusion with the animals' own shed blood [23]. A related product is currently in clinical Phase II trials in patients undergoing surgical procedures.

Conclusion

Trauma is the dominating cause of death in individuals below 40–45 years of age in the industrialized world. Much of the mortality and morbidity in trauma is due to hemorrhagic shock and the following hypoxia on the cellular level. Shock treatment on the scene of accident often consists of i.v. administration of crystalloid and/or colloid resuscitation fluids. Such fluids can support circulating blood volume, but can not deliver oxygen to hypoxic tissues and cells. At the hospital level, bank blood can be given to treat hemorrhagic shock. There is in many parts of the world a lack of donor blood. Even in developed countries blood for transfusion is not always as readily available as one could imagine. Furthermore, there is always a certain risk of transmission of contagious diseases (hepatitis, HIV) inherent in blood transfusions. Consequently, there is a place for suitable AOC in treatment of hemorrhagic shock in trauma, maybe both on scene and at the hospital. Even if there has been disappointment in the outcome of some previous clinical trials, promising novel products have been developed. Some of these are already in clinical trials. Furthermore, a limited number of AOC are approved for clinical use in a couple of countries today.

Conflict of Interest Statement. Dr. B. Thomas Kjellström is a member of the scientific advisory board of Sangart, Inc.

Acknowledgments. Financial support was received from The Swedish Defense Research Agency, Stockholm, Sweden (Grants E 5054 and E 46903) and from Sangart, Inc., San Diego, CA, USA.

References

1. Trunkey DD (1983) Trauma. Sci Am 249:28–35
2. Brismar B (1996) Trauma care organization in Sweden. In: Risberg B (ed) Trauma care—an update. Pharmacia & Upjohn, Göteborg, pp 3–4
3. Wladis A (2001) Hypothermia and trauma. Thesis, Karolinska University Press Stockholm, Sweden, pp 10–14
4. Regel G, Tscherne H (1996) Trauma care organization in Germany. In: Risberg B (ed) Trauma care—an update. Pharmacia & Upjohn, Göteborg, pp 12–17
5. MacKenzie EJ, Siegel JH, Shapiro S, et al (1988) Functional recovery and medical costs of trauma: an analysis by type and severity of injury. J Trauma 28:281–297
6. Kreimeier U, Messmer K (1996) Regional blood flow and oxygen delivery in shock. In: Risberg B (ed) Trauma care—an update. Pharmacia & Upjohn, Göteborg, pp 104–117
7. Haljamäe H (1996) Crystalloids vs colloids. In: Risberg B (ed) Trauma care—an update. Pharmacia & Upjohn, Göteborg, pp 129–141
8. Mattox KL, Maningas PA, Moore EE, et al (1991) Prehospital hypertonic saline/Dextran infusion for post-traumatic hypotension. Ann Surg 213:482–491
9. Wade CE, Kramer GC, Grady JJ, et al (1997) Efficacy of hypertonic 7.5% saline and 6% Dextran-70 in treating trauma: a meta-analysis of controlled clinical studies. Surgery 122:609–616
10. Riddez L, Drobin D, Sjöstrand F, et al (2002) Lower dose of hypertonic saline dextran reduces the risk of lethal rebleeding in uncontrolled hemorrhage. Shock 17:377–382

11. Kjellström BT (2003) Blood substitutes: where do we stand today? J Int Med 253:495–497
12. Squires JE (2002) Artificial blood. Science 295:1002–1005
13. Chang TMS (1997) Blood substitutes: principles, methods, products and clinical trials. vol. 1. Karger, Basel, pp 82–87
14. Chang TMS (1997) Blood substitutes: principles, methods, products and clinical trials. vol. 1. Karger, Basel, pp 9–31
15. Ivanitsky GR (2001) Biophysics at the turn of the millennium: perfluorocarbon media and gas-transporting blood substitutes. Biophysics 46:1–31
16. Edwards G, Levien L, Benn C (2003) Oxygen therapeutic Hemopure in breast cancer reconstructive surgery. Artif Blood 11:38
17. Kreimeier U, Thiel M, Messmer K (1996) Hypertonic-hyperoncotic solutions. In: Risberg B (ed) Trauma care—an update, Pharmacia & Upjohn, Göteborg, pp 142–153
18. Sloan EP, Koenigsberg M, Gens D, et al (1999) Diaspirin cross-linked hemoglobin (DCLHb) in the treatment of severe traumatic hemorrhagic shock. A randomized controlled efficacy trial. JAMA 282:1857–1864
19. Winslow RM (2000) αα-Crosslinked hemoglobin: was failure predicted by preclinical testing? Vox Sang 79:1–20
20. Migita R, Gonzales A, Gonzales ML, et al (1997) Blood volume and cardiac index in rats after exchange transfusion with hemoglobin-based oxygen carriers. J Appl Physiol 82:1995–2002
21. Winslow RM, Gonzales A, Gonzales ML, et al (1998) Vascular resistance and the efficacy of red cell substitutes in a rat hemorrhage model. J Appl Physiol 85:993–1003
22. Vandegriff KD, Lohman JM, Tsai AG, et al (2000) Hemospan, a non-hypertensive, high-blood flow red cell substitute. Proc VIII Internat'nl Symp Blood Subst, San Diego, USA, p 23
23. Drobin D, Lohman J, Malm E, et al (2003) Increased survival time during second hemorrhage when first hemorrhage is resuscitated with Hemospan compared to blood or colloid. Artif Blood 11:89
24. Kjellström BT, Drobin D, Malm E, et al (2003) Hemodynamic and metabolic changes after administration of PEG-Hb in hemorrhagic shock in swine. Artif Blood 11:70
25. Drobin D, Kjellström BT, Malm E, et al (2004) Hemodynamic response and oxygen transport in pigs resuscitated with maleimide-polyethylene glycol-modified hemoglobin (MPH). J Appl Physiol 96:1843–1854

Clinical Needs for Artificial Oxygen Carriers in Anaesthesia

Robert G. Hahn

Summary. Transfusion of blood is associated with high costs in the anaesthesia department. Immunological testing and/or cross-matching is routinely done before many operations entailing only a small risk of major haemorrhage. The introduction of artificial oxygen substitutes would save not only the cost of the erythrocytes but also of the extensive blood testing. In operations with an expected large blood loss, competition with donated blood will probably be focused largely on the potential prevention of adverse effects and infection. In the intensive care unit, a beneficial influence on blood rheology is more important than during surgery, and it must be possible to evaluate oxygen delivery after administration of the artificial oxygen substitute. For trauma outside hospital, artificial oxygen substitutes compete with fluid resuscitation as donated blood is rarely an option. Surprisingly, it is currently unclear where and when fluid resuscitation should be provided in the prehospital setting. Long transport times and head trauma are currently the most apparent indications. Artificial oxygen substitutes should be available at short notice, i.e., not requiring thawing, in order to be successful products. Here, volume expansion is a desired property along with improvement in oxygen-carrying capacity.

Key words. Artificial oxygen carriers, Hemodilution, Fluid resuscitation, Prehospital care, Red blood cells, Transurethral resection of the prostate

---

Department of Anesthesiology, Söder Hospital, S-118 83 Stockholm, Sweden

Introduction

Anaesthesia is a medical speciality in which there is much interest in the development of artificial oxygen carriers. Anaesthetists will certainly be important purchasers of these products regardless of which ones will eventually appear on the market. The anaesthetist works in four areas, and the focus might be slightly different depending on the country studied. They are: (1) in the operating theatre, (2) the intensive care unit, (3) on the prehospital scene, and (4) in the pain clinic. The following presentation is focused on explaining the prerequisites for marketing artificial oxygen carriers in the first three of these areas.

Small Risk of Surgical Bleeding

Many surgical operations that are performed today carry only a moderate risk of blood loss requiring transfusion of erythrocytes. In such cases, the cost of the erythrocytes that are eventually given is exceedingly high. The rationale for this view is that all patients at risk need to undergo blood grouping followed by immunological testing and sometimes cross-matching of each transfused bag of erythrocytes (if irregular antibodies are present). The cost of this procedure is substantial, for both analyses and blood sampling, as well as for the involved logistics.

Transurethral resection of the prostate (TURP) can be used as an example. This operation is still one of the most common operations in the Western world. In a series of 1,034 patients operated on at Söder Hospital, the median blood loss was only 300 ml. However, the bled volume exceeded 1 litre, which is often treated with erythrocytes in elderly males, in 14% of the patients [1] (Fig. 1). The risk of a blood loss requiring erythrocyte transfusion makes it necessary for the hospital to test all TURP patients as if they were to receive blood. This practice is logical since one never knows who is going to bleed. However, nearly all of this testing is meaningless as only a few actually benefit from the result. Operations which carry a risk of only 1% for requiring erythrocytes would not normally require preoperative testing, but operations with a 10% risk do.

An artificial oxygen carrier would be very cost-effective in TURP patients with excessive bleeding as not only the costs for the transfused erythrocytes can be saved but also for the blood testing of the vast majority of patients who do not require erythrocytes.

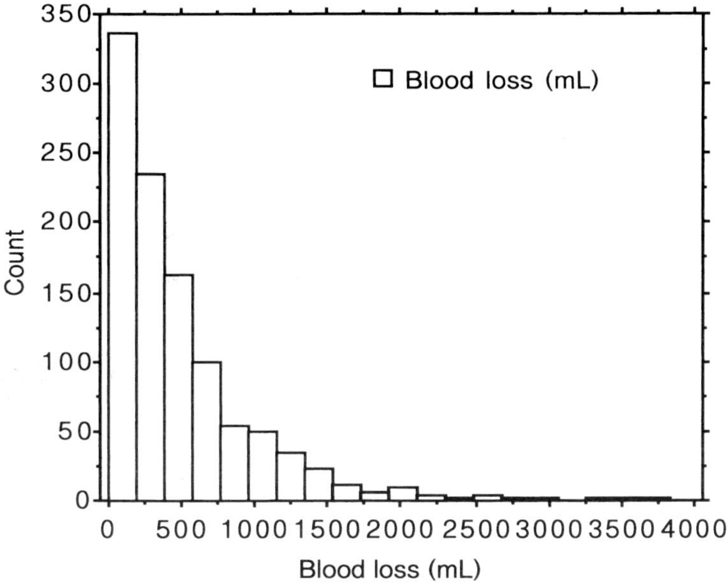

FIG. 1. The blood loss in 1,034 transurethral prostatic resections. Although the median blood loss is only 300 ml, it exceeded 1,000 ml in 14% of the patients. The existence of transfusion-requiring operations necessitates blood group and immunological testing/cross-matching in all patients. The use of artificial oxygen carriers saves not only the cost of the transfused erythrocytes in the small group with extensive haemorrhage, but also the extensive blood testing in the entire group

Expected Major Bleeding

Patients who undergo major surgery are routinely subjected to normovolaemic haemodilution. This means that the blood loss is treated with infusions of salt solutions to maintain the blood volume. Such infusions dilute the blood Hb concentration, and the artificial oxygen carrier then only needs to treat the reduced Hb level without the influence of hypovolaemia. The body has sophisticated compensatory mechanisms to deal with an acute lowering of Hb, the most important one being an increase in stroke volume to maintain oxygen delivery. Another mechanism consists in an increase in the peripheral extraction of oxygen. At a certain point, however, the compensatory mechanisms simply are not sufficient for the body's needs of oxygen, which limit is called the "anaerobic threshold". If Hb is further reduced, the delivery of oxygen to the tissues becomes too small, lactate production increases and the patient becomes acidotic.

Many efforts have been made to find the Hb level that signifies the anaerobic threshold. This Hb level is called the "transfusion trigger". Ethical difficulties in performing experimental research to find the transfusion trigger on humans are apparent. The truth is that each individual has a different capacity to deal with a low Hb. In old age, the cardiac capacity is reduced and this limits the ability to increase the stroke volume. The heart itself might also be susceptible to ischaemia. Young healthy people tolerate a low Hb, even down to 50–55 g/l, much better [2].

The consensus in this field is that the transfusion trigger should range between 60 and 100 g/l (6–10 g/dl) and what the trigger should be in individual patients must be determined by sound clinical judgement [3]. If a lower Hb level is reached, the patient should be transfused with erythrocytes.

A concept in normovolaemic haemodilution is the "allowable blood loss". This represents the volume of blood that can be lost before the transfusion trigger is reached. If the Hb concentration is the same in all blood that is lost, the allowable blood loss and the fall in Hb from before surgery to the transfusion trigger would be directly proportional. This is not the case, however, because the blood volume is constantly kept normal by infusions of salt solution. The last portion of the bled volume during a haemodilution process will therefore reduce Hb at a slower rate than the first portion. The following logarithmic equation by Bourke and Smith [4], which is widely used to estimate how large a bleed can be allowed, is based on the estimated blood volume at baseline (BV_o), the Hb level before the operation (Hb_o) and the transfusion trigger ($Hb(t)$) which is reached at time (t):

$$\text{Allowable blood loss} = BV_o\,[\ln Hb_o - \ln Hb(t)]$$

This equation assumes that the Hb level is always lowered in direct proportion to the blood loss. Erroneous estimations will ensue if the haemodilution does not catch up with the bleeding at all times. This is a very common mistake.

An alternative to the use of the haemodilution equation of Bourke and Smith [4] is to measure Hb in the operating theatre (remember that what we only want to find out is whether the "target" Hb has been reached). Today, good equipment is available at low cost.

One may also compare the results of the haemodilution equation with the loss of Hb molecules in order to estimate how much the blood volume has changed, if at all. Such calculations are based on simple mathematical relationships between blood volume, the amount of Hb lost and the Hb level. Here, we must involve the Hb mass in the body, which is slightly less than 1 kg [5]:

$$\text{HB mass}_o = BV_o * Hb_o$$

$$BV(t) = \frac{\text{Hb mass}_o - \text{loss of Hb mass}_{(t-0)}}{\text{Hb}(t)}$$

Thus, alterations in blood volume can be estimated from the Hb level in whole blood provided that the loss of Hb through bleeding is known. Such simple equations, which, in contrast to the equation of Bourke and Smith [4], are insensitive to how well the fluid therapy has been managed, can be used to examine whether the haemodilution has indeed been performed in a normovolaemic patient [6]. Since hypovolaemia is a serious condition in that it reduces the cardiac output, a low blood volume is certainly a confounder in many (perhaps most) studies attempting to define the transfusion trigger. Therefore, ideally, studies that draw conclusions about the consequences of haemodilution during surgery should check that the blood volume is normal at the end of the experiments.

The well-controlled environment in which normovolaemic haemodilution is performed puts a slightly different emphasis on the need for artificial oxygen carriers. Here, the arguments for such products are to be found in the profile of adverse effects. Erythrocytes carry a risk of viral infection, and bank blood might impair the microcirculation. Immunomodulation (TRIM) is a known consequence, even to the extent that organ dysfunction (TRALI) may develop. Septic reactions may occur, although such problems are more common when platelets are transfused.

Verification that artificial oxygen carriers entail smaller risks of adverse effects would open up this market. The products will sometimes be used when very large transfusions are required simply because the hospital has run out of blood. However, public opinion is likely to be crucial. If the patients prefer artificial oxygen carriers, the hospitals may have to use them even if they are more expensive than coventional donated blood.

Various erythrocyte-saving techniques are used in the clinic today, but they cannot replace the transfusion of erythrocytes. Predonation of autologous blood which is given back to the patient during the operation emerged during the 1990s, but its use is limited in most countries because of the high cost. In some hospitals, predonation remains a service for the interested. Autotransfusion of blood from wounds can indeed be useful during extensive surgery. The lost blood is suctioned into an apparatus (such as the Cell Saver) where it is anticoagulated, washed, filtrated and retransfused directly in the operating theatre. One problem is the high cost of this technique as well. Just the sterile tubes needed for each operation may cost as much $1,000. Blood that is retransfused without being washed presents the problem of being "activated", i.e., it contains high concentrations of cytokines and other substances that may affect the patient [7]. There are also groups of patients, such as cancer patients, in whom retransfusion is unsuitable. These blood-saving techniques will certainly remain in the future and should be regarded as a complement to artificial oxygen carriers.

Intensive Care

The need for artificial oxygen carriers in intensive care is governed by the often quite long period of care for certain patients (1–2 months), during which time the oxygen demand might be increased owing to such conditions as sepsis and burns. Moreover, blood sampling is usually extensive and often amounts to one erythrocyte bag per week.

The severity of the patient's disease usually prompts the use of a high transfusion trigger. A widely used Hb level is 100 g/l. One study supporting this transfusion trigger was conducted by Hebert et al. [8], who studied 4,470 critically ill patients with cardiac disease and found a trend to an increased mortality when Hb was below 95 g/l. However, divergent results have also been obtained, even by the same author [9].

Intensive care patients are immobilised for long periods of time, so the rheological properties of any artificial oxygen carrier will be important in this setting. Any improvement in the peripheral blood flow without increasing the bleeding tendency is beneficial. Moreover, oxygen delivery needs to evaluated more or less continuously in these patients, and it is important that any modification of the transfusion trigger with respect to the oxygen carrier is clearly described. For example, frequently used equations for oxygen delivery probably need to be redefined. Such efforts may include placement of a device for measuring plasma Hb in the intensive care unit.

Prehospital Care

Haemorrhage is an important cause of death in the prehospital trauma victim. One third of the deaths that occur outside hospital following major trauma are caused by exsanguination [10]. Owing to logistical difficulties, erythrocytes are hardly ever transfused. Although hypovolaemia is a major issue, it is unclear how and when hypovolaemia should be treated. One criticism is that fluid resuscitation requires a few minutes to initiate and, in the larger cities, it might not take much longer to reach hospital. When the transport time is less than 30 min the patient is probably better off if rushed directly to hospital without receiving volume resuscitation. Salt solutions should be given. When there is a long distance to hospital or the patient is stuck in a car and cannot be readily extricated. Another situation is head trauma, where the mean arterial pressure must be kept higher than 80 mmHg to maintain adequate cerebral perfusion.

One reason why prehospital fluid resuscitation has not been successful in the final analysis may be that the blood vessels are dependent on a low blood flow and pressure to repair a major injury. If fluid is infused at a high rate, immature blood clots will be disrupted and this results in rebleeding and increased mortality [11,12]. This phenomenon is best described in animals, while little data is available on humans. The anticipated danger of uncontrolled haemorrhage has prompted a strategy called "hypotensive resuscitation", which implies that fluid therapy is not aimed at completely restoring the blood pressure. However, a recent study did not demonstrate any benefit of hypotensive resuscitation as compared to standard care [13].

Blood is intuitively better to give than salt solution in cases of major haemorrhage outside hospital. Artificial oxygen carriers do not compete with donated blood on the prehospital scene, but with fluid resuscitation. As it is still unclear in what circumstances intravenous salt solutions are indicated, the benefit of the artificial oxygen carrier needs to be demonstrated specifically in the prehospital setting. A marked volume expansion elicited by the product is helpful, and the product does not even have to be as effective as donated blood to be valuable. Regardless of the uncertainties described here, the potential market for artificial oxygen carriers is very large in prehospital medicine. It is important that large amounts of the product can be available at short notice, preferably without needing to be thawed.

Conclusions

In the hospital, artificial oxygen carriers have a market when there is both a moderately high and a high risk of haemorrhage that would require transfusion with erythrocytes. In the first case, its use may be very cost-effective because blood testing of large populations of patients can then be abandoned. In the latter case, competition with donated erythrocytes is more clear-cut, and attention will be very much focused on the profile of adverse effects. In intensive care, improved rheology is an issue, as well as valid instructions for how to evaluate oxygen delivery after an artificial oxygen carrier has been administered. In the prehospital setting, an artificial oxygen carrier must mimic what fluid resuscitation can do, but still improve oxygen delivery. Here, donated erythrocytes are not an option.

References

1. Ekengren J, Hahn RG (1993) Blood loss during transurethral resection of the prostate as measured with the HemoCue photometer. Scand J Urol Nephrol 27:501–507

2. Leung JM, Weiskopf RB, Feiner J, et al (2000) Electrocardiographic ST-segment changes during acute, severe isovolemic hemodilution in humans. Anesthesiology 93:1004–1010
3. Stehling L, Doherty DC, Faust RJ, et al (1996) Practice guidelines for blood component therapy. A report of the American Society of Anesthesiologists Task Force on Blood Component Therapy. Anesthesiology 84:732–747
4. Bourke DL, Smith TC (1974) Estimating allowable blood loss. Anesthesiology 41:609–612
5. Hahn RG (1989) Estimating allowable blood loss with correction for variations in blood volume. Acta Anaesthesiol Scand 33:508–512
6. Hahn RG (1987) A haemoglobin dilution method (HDM) for estimation of blood volume variations during transurethral prostatic surgery. Acta Anaesthesiol Scand 31:572–578
7. Kristiansson M, Soop M, Saraste L, et al (1995) Cytokine and coagulation characteristics of retrieved blood after arthroplasty. Int Care Med 21:989–995
8. Hébert PC, Wells G, Tweeddale M, et al (1997) Does transfusion practice affect mortality in critically ill patients? Transfusion requirements in Critical Care (TRICC) Investigators and the Canadian Critical Care Trials Group. Am J Respir Crit Care Med 155:1618–1623
9. Hébert PC, Wells G, Blajchman MA, et al (1999) A multicenter, randomized, controlled clinical trial of transfusion requirements in critical care. Transfusion Requirements in Critical Care Investigators for the Canadian Critical Care Trials. N Engl J Med 340:409–417
10. Shackford SR, Mackersie RC, Holbrook TL, et al (1993) The epidemiology of traumatic death. A population-based analysis. Arch Surg 128:571–575
11. Stern SA, Dronen SC, Birrer P, Wang X (1995) Effect of blood pressure on hemorrhage volume and survival in a near-fatal hemorrhage model incorporating a vascular injury. Ann Emerg Med 22:155–163
12. Riddez L, Johnsson L, Hahn RG (1998) Central and regional hemodynamics during fluid therapy after uncontrolled intra-abdominal bleeding. J Trauma 44:433–439
13. Dutton RP, Mackenzie CF, Scalea TM (2002) Hypotensive resuscitation during active hemorrhage: impact on in-hospital mortality. J Trauma 52:1141–1146

Studies on Red Cell Substitutes in Japan and Future Perspectives

Masuhiko Takaori

Key words. Artificial blood, Chemical property, Preclinical assessment, Clinical trial, Clinical efficacy

In 1966 Toyoda [1] at the Department of Surgery, Tokyo University School of Medicine, synthesized polystyrene encapsulated hemoglobin vesicles as artificial red cells and infused them in rabbits intravenously. However, they could not confirm whether or not those vesicles actually transported oxygen to the tissues. In 1979, Naito and Yokoyama [2] of Green Cross, Japan, produced Fluosol DA (Green Cross, Osaka, Japan), mixture of perfluorodecalin and perfluorotripropylamine, which looked like milk and was called "white blood". They performed some clinical trails in Japan. We used this product for a patient who suffered from unexpected massive bleeding and could not get proper blood for transfusion. The patient recovered uneventfully. However, it could be certain whether the Fluosol DA (Green Cross) was absolutely effective for oxygen transport, as it failed to transport sufficient amounts of oxygen to the tissues under normal atmospheric pressure without a high concentration of Fluosol DA [3].

Pharmaceutical companies such as Baxter, Biopure, Hemosol, and Alliance developed various artificial blood products in the past [4]. Data from some of the clinical trials which were performed in Europe [5] and the USA [6] have been published; however, none of the products progressed to clinical use. Nevertheless, the development of artificial blood for clinical use remains an urgent problem, particularly in the face of an expected shortage of blood for transfusion in the near future. In Japan we already occasionally experience

East Takarazuka Sato Hospital, 2-1 Nagao-cho, Takarazuka, Hyogo 665-0873, Japan

shortfalls in blood supply for transfusion, and anticipate a very severe shortfall in the future. Watanabe et al. [7] demonstrated that demand for blood will exceed supply by 2005. We are collecting outdated blood and extracting hemoglobin (Hb) for storage now as a possible solution. We hope to convert the collected blood products into artificial blood for use as a supplement for blood for transfusion in the future.

Recent Progress in Artificial Blood

Since 1990 the research group at Waseda University has developed a liposome encapsulated hemoglobin vesicle (HbV) as a substitute for red blood cells. In 1995 the Terumo company, which was associated with Waseda's scientific research, produced a similar HbV called the Neo Red Cells (NRC) (Terumo, Tokyo, Japan). We tested this product in animal experiments and found that it could transport oxygen to the tissues [8]. Under hemodilution, in which the animal's hematocrit value decreased to about 12%, the mixed venous oxygen saturation could be maintained at mostly normal with NRC's (Terumo) infusion but not with a plasma substitute such as hydroxyethyl starch (HES) solution. Oxygen consumption was maintained sufficiently with NRC (Terumo) but not with HES solution (Table 1).

Similarly Motoki et al. [9] noted that NRC (Terumo) released a greater amount of oxygen in the peripheral tissues compared with autologous blood transfusion (Fig. 1). Cardiac output in our study [6] was maintained satisfactorily with NRC (Terumo). Furthermore, it was noted that the circulating blood volume in the same situation could be maintained at a normal level without adverse effects, particulary life-threating complications. Therefore we believe that NRC can be used in practice.

Yoshizu et al. [10] at Keio University hemodiluted rats in which the hematocrit value was decreased to around 20% with either albumin solution or NRC. They measured tissue oxygen tension in the kidney polarographically and noted that NRC could maintain oxygen tension higher than the albumin solution or autologous blood transfusion did. A similar trend was also noted in skeletal muscle.

Subsequently the Waseda and Keio groups improved the efficiency of HbV for oxygen transport, and recently presented the physicochemical properties [11] (Table 2).

In the meantime, Nishi and Kida [12] at the University of Kumamoto, School of Medicine, Department of Pharmacology, formed pyridoxal phosphate polyethylene conjugated hemoglobin dimer (Fig. 2) as artificial red cells and used them for organ perfusion. This product obtained 24 h half life in the circulation of rats. It was noted, however, that this product scavenged nitric

Table 1. Changes in oxygen partial pressure (PvO_2), oxygen saturation (SvO_2), oxygen content (CvO_2) in mixed venous blood and oxygen consumption (VO_2) following hemodilution with Neo Red Cell and HES (hydroxyethyl starch) solution

		Initial	4× hemodilutions	8× hemodilutions	1 h after hemodilution	2 h after hemodilution
PvO_2	H	62 ± 5	52 ± 4	46 ± 6	41 ± 7	41 ± 7
mmHg	N	64 ± 3	50 ± 4	45 ± 4	42 ± 6	42 ± 5
SvO_2	H	73 ± 4	66 ± 5	41 ± 4	38 ± 6	37 ± 9
%	N	73 ± 5	67 ± 6	51 ± 6**	55 ± 6**	52 ± 5**
CvO_2	H	14.7 ± 0.7	8.2 ± 0.4	2.2 ± 0.4	2.4 ± 0.5	2.4 ± 0.4
ml/dl	N	15.1 ± 0.5	8.0 ± 0.5	3.2 ± 0.4**	3.2 ± 0.6**	2.9 ± 0.5**
VO_2	H	91.4 ± 7.4	68.4 ± 5.3	56.2 ± 5.9	46.3 ± 7.5	42.4 ± 6.2
ml/min	N	94.9 ± 7.3	74.3 ± 8.6	74.1 ± 8.4**	77.2 ± 6.1**	80.5 ± 6.9**

mean ± SD.
H, hydroxyethyl starch group; N, Neo Red Cells group.
Source: Takaori M, Fukui A (1996) Treatment of massive hemorrhage with liposome encapsulated hemoglobin (NRC) and hydroxyethyl starch (HES) in beagles.
Artif Cells Blood Substs Immunob Biotechnol 24; 643–653.
Comparison between groups **: $p < 0.01$.

TABLE 2. Physicochemical Properties of HbV

Hb	10.0 g/dl
Hb/Lipid	1.7
PEG-DSPE	0.3 mol %
diameter	247 µm
allosteric effector (Pyridoxal Phosphate/Hb)	2.5 mol/mol
P50	33 mmHg
MetHb	<1.0%
HbCO	<2.0%
Suspension	Saline

Hb, hemoglobin; PEG-DSPE, polyethylene glycole; MetHb, methemoglobin; HbCO, carboxylhemoglobin.

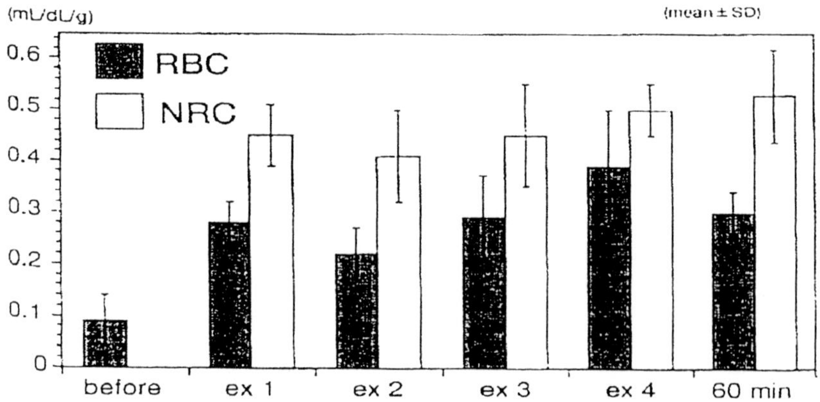

FIG. 1. AV (arteriovenous) oxygen content difference/Hb. Source: Usuba et al. [7]

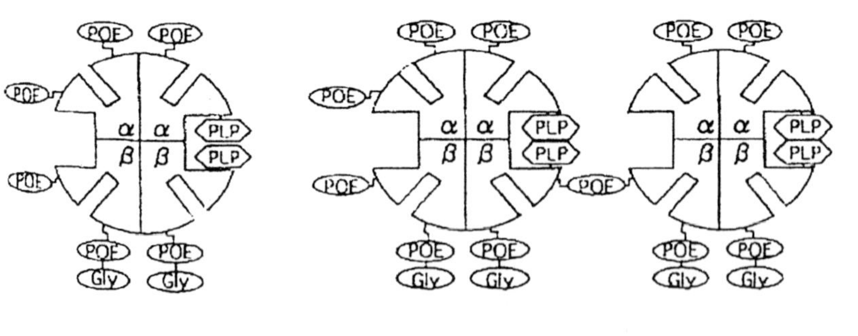

FIG. 2. Molecular structure of PHP. Source: Nishi and Kida [9]. *POE*, polyoxyethylene; *Gly*, glycine; *PLP*, phosphoenolpyruvate

oxide from the endothelium. Therefore, this product was excluded from clinical application.

Design of Artificial Red Cells

Although a search has been attempted for a substance which transports oxygen and releases it at the peripheral tissues more efficiently than hemoglobin, no such substance has yet been found. Therefore we concluded that natural Hb is best for this purpose at the present time.

We were concerned which type of artificial red cell is better, the cellular or acellular type. We concluded that the cellular type is superior to the acellular type for the following reasons:

1. Some substances, for example allostetic substances, such as pyridoxal phosphate as a substitute for 2.3 DPG (diphosphoglycerol), and a reductive substance such as homocysteine as substitute a for methemoglobin reductase, can be encapsulated in a vesicle accompanied with hemoglobin.
2. Greater blood flow may be maintained in the coronary and peripheral minute vessels, since the fluid contained in cellular particles can maintain a more similar blood viscosity, even under high-graded hemodilution.
3. Longer persistence of the artificial red cell in the circulating blood can be obtained with a cellular type. Rapid excretion in urine and in exhaled air, as seen with conjugated hemoglobin and with perfluorocarbon emulsion, respectively, will not occur with the cellular type.
4. Encapsulated Hb can be kept from direct contact with surrounding tissues, such as the endothelium and circulating blood cells, meaning the oxygen-carrying substance is protected and does not affect the surrounding tissues.

The Waseda research group enclosed pyridoxal phosphate in HbV and controlled P50 of hemoglobin at 33 mmHg (Table 2).

It has been found that extremely severe hemodilution with less than 10% of hematocrit value causes an increase in pulse pressure even when systolic pressure decreases slightly. Diastolic pressure is decreased markedly at 40 mmHg, which approaches the critical pressure for corony perfusion. However, when hemodilution can be done, with artificial blood which contains cellular type red cells and viscosity that can be maintained similarly to physiological blood, the perfusion pressure that will be created from peripheral vessel back pressure will be normal.

Retention time of artificial red cells in circulation after infusion needs to be longer than 24 h. If not, oxygen transport to the tissues will be reduced sharply. Since some physiological adaptation is needed, such as hematopoiesis

(2 ml/kg per day for red cell mass), an increase in 2,3 DPG in the red cells would need to be induced in accordance with gradual extravasation of the artificial red cells. Thus we can not safely use artificial blood with a short half life in clinical practice. The half-life of HbV is estimated as 16–18 h by the Waseda study in the rat [11] (Fig. 3). In addition, Tsutsui et al. [13] (Fig. 4), reported that the half-life is about 16–18 h in rats. However, we were recently informed that the half-life of HbV was 36–40 h in a primate (personal/communication, Ogata, Terumo).

Both the above studies present the perplexing problem of the rapid conversion from hemoglobin to metHb in vivo. To address this problem Waseda's investigators tried to encapsulate catalase, as reductase, in the vesicle. They encapsulated various doses of catalase in the vesicle, and found that encapsulation of catalase of 6000 unit/ml reduced the conversion of Hb to MetHb to $\frac{1}{3}$ of that of homocysteine alone. They observed that the suppresion of conversion seemed to be dose dependent and its optimum dose has not yet been decided [11].

With regard to direct contact of Hb with the surrounding tissues, Waseda and Keio's investigators bled 50% of circulating blood from rats and left the

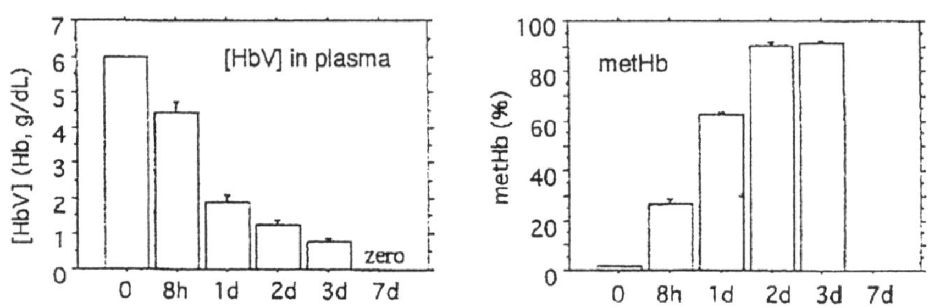

Fig. 3. Retention volume of HbV in plasma and metHb content. Source: Sakai et al. [12]

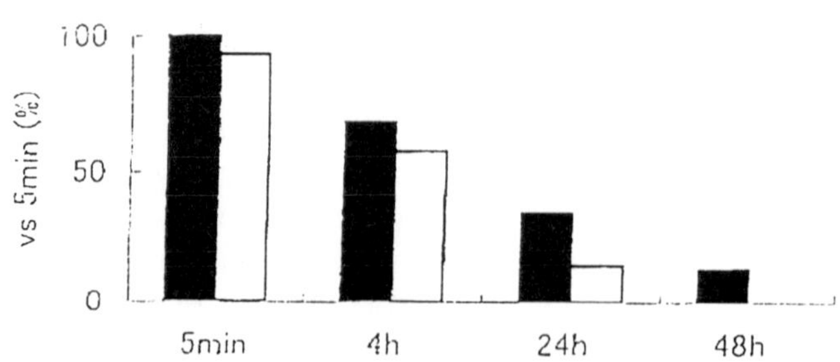

Fig. 4. Blood concentration of NRC on topload model. *Shaded*, total NRC-crit (%. vs 5 min); *unshaded*, NRC-crit with function estimated by NRC-crit and methemoglobin ratio (%. vs 5 min of total NRC-crit). Source: Tsutsui et al. [13]

blood in place for 15 min. They then replaced the blood loss with the withdrawn blood, human albumin solution, and the HbV suspended in 5% human albumin. They noted that no increase in blood pressure occurred immediately after the infusion of HbV (Fig. 5). It is suggested that encapsulation of Hb with liposome membrane blocked nitric oxide scavenging and prevented vasoconstriction [12]. Incidentally, rats treated with the HbV or autologous blood all survived but rats treated with albumin solution did not. In addition, blood lactate levels elevated transiently in a shock state and recovered rapidly after the infusion of HbV and autologous blood. However, lactate levels with the infusion of human albumin recovered in surviving animals, but may remain or elevate in nonsurvival.

On the other hand, some objections could be made against our recommendation for cellular types such as:

1. The complexity of production process. Many processes for the encapsulation of hemoglobin, allostetic substances and metHb reductase, PEGylation, such as coating the surface of HbV with polyethylene glycol, and the extraction of carbon monoxide are required.
2. The cost for cellular artificial red cells would be higher than that of acellular types.
3. Apprehension about phagocytotic tissue retention of the HbV and subsequent immunosuppression is not excluded.

Waseda's investigators observed microscopically that HbVs were captured in microphages and bone marrow cells. Therefore the weight of the liver and spleen was increased respectively. They noted a paradoxical phenomenon that phagocytotic activity for carbon particles infused intravenously increased temporarily after infusion of HbV but recovered completely 7 days later.

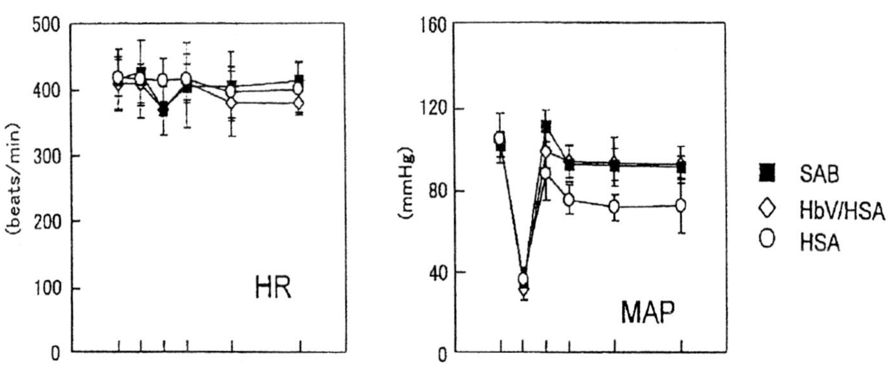

FIG. 5. *HR*, heart rate; *MAP*, mean arterial pressure; *SAB*, autologous blood; *HbV/HSA*, HbV/human albumin; *HSA*, human albumin. Source: Sakai et al. [12]

Abe et al. [15] at the Hokkaido Blood Supply Center tested the effect of HbV on complement hemolytic activity and the complement killing activity of bacteria. They noted that infusion of HbV reduced the hemolytic activity in a dose-dependent manner, and that HbV infusion suppressed the bacteria-killing activity with complements. However, they concluded that the human defense system against bacterial infection would be little influenced [15].

Yanagida et al. [16] noted a severe decrease in immunoglobulins after hemodilution with NRC, in which animal hematocrit was decreased to 7.1%. However, circulating neutrophils and lymphocytes increased after the hemodilution. These changes are similar to those we observed in severe hemodilution with dextran and HES [17]. Therefore, changes observed seem unlikely specific responses to NRC. Incidentally, changes in immunoglobulins and leukocytes recovered within a few days.

Hoka et al. [18] of the Kitazato University School of Medicine, Department of Anesthesiology, studied the effect of HbV on interaction between the neutrophil and the endothelium. Under vital microscopic observation they found in the golden hamster that the migration of the neutrophil through the endothelium layer of the buccal mucous pouch was markedly attenuated with infusion of HbV.

Safety and Efficacy of Artificial Blood

In accordance with the accumulation of data about the safety and efficacy of HbV in pre-clinical studies, a project team supported by the Japanese Ministry of Health and Welfare, sought to make safety and efficacy criteria for the clinical use of HbV.

Several studies referring to chemical and biological safety have been reported [19–22]. However, particularly with HbV, we proposed several measures recently. In the process of encapsulation of Hb in liposome vesicles, it is necessary convert Hb to carbon monoxide Hb. Therefore, it must be confirmed whether or not there will be residual carbon monoxide Hb and carbon monoxide in the solution. Likewise there must be checks to see if excess phospholipid of lipsosome or polyethylene glycol remain in the solution. Obviously endotoxin contamination cannot be allowed. It must be also kept absolutely sterile during storage. The physicochemical properties of HbV as shown in Table 2 have been tested and guaranteed to be absolutely safe.

Concerning the clinical safety of artificial blood, several studies have reported as above. However, a check list for finding adverse effects of HbV on vital functions is shown in Table 3.

Most of those have been tested in pre-clinical studies. However, due to present inability to mass produce HbV, a few items remain to be tested in the

TABLE 3. Safety of HbV solution

Clinical Assessment	
Psychological function and behavior	Mental and nervous function
Tendon and muscle function	Heart and circulartory function
Respiratory and gas exchange function	Hepatic function
Body fluid buffering capacity	Serum electrolyte composition
Renal function	Digestive function
Hemostatic and fibrinolytic function	Hematopoietic function
Endocrine functions	Defensive and immune function
Reproductive function	Teratogenicity
Tumorigenicity	Interaction with commonly used drugs

near future. Incidentally, the criteria of the Japanese Ministry of Health and Welfare regarding the severity of adverse effects should be applied in preclinical studies and clinical trials.

Regarding the efficacy of artificial blood, however, few criteria have been established. As with the safety criteria, efficacy of HbV as artificial blood should be evaluated from physicochemical activity and clinical efficacy points of view. The following should be considered: (1) oxygen-deliverying capacity, which is mainly controlled by the amount of Hb and the oxygen dissociation curve of Hb inside of the vesicles; (2) conversion rate of Hb to metHb during storage and in vivo after infusion; (3) dispersibility of the vesicles in the solution and blood; (4) size of the vesicle; (5) viscosity of the solution; (6) homogeneity and stability of the vesicles in the solution; and (7) pH of the solution.

The most important property in clinical efficacy is an ability for the oxygen supply to reach tissues. It depends on good pulmonary oxygenation, oxygen extraction in the tissues, a lower conversion rate from Hb to metHb, and having a cardiac output associated with normal circulating blood volume after infusion for blood loss. Finally it depends on adequate retention of the vesicles in the circulation.

After confirmation of safety and efficacy, clinical trials must be performed before use in practice. The Society of Blood Substitutes, Japan, provided guidelines for clinical trials of artificial blood 6 years ago. We intend to follow those guidelines to clinical trial.

Design of Clinical Trials

Clinical trials should satisfy the following two points: (1) good design to obtain definite results for evidence, and (2) obtaining proper informed consent from subjects.

TABLE 4. Ethical considerations for clinical trials

Clinical trials should be done for the treatment or therapy for patients
Clinical trials should be equivalent or superior to conventional treatment or therapy
Clinical trials must be performed with informed consent

TABLE 5. Criteria for selection for clinical trial

Replacement of surgical blood loss (15–20 ml/kg)
Hemodilutional autologous blood transfusion
Blood transfusion for unexpected intraoperative bleeding
Blood transfusion for emergent surgery without proper blood
Transfusion for patients with uncommon blood types whose surgery is relatively urgent

Limit to anticipated blood loss of 15–20 ml/kg.

For achievement of definite satisfactory results, four items should be prepared, namely: (1) proper setting of controls for the procedure or treatment, (2) establishing control measures before the procedure or treatment begins, (3) application of routine laboratory tests and simple procedures, and (4) exclusion of subjects with severe illness or subjects with complicated or unstable conditions.

Regarding medical ethics, we must recognize and observe three items listed in Table 4, namely: (1) clinical trials should be performed for treatment or therapy of the patient, (2) the treatment or therapy in clinical trials should be equivalent or superior to conventional treatment or therapy, and (3) clinical trials must be done with the proper informed consent of the patient.

Considering the above restrictions, we designed a clinical trial (Table 5). It will be limited to treatment of 15–20 ml/kg blood loss, such as hemodilutional autologous blood transfusion, transfusion for unexpected surgical bleeding, transfusion in emergent surgery without proper blood preparation, and transfusion for patients with an uncommon blood type whose surgery is relatively urgent.

Some other applications might be proposed (Table 6). We would like to avoid other applications in the first clinical trial, since pathological conditions or illness influence procedures for measurement and accuracy, and so data obtained from those patients would skew the results.

Conclusions

Further assessment and confirmation remain to be done for the safety of HbV. Further improvement of the physicochemical properties of HbV and its mass production should be done in the near future. For example, a fine filter with

TABLE 6. No program projected first clinical trial for new artificial blood

Post-traumatic hypovolemia
Hemorrhagic shock
Myocardial and cerebral ischemia
Supplemental treatment for idiopathic anemia
Priming for extraorporeal circuit
Superoxygenation for malignant neoplasma therapy
Liquid ventilation
Perfusion and preservation for organ transplantation

TABLE 7. Social needs for artificial blood

Disaster use	long-term shelf storage
Emergent use	before arrival of matched or O-blood
Shortage of blood for transfusion	
Recycle use of hemoglobin from donated blood	
Application as universal blood	
Avoiding transfusion complications and human errors	
Transfusion for patients with uncommon blood type or with refusal of donated blood	

0.2 μ diameter is used for elimination of bacteria from the product at the present time; however more definite methods for asepsis such as carbon dioxide replenishment or gamma radiation, should be introduced.

Social needs for artificial blood are shown in Table 7. They are all urgent. In my view, blood transfusions as routinely performed in practice today do not fit well with sophisticated medicine. It seems that, in the future, transfusion medicine, particularly red cell transfusion, will be replaced by infusion of artificial blood. Therefore I earnestly hope for great development of artificial blood and its use in clinical practice in the near future.

References

1. Toyoda T (1966) Preclinical studies of artificial blood. J Jpn Soc Surg 1:36–57 (in Japanese)
2. Ohyanagi H, Toshima K, Sekita M, et al (1979) Clinical studies of perfluorochemical whole blood substitutes: Safety of Fluosol-DS (20%) in normal human volunteers. Clin Ther 2:306–312
3. Motoki R, Usuba A (1996) Artificial oxygen-carrier from view point of surgery. Artif Blood 4:56–64
4. Takaori M (2002) Designs for clinical trial of artificial blood (HbV) for evaluation of its efficacy and safety. Artif Blood 10:99–106

5. Spahn DR, van Brempt R, Theilmeier G, et al (1999) Perflubron, emulsion delays blood transfusions in orthopedic surgery. Anesthesiology 91:1195–1208
6. Sloan EP, Koenigsberg M, Gens D, et al (1999) Diaspirin cross-linked hemoglobin (DCLHb) in the treatment of severe traumatic hemorrhagic shock: a randomized controlled efficacy trial. JAMA 282:1857–1864
7. Watanabe Y, Takahashi K, Kakegawa H, et al (1998) Extrapolation of demand and supply of blood for the next 30 years in Japan based on published goverment demographic projection. Jpn J Transf Med 44:328–335
8. Takaori M, Fukui A (1996) Treatment of massive hemorrhage with liposome encapsulated hemoglobin (NRC) and hydroxy Ethyl starch (HES) in beagles. Artif Cells Blood Substit Immmobil Biotechnol 24:643–653
9. Usuba A, Motoki R, Fukui H, et al (1996) Effect of liposome encapsulated hemoglobin "Neo Red Cells" as a resuscitation fluid for severe hemorrhagic shock. Artif Blood 4:69–78
10. Yoshizu A, Yamahata T, Izumi Y, et al (1997) The oxygen-transporting capability of hemoglobin vesicle, as an artificial oxygen carrier, evaluated in a rat hemorrhagic shock model. Artif Blood 5:18–22
11. Sakai H, Takeoka S, Tsuchida E (2002) Retention volume of HbV in plasma and metHb content. The project study of Japanese Ministry of Health and Welfare reported on April 25th, 2002 Tokyo
12. Nishi K, Kida Y (1996) Effects of hemoglobin-based oxygen-carrying artificial blood substitutes on the circulatory system. Artif Blood 2:82–93
13. Tsutsui Y, Kimura T, Ishizuka T, et al (2002) Duration of efficacy NRC (Neo Red Cell) in a rat hemodilution model. Artif Blood 10:36–41
14. Sakai H, Takeoka S, Tsuchida E (2002) Changes in arterial blood pressure following infusion of HbV for treatment of hemorrhagic shock. The project study of Japanese Ministry of Health and Welfare reported on April 25th, 2002 Tokyo
15. Abe H, Azuma H, Ikeda H (2002) Serum complement hemolytic activity after infusion of HbV. The project study of Japanese Ministry of Health and Welfare reported on April 25th, 2002 Tokyo
16. Yanagida N, Kawamura A, Tanaka M, et al (2001) Study on immune state of high grade blood exchange (Hemodilution Hct 43.5 $\rightarrow$ 7.1) using NRC in rats. Artif Blood 9:42–45
17. Lewis J, Szeto ILF, Bayer WL, et al (1966) Severe hemodilution with hydroxyethyl starch and dextrans. Arch Surg 93:941–950
18. Hoka S, Ozawa A, Nara Y (2003) Effect of artificial oxygen carrier on neutrophil movement in the microvasculature of hamster cheek pouch. Artif Blood 11:67
19. Center for Biologic Evaluation and Research (1991) Points to consider in the safety evaluation of hemoglobin-based oxygen carriers. Transfusion 31:369–371
20. Center for Biologic Evaluation and Research (1994) Points to consider in the safety evaluation of hemoglobin-based and perfluorocarbon-based oxygen carriers. Transfusion 34:712–713
21. Przybelski RL, Daily EK, Stern KN, et al (1997) A grade scale for assessment of safety of blood substitutes. Transfusion 37:749–751
22. Fratantoni JC (1998) Red cell substitutes: evolution of approaches for demonstrating efficacy. In: Tsuchida E (ed) Blood Substitutes—Present and Future Perspectives. Elsevier, Amsterdam, pp 33–39

Key Word Index